Urbanization and Public Health in China

Urbanization and Public Health in China

Editors

Mu Li

The University of Sydney, Australia

Yang Feng Wu

Peking University Health Science Center, China

ICP

Imperial College Press

Published by

Imperial College Press
57 Shelton Street
Covent Garden
London WC2H 9HE

Distributed by

World Scientific Publishing Co. Pte. Ltd.
5 Toh Tuck Link, Singapore 596224
USA office: 27 Warren Street, Suite 401-402, Hackensack, NJ 07601
UK office: 57 Shelton Street, Covent Garden, London WC2H 9HE

Library of Congress Cataloging-in-Publication Data
Names: Li, Mu (Professor of public heath)
Title: Urbanization and public health in China / Mu Li & Yang Feng Wu.
Description: New Jersey : Imperial College Press, [2015]
Identifiers: LCCN 2015027305 | ISBN 9781783268542 (alk. paper)
Subjects: LCSH: Urban health--China. | City planning--Health aspects--China.
Classification: LCC RA566.5.C6 U73 2015 | DDC 362.1/0420951--dc23
LC record available at http://lccn.loc.gov/2015027305

British Library Cataloguing-in-Publication Data
A catalogue record for this book is available from the British Library.

In-house Editors: Mary Simpson/Dipasri Sardar

Typeset by Stallion Press
Email: enquiries@stallionpress.com

Printed in Singapore by B & Jo Enterprise Pte Ltd

Contents

Foreword

Since my first visit in 1974, I have returned to China many times, in both an official capacity and as a private individual. I have therefore had the privilege of observing dramatic changes, particularly since the reforms and the opening of China in late 1970s. These changes have demonstrated the vision of the Chinese government and the outstanding spirit of its people. The living standards of 1.3 billion Chinese people have been elevated, from large-scale poverty to improved nutrition, housing and to a strong economy.

Among major changes, China has experienced an unprecedented pace of urbanization in recent decades. In 2011, for the first time, more than half of Chinese people lived in urban areas, compared with only 19.4% in 1950. By comparison, the world population living in cities increased to 51.6% from 42% over the same period. The urban environment can provide people with dreams, hopes and especially with opportunity; it can also have a profound impact on human behavior and health. Over the coming ten years, China's urban population rate is expected to grow to 60%. This tremendous change in the distribution of the world's largest population, together with its associated challenges and opportunities for both the government and the whole society certainly deserves the attention of researchers.

Urbanization and Public Health in China presents a cross section assessment of many public health issues and their association with urbanization. It presents viewpoints by researchers from The University of Sydney and many universities in China in their areas of expertise. One topic discussed in the book relate to a change in the burden of disease pattern from infectious diseases to non-communicable diseases, which now dominate the major challenges. Many communicable diseases are still posing a threat to public health due to increased people movement, climate change or overcrowded housing.

Other important issues discussed include the growing concerns regarding childhood obesity, access to and the need for health services of the tens of thousands of rural-to-urban migrants, and those who remain in the rural areas. The struggle of the health system and society more broadly, to cope with a rapidly aging population is also addressed. These issues not only affect the people's daily life and wellbeing, but also have long-lasting social and economic effects on the nation, if not addressed effectively.

Although the public health problems associated with urbanization, as revealed in the various chapters, seem daunting, considerable effort has been made to prevent or reduce those problems. Government and non-government initiatives and programs that are addressing the problems are discussed, research results are shared and future research needs are identified. An interesting and exciting quality is that the book presents some positive perspectives on how certain problems are being tackled. Examples include building environmentally friendly and sustainable eco-cities to balance environment, eco-system and human health needs, and promoting active urban transport, increasing opportunities for physical activity, and the reduction of air pollution and traffic congestion in cities. Through reforming the government-run health system and allowing private providers to play a role, the provision of health and aged-care services can be improved.

Many of the issues presented in the book are not unique to China. We all share similar major challenges in the 21st century, including globalization and urbanization, population aging, and climate change. This book is therefore a timely contribution to knowledge on urbanization and public health. It is particularly relevant to many low-middle income countries which are experiencing rapid urbanization and health transition.

It is particularly pleasing to note that several students undertaking advanced studies for doctorates, are among the contributors of the book. Research education above all must nurture young minds and thus promote future leaders.

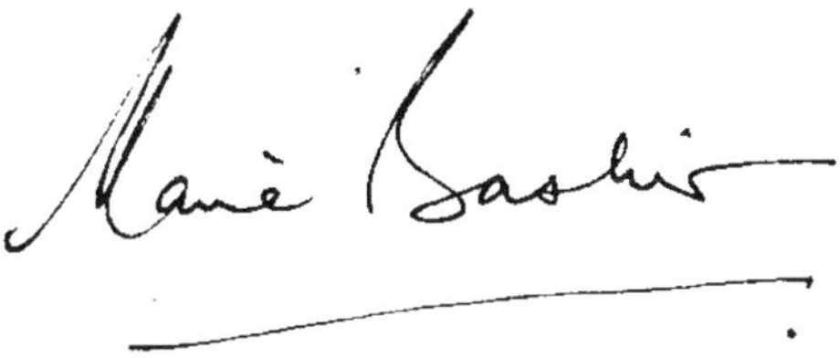

Professor the Honourable Dame Marie Bashir AD CVO

Gordon G. Liu, Yangtze River Scholar and Professor of Economics at the National School of Development, Peking University, and Director of Peking University China Center for Health Economic Research, China

Duan Fang Lu, Associate Professor in the Faculty of Architecture, Design and Planning at the University of Sydney, Australia

Feng Lu, Researcher at the Institute of Population Research, Peking University and Institute of Environmental Health and Related Product Safety, Chinese Centre for Disease Control and Prevention, China

Ji Xiang Ma, Deputy Director of the National Center for Non-communicable Disease Control (NCD) and Prevention, Chinese Center for Disease Control and Prevention, China

Wei Ma, Associate Professor at the School of Public Health, Center for Climate Change and Health, Shandong University, China

Phil McManus, Professor of Urban and Environmental Geography, and the Head of School of Geosciences, The University of Sydney, Australia

Monika Nitschke, Principal Scientific Officer at the South Australian Government Department of Health, Australia

Jay Pan, Associate Professor of Health Policy and Economics at the West China School of Public Health, Sichuan University, China

Li Hua Pang, Associate Professor at the Institution of Population, Peking University, China

Zhu Jun Shao, Professor and Director of the Department of Respiratory Infectious Disease, National Institute for Communicable Disease Control and Prevention, Chinese Center for Disease Control and Prevention, China

Qiang Zheng Sun, Research Fellow at the State Key Laboratory for Infectious Disease Prevention and Control, National Institute for Communicable Disease Control and Prevention, Chinese Center for Disease Control and Prevention, China

Hao Chen Wang, PhD candidate in demography at the Institute of Population Research, Peking University, China

Jia Zheng Wang, Researcher from the State Key Laboratory for Infectious Disease Prevention and Control, National Institute for Communicable Disease Control and Prevention, Chinese Center for Disease Control and Prevention, China

Jin Nan Wang, Lecturer and PhD candidate in Environmental Health, at the School of Public Health at Shandong University, China

Quan Yi Wang, Professor of Epidemiology and Director of Infectious Diseases Institute, Beijing Center for Disease Prevention and Control, China

Li Ming Wen, Adjunct Associate Professor at the Sydney Medical School, The University of Sydney, Australia; Professor at Shanghai 10th People's Hospital, Faculty of Medicine, Tongji University, China

Yang Feng Wu, Professor of Epidemiology, Peking University School of Public Health; Executive Associate Director, Peking University Clinical Research Institute; Senior Director, the George Institute for Global Health at Peking University Health Science Center, China

Xiao Yu Wu, Associate Professor of Economics at the China Academy of Public Finance and Policy, Central University of Finance and Economics, China

Hui Lan Xu, PhD candidate at the Sydney Medical School, University of Sydney, Research and Evaluation Officer in the Health Promotion Service, South Western Sydney and Sydney Local Health Districts, Australia

Jian Guo Xu, Director and Professor of the National Institute of Communicable Diseases Control and Prevention, Chinese Center for Disease Control and Prevention, and Director of State Key Laboratory for Infectious Diseases Prevention and Control, China

Gang Zhang, Assistant Researcher at the China Population and Development Research Center and PhD candidate at the Institute of Population Research, Peking University, China

Tuo Hong Zhang, Professor in the School of Public Health, Peking University Health Science Centre, China

Ying Zhang, Senior Lecturer at the School of Public Health and China Studies Centre, The University of Sydney, Australia

Xiao Ying Zheng, Professor and Director at the Center of Chinese Population Health and Development, Institute of Population Research/WHO Collaborating Center for Reproductive Health and Population Science at Peking University, China

Introduction

Mu Li and Yang Feng Wu

Urbanization (*cheng zhen hua*) is transforming China and the lives of the Chinese people. Urbanization in China has been a topic of research interest across many disciplines, such as economics, social and political science, urban planning, and public health. The United Nations defines urbanization as the "movement of people from rural to urban areas", or a population increase in urban as opposed to rural areas, and the level of urbanization is measured by the proportion of the total population living in urban areas (United Nations Department of Economics and Social Affairs, 2014). This widely accepted definition will be used in this Introduction, and, to a large extent, throughout this book.

As the longest continuous civilization in the world, and a society deeply rooted in agriculture, China recently passed a key milestone in its urbanization process. In January 2012, for the first time, there were fewer Chinese people living in rural areas than in urban areas, that is, in cities and towns. One of the key features of urbanization in China is that it started from a relatively low point, and is developing at a much faster speed compared with the global trend. The proportion of the world's population living in urban settings reached 50% in 2008, up from 30% in 1950, while the comparable figures for China increased from about 11% to close to 50% over the same period. In particular,

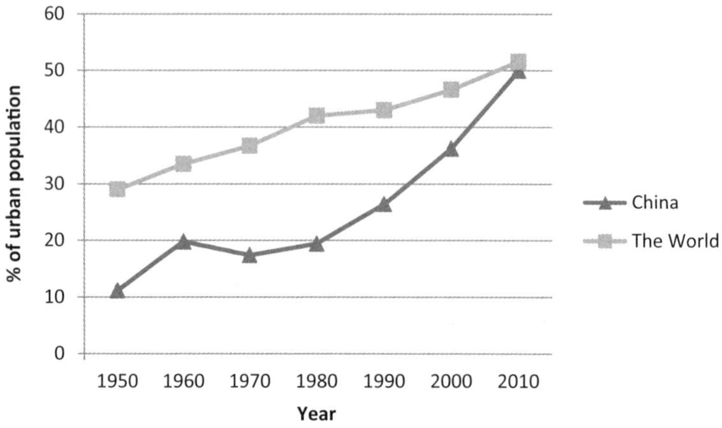

Figure 1. Urban population growth in China and the World 1950–2010 (United Nation).

between 1978 and 2013 — since the economic reforms and the 'Open Door' policy that is to open up to the outside world, relaxing the import and export control and allowing foreign investment to come in China — the proportion of urban long-term residents increased from 17.9% to 53.7%, with an average annual rate of increase of 1.02% (Ministry of Land and Resouces, 2014). Figure 1 illustrates the pace of urbanization in the world and in China according to the growth in the percentage of the urban population.

It is projected that by the mid-twenty-first century, two thirds of the world's population will be living in cities. The Ministry of Land Resource's *National New Urbanization Integrated Plan (2014–2020)* indicates that 'by 2020 the long-term urban population in China will reach approximately 60%' (Ministry of Land and Resouces, 2014). This increase in urban population is accompanied by a spatial expansion of urban areas. Based on the Sixth Census data, the number of Chinese cities increased from 193 in 1978 to 658 in 2013, with 140 cities having a population exceeding one million, and a further 138 with between 500,000 and one million people (Table 1).

As early as 1979, about the time the urbanization was about to take off in China, Bartrand Renaud (1979) defined some key

Table 1. The changes of number and size of cities and townships between 1978 and 2010

	1978	2010
Total number of cities	193	658
city size by population		
>10,000,000 people	0	6
5,000,000–10,000,000	2	10
3,000,000–5,000,000	2	21
1,000,000–3,000,000	25	103
500,000–1,000,000	35	138
<500,000	129	380
Total number of townships	2,173	19,410

Source: Ministry of Land and Resouces (2014).

determinants of urbanization and population concentration in urban areas:

- The rate of development and the structure of the agricultural sector, which is influenced by the distribution of land holdings.
- The rate of growth and sectoral pattern of industrialization and location decisions, which affect the distribution of manufacturing and therefore of services and activities among cities.

Historically, population redistribution and migration are the results of employment opportunities. Cities have always drawn hundreds of millions of people to seek employment and a better life. However, the speed of the expansion of existing Chinese cities and the creation of new ones is unprecedented. The key driving forces of large scale internal migration and rapid urbanization in China have been attributed to a set of 'pull' and 'push' factors (Gong *et al.*, 2012). These have been particularly relevant in the 'stable development stage' (1978–1995) and the 'rapid development stage' (1996–2012) of the urbanization (described here in Chapter Two). High demand for a workforce in the construction and manufacturing sectors, plus favorable policies (such as relaxing the household registration system from the late 1970s to mid-1980s), attracted people from rural areas to the cities (pull factors). On the other hand, the increasing gap in income levels between urban and rural communities, and the loss of arable land in rural communities to urban development, resulted in a labor surplus in the agricultural sector, with people pushed off the land subsequently moving to cities for work (push factors).

Defining urban areas, both their boundaries and the actual urban population size in China has proven to be complex and challenging. Firstly, from the administrative division point of view, China has a hierarchical structure. From the top down, the structure consists of five levels — central, provincial/autonomous regional, prefectural, county and township (China Internet Information Centre, 2014). Urban areas, in the Chinese context, include cities (*Shi*) and townships (*Zhen*). Typically, cities are divided into urban districts plus surrounding rural or semi-rural counties, or 'peri-urban' districts. That means that some rural areas on city fringes are reclassified as urban areas due to rezoning, or as the result of changing administrative levels. The people living in those areas can either retain their rural agricultural resident status or they can change their status to urban residents; however, they still do not have the same rights as those long-term urban residents — this is discussed further later in this Introduction.

Increasingly, there are more prefectural level cities and county level cities, the status often determined by the level of development or population size. When a township is reclassified as a city, or when a city moves up one level in the administrative hierarchy, it often means not only more financial resources and investment opportunities, but also greater decision-making power on the part of local government, for example raising local taxes (Chan, 1994).

Secondly, under current law, each citizen is required to register in only one place of permanent residence in the Chinese household registration system (*Hukou*). The *Hukou* is classified into two categories, agricultural and non-agricultural, to segregate the rural and urban populations. This *Hukou* system has kept a tight lid on the internal movement of the population and restricted the pace of urbanization (Chan, 1992). Although it has become much easier for people to travel internally since the economic reform in 1978, the *Hukou* system still has a strong foothold in modern Chinese society (Chan, 2010). It was and still is difficult for an agricultural *Hukou* holder to be reclassified as non-agricultural. There is, therefore, often a huge discrepancy between the census data and population statistics of a city based on household registration. The latter does not represent the real size of the population living in the city, as it does not include migrants, often known as the 'floating population', whose *Hukou* remains in their rural community of origin. In 2012 the inconsistency in population data based on residential address and household registration was 279 million; of these 236 million were 'floating population' (National Bureau of Statistics of China, 2014).

The *Hukou* defines people's rights and eligibility for welfare and services such as public education, housing and health services, including the type of health insurance they can or cannot have. From a city government's perspective the number of people with a permanent household registration status — i.e. *Hukou* — in its jurisdiction, is the population that counts and for whom it has a responsibility to provide public services, including health and education. This discrepancy in "head counting" not only creates confusion but also underlies inequalities and inequities for migrants accessing government services (Chan, 2010).

Renaud (1979) foresaw some major imbalances as the result of urbanization, notably:

- imbalances between rural and urban sectors
- imbalances between the level of development of different regions
- imbalances between cites of different sizes
- imbalances between social groups within cities

The levels of urbanization in the world and in China are, indeed, uneven. For example, in North America and many European countries more than three quarters of the population are now living in cities. In eastern China the urban population rate is already as high as 62%, while in central and western China it is 48.5% and 44.8%, respectively. This unevenness of urbanization is a manifestation of the uneven level of economic development. For example, the Beijing – Tianjin – Hebei Metropolitan Region, the Yangtze Delta Economic Zone and the Pearl River Delta Economic Zone in the eastern and southeastern parts of China account for 18% of the total Chinese population, but contribute 36% of the Chinese GNP (Ministry of Land and Resouces, 2014). The labor provided by rural-to-urban migrants has, to a large extent, underpinned this economic output. This unevenness in the level of development has also caused uneven distribution of resources, including health services, between east and west, and between urban and rural areas.

There is no sign that urbanization is slowing down; in fact just the opposite. Why does China need to push so hard on urbanization? In the *National New Urbanization Integrated Plan (2014–2020)*, the importance of urbanization to China is expressed unequivocally (Ministry of Land and Resouces, 2014). Urbanization:

- is the natural pathway of the country towards modernization
- is the engine for ensuring healthy and sustainable economic development
- provides leverage for industrial transformation and elevation
- is the solution for issues regarding rationalized land use, scaled agricultural production and improved living standards for the rural population.
- is the foundation of coordinated regional development
- is essential for promoting the advancement of the whole society

Urbanization and migration in other developing countries have often resulted in shantytowns and slums, which become centers of public health and other social problems. This has not been the case in China. Although the provision of housing, and other public services, is not keeping pace with population growth, the basic urban development indicators presented in Table 2, nevertheless, demonstrate the government's efforts in providing essential services, through policies such as a low-rent housing scheme to provide a safeguard for the housing problems of the urban poor, and the affordable housing schemes aimed at facilitating private ownership of houses (Deng *et al.*, 2009).

Table 2 Changes in relevant urban facilities between 2000 and 2012

Indicators	2000	2012
Road per person (m^2)	6.1	14.4
Housing per person (m^2)	20.3	32.9
Waste water treatment (%)	34.3	87.3
Green park land per person (m^2)	3.7	12.3
Ordinary middle schools	14,473	17,333
Hospital beds (×10,000)	142.6	273.3

***Source*: Ministry of Land and Resouces (2014).**

In China's context, urbanization could mean opportunities for better health infrastructure and access to healthcare services, hence improved health outcomes for all urban residents. It is, however, increasing the risk to people's health due to changing diets, changing work conditions and lifestyle, and deteriorating air quality. For example, in a large study involving close to 50,000 men and women, urban living was found to be an independent risk factor for pre-diabetes and diabetes (Yang *et al.*, 2010).

While not intended to encompass every public health-related issue, this volume takes a wide-angled look at some of the contemporary public health issues in China in the context of urbanization. The first six chapters examine the demographic and health transitions since the founding of the People's Republic of China in 1949, with a focus on the nearly four decades since the economic reforms of 1978 and the rapid urban developments and urbanization which has followed.

For instance, one of the key features of the demographic change is the improvement in life expectancy and consequent aging of the population. This presents a set of pressing issues in terms of being able to care for its elders, as society gets old before it gets rich. The volume also explores the increasing disease burden from non-communicable diseases and road traffic injuries; and the pattern and risk factors for communicable diseases, which are still evolving and still affect many people, particularly the poor and vulnerable. Another public health problem that could potentially have a significant impact on the future health of the nation, productivity and the economy is childhood obesity, which is also considered.

In Chapter One, Zheng and Guo focus on the changes in some of the most important demographic variables, such as birth and fertility, mortality and life expectancy, and age structure, since the founding of the People's Republic of China in 1949. It also explores the transition of health patterns, based on changes in the 'cause-of-death' data among the Chinese population, during this period of rapid urbanization.

The Chinese population aged 65 or above has nearly doubled in the past 30 years, from 4.9% in 1982 to 9.2% in 2012 (National Bureau of Statistics of China, 2014). In Chapter Two, Chen and Zhang explore the population aging issues that the Chinese government and society are facing, in terms of economic impact, health service delivery, long term care and social security support. The chapter highlights some recent government regulations, and the development of elderly friendly environments, to tackle the challenge of population aging.

The rapid rise of non-communicable diseases (NCDs), driven by urbanization and rising incomes, has made them the leading cause of death in China, accounting for close to 70% of the overall disease burden and over 80% of total mortality (Yang *et al.*, 2013). The four leading NCDs in China are cardiovascular diseases (CVDs), diabetes, cancer and chronic obstructive pulmonary diseases (COPDs). This is compounded by a large aging population, with a higher prevalence of NCDs, who need more health services and long-term care. Ma and co-authors dedicate Chapter Three to describing trends and key behavioral risk factors of NCDs in the new era of urbanization. These analyses provide strong evidence for policymakers and public healthcare providers to shape policies and programs to address these risk factors.

In the *Global Burden of Diseases, Injuries, and Risk Factors Study 2010*, road traffic injury moved from the tenth highest ranked cause of premature death in 1990 the fourth place in 2010, after cerebrovascular disease, ischemic heart disease, and chronic obstructive pulmonary disease (Institute for Health Metrics and Evaluation, 2010). In Chapter Four, Li Ping Li examines these trends in road traffic injury. With continuing urban development and the concentration of people in cities, the road network capacity cannot meet the demands presented by social development. At the same time, the paper highlights that the structure of most urban transport systems is unbalanced; coordinated management and utilization of the traffic system, and development of a life protection mechanism should be prioritized.

In the process of rapid urbanization, with increasing population density and human movement, and increasing trade in fresh agricultural produce, infectious diseases continue to be a major threat to health. In Chapter Five, Wang and co-authors highlight these threats by analyzing the changing epidemiological patterns of infectious disease in China in recent decades, that is, changes in disease morbidity in relation to respiratory tract infection, diarrhea and zoonotic diseases. Changes in the prevalence of other infectious diseases, as a result of changes in social behavior, are also discussed.

As recently as 1990, nearly one-third of Chinese children under the age of five years were 'stunted', meaning they had low height for their age; and one in seven children under five years old was underweight, meaning their body weight was low for their age (United Nations Children's Fund, 2013). A 2010 inter-country study showed that young Chinese children (at six years) experienced larger increases in body mass index — a measure of fatness — compared with their counterparts in the United Kingdom, the United States of America and Australia (Popkin, 2010). This change in children's nutritional status coincides with China's nutrition transition. Li and Baur's chapter on Childhood Obesity: Chinese Perspective, postulates that obesity is being driven up by increased household income, resulting from economic development and urbanization, as demonstrated by the gradient of childhood overweight and obesity prevalence between large eastern coastal cities and western inland rural areas, which shows a declining pattern coincident with the level of economic development.

In the remaining chapters of the volume, the authors take a closer look at some underlying social issues, such as the inequalities and inequities in health services provided for the underprivileged, in both urban and rural settings, and people's perception of resettlement in urbanized new villages occurring at city fringes, highlighting possible implications for their health and social interaction. They also cover awareness and utilization of health services among rural-to-urban migrant workers, using reproductive health as an example, as well as the environmental costs of urbanization. These chapters attempt to make the connection between these social issues and public health, with urbanization as the backdrop.

In Chapter Seven, Carrillo Garcia highlights the widening socio–economic gap between rich and poor, manifested in the inequality of access to health services endured by under-privileged urban dwellers, laid-off government enterprise employees, rural-to-urban migrants and people living in rural and remote areas.

When urbanization and health is discussed, the focus is often fixed on the health of, and provision of health services to, the urban population, existing or new, described by the term 'urban health' (Chan, 2011). The reality is that when young people, including some of the healthy workforce, move from rural areas to cities and towns, there are still many people remaining in rural and remote areas. These 'left behind' groups comprise mainly children, the elderly and people with physical or mental disabilities. In Chapter Eight, Yang Feng Wu focuses our attention on the inequities in access to health services for the rural poor, particularly the elderly, who encounter an under-resourced health system whilst carrying a larger burden of chronic diseases.

China's rapid urbanization has led to a substantial reduction in farmland, and the rapid expansion of land use for urban and rural construction. The introduction of government policies coordinating urban and rural construction in recent years has given rise to intensive local initiatives of rural relocation and combination (*chai cun bing ju*) (Huang *et al.*, 2013). Under this policy, numerous villages with long histories have been razed to the ground, and turned into cultivable land. In Chapter Nine, Lu and Dang critically examine changes surrounding China's rural resettlement program on urban fringes, that is, in the areas where the city ends and countryside begins. This does not only change the farmers' living environment, often with improved water and sanitation facilities, but also involves changes in the way people live and their interaction with each other, the social fabric of rural society and rural health. The research presented here focuses on peasant experiences and their perceptions of the resettlement program, and the spatial effects of the new villages.

As the majority of rural-to-urban migrants are young people, women's reproductive health is one of the most prominent public health issues they encounter (Liu and Griffiths, 2011). Based on two large, nationally representative surveys Guo and co-authors report in Chapter Ten that the migrants — in this case unmarried youth and married women of childbearing age — tend to have less understanding of the need for, and less access to, reproductive health services in cities, their adopted residential location.

China's rapid urbanization has come with considerable environmental costs, in terms of air, water, soil, and noise pollution, and the 'heat island effect' in major cities. These have the potential to affect people's health adversely. In Chapter Eleven, Wang and co-authors critically review the impact on the environment of urbanization. They also explore how environmental factors influence people's health. The authors attempt to provide some suggestions, based on their analysis, that could minimize the environmental impact of the urbanization process and make it more sustainable.

Many issues in public health interconnect with other pressing concerns. For example, promoting awareness of and preparedness for climate change could help to mitigate its effects on health, particularly among elderly people who represent one of the groups most vulnerable to extreme climate events. Further, promoting active transport could prevent NCDs by increasing physical activity, as well as reducing greenhouse emissions and road accident injuries. These topics are discussed in the next two chapters.

Aging and climate change are two of the biggest challenges the world is facing in the 21st century. Zhang and co-authors argue that elderly people are more vulnerable to climate change related health effects, especially since many may suffer from chronic diseases, exacerbated by extreme weather in their local geographic area. Awareness of the problem on the part of the elderly, and an understanding that they can protect themselves through mitigating the impact of climate change, are both vitally important.

Another example of the complexity of interconnected issues in relation to urbanization and health is the increased dependency on motor vehicles for commuting. This response to expanding cities has health consequences in relation to non-communicable diseases. Major adverse effects of this dependency include increased potential for road traffic injury; declining levels of active transport such as walking and riding bicycles (once the main modes of transportation in China), thus reducing physical activity; and increased carbon emissions and deteriorating air quality, which again have significant adverse effects on health and mortality. In Chapter Thirteen, Wen and Xu critically examine international literature on active transportation, and provide some insightful suggestions for China based on experiences from other countries.

The volume concludes with an account of an exciting pilot eco-city project that could be a model for future cities, and insightful critiques on health reforms, intended to address the mismatch between the demand and the supply of health services.

McManus provides an historical recount of urban reform and explores the context, origins, progress and potential future of the Sino-Singapore Tianjin eco-city, a purpose-built city for an ecologically sustainable future, which seeks to balance environmental, social and economic health in one of the cities of the Beijing–Tianjin–Hebei Metropolitan Region. This could be a model for the future planning, and design of healthy urban living in China and elsewhere.

Public health problems in China, driven by or as a side effect of urbanization are real. However, it will be ineffective, indeed impossible, for the public health sector alone to provide solutions. There are some positive developments, and governments at different levels are playing a key role. At the central level, health reform, begun in 2009, is one of the Chinese Government's priorities. For example, health insurance for both urban and rural residents has achieved near universal coverage, reaching 95.7% in 2011, up from 29.7% in 2003 (Lancet, 2012). In Chapter Fifteen, Liu and colleagues provide an empirical analysis of how urbanization affects people's health, and critique health reforms in relation to health policies which are likely to shape how population health will be managed as urbanization progresses in China. Other initiatives — such as slowing climate change by reducing greenhouse emissions — also depend on strong political will. Recently, China set the target to 'increase the non-fossil fuel share of all energy to around 20% by 2030' (Lan, 2014).

A recent joint report by the World Bank and the Development Research Center of China's State Council, *Urban China: Toward Efficient, Inclusive and Sustainable Urbanization* (World Bank and Development Research Center of the State Council of the People's Republic of China, 2014), highlights six priority areas for a new model of China's urbanization in coming years:

1. **Reforming land management and institutions**: Most urban expansion to date has been at the expense of converted rural land. More efficient use of land requires stronger property rights for farmers, and new mechanisms for converting rural construction land to urban uses with strong legal limits.
2. **Reforming the *Hukou* household registration system to provide equal access to quality services for all citizens and to create a more mobile and versatile labor force**: The system should remove barriers to labor mobility from rural to urban areas and between cities; this will help close the gap of workers' wages.
3. **Placing urban finances on a more sustainable footing, while creating financial discipline for local government**: This requires moving to a revenue system that ensures a higher portion of local expenditure is financed by local revenues, such as property taxes, and fees and charges for using urban public services.
4. **Reforming urban planning and design**: More effort is needed to make better use of existing urban land, leading to more efficient urban development. Further, linking transport infrastructure to urban centers, and promoting coordination among cities, would encourage better management of traffic congestion and reduced air pollution.

5. **Managing environmental pressures**: While China has already developed tough environmental laws, regulations and standards, the most important and urgent task for achieving greener and healthier urbanization is strengthening law enforcement to protect the environment.
6. **Improving local governance**: This can be achieved by enhancing the performance evaluation system of local officials, giving a greater incentive for a more efficient, inclusive and sustainable urbanization process.

The effects of urbanization on public health require strong and innovative policies. This set of guiding principles and reform priorities have great relevance to the issues discussed in this book. For example, reforming the *Hukou* system will improve the equality of legal status, and therefore rights of access to housing, education and health services in cities, the adopted home of hundreds of millions of rural-to-urban migrants. Reforming urban planning and design, along with management of environmental pressures, will have strong public health benefits by providing an enabling environment for outdoor physical activity and active transportation, thus reducing air and water pollution, and road traffic injuries. This will provide a great opportunity for researchers to be involved, particularly in gathering scientific evidence through empirical investigation, and evaluating the effectiveness of government priorities.

Finally, we would like to express our gratitude to the contributors. Among them, there are world renowned leaders in their respective research fields, mid-career researchers who are at the most productive phase of their careers, and early career researchers, including PhD students, who are on the trajectory of making a big impact in future research in this area. We are honored to have so many colleagues willing to share their thoughts and new research with us in this volume.

References

Chan, K. (1992). Economic Growth Strategy and Urbanisation Policies in **China**, 1949–1982, *International Journal Urban and Regional Research* **16:** 275–305.

Chan, K. (1994). Urbanisation and Rural-Urban Migration in China Since 1982: A New Baseline, *Modern China* **20**(3): 243–281.

Chan, K. (2010). The Household Registration System and Migrant Labor in China: Notes on a Debate, *Population and Develpment Review* **36**(2): 357–364.

Chan, M. (2011). Introduction, Vlahov, D., Boufford, J., Pearson, C., *et al.* (eds), *Urban Health: Global Perspectives*, Jossey-Bass. San Francisco.

China Internet Information Centre (2014). Administrative Division System. Available at http://www.china.org.cn/english/feature/38436.htm# [Accessed 2 March 2015].

Deng, L., Shen, Q. and Wang, L. (2009). *Housing Policy and Finance in China: A Literature Review*, US Department of Housing and Urban Development. Available at http://www.chinaplanning.org/Publications/Lan%20Deng%20-%20Housing%20Policy%20and%20Finance%20In%20China.pdf [Accessed 2 March 2015].

Gong, P., Liang S., Carlton, E.J., *et al.* Remais (2012). Urbanisation and Health in China, *The Lancet* **379**(9818): 843–852.

Huang, C., Deng, L., Gao, X., *et al.* (2013). Rural Housing Land Consolidation and Transformation of Rural Villages under the "Coordinating Urban and Rural Construction Land" Policy: A Case of Chengdu City, *China* **4**(3): 95–103.

Institute for Health Metrics and Evaluation (2010). 'Global Burden of Diseases, Injuries, and Risk factors Study 2010', Institute for Health Metrics and Evaluation, Washington DC.

Lan, L. (2014). China, US promise to reduce emissions. Available at http://www.chinadaily.com.cn/china/2014-11/13/content_18904652.htm [Accessed 2 March 2015].

Lancet (2012). What Can be Learnt from China's Health System?, *The Lancet* **379**(9818). 777.

Liu, S. and Griffiths, S. (2011). From Economic Development to Public Health Improvement: China Faces Equity Challenges, *Public Health* **125**(10): 669–674.

Ministry of Land and Resouces (2014). *National New Urbanisation Integrated Plan. Beijing, Ministry of Land and Resouces*, Government of the PRC, Beijing.

National Bureau of Statistics of China (2014). *China National Statistical Yearbook 2013*, National Bureau of Statistics of China, Beijing.

Popkin, B. (2010). Recent Dynamics Suggest Selected Countries Catching Up to US Obesity, *American Journal of Clinical Nutrition* **91**(1): 284S–288S.

Renaud, B. (1979). *National Urbanisation Policies in Developing Countries*, World Bank, Washigton DC.

United Nations Children's Fund (2013). *Improving Child Nutrition: The Achievable Imperative for Global Progress*, United Nations Children's Fund, New York.

United Nations Department of Economics and Social Affairs (2014). World Urbanisation Prospects. Available at http://esa.un.org/unpd/wup/ [Accessed 2 March 2015].

World Bank and Development Research Center of the State Council of the People's Republic of China (2014). *Urban China : Toward Efficient, Inclusive, and Sustainable Urbanization*, World Bank, Washington, DC.

Yang, G., Wang, Y., Zeng, Y., *et al.* (2013). Rapid Health Transition in China 1990–2010: Findings From the Global Burden of Disease Study 2010, *The Lancet* **38**(9882): 1987–2015.

Yang, W.Y., Lu, J.M., Weng, J.P., *et al.* (2010). Prevalence of Diabetes among Men and Women in China, *New England Journal of Medicine* **362**(12): 1090–1101.

Chapter One

Demographic and Health Change in the Context of Urbanization in China

Xiao Ying Zheng and Chao Guo

Abstract

Population change is one of the basic features of urbanization. This chapter discusses demographic and health issues in the context of urbanization in China since the People's Republic of China was established in 1949. It focuses on changes in some of the most important demographic variables, such as birth and fertility, mortality and life expectancy, and age structure and aging. It further explores transitions in patterns of health related to changes in the 'cause-of-death structure' among the Chinese population during the 'rapid development' period of urbanization.

1.1 Introduction

Joseph Stiglitz, a Nobel laureate in Economics, has said that there will be two major events affecting human civilization in the 21st century: the new technological revolution led by the United States, and China's urbanization (Zhao and Li, 2009). Urbanization is, in essence,

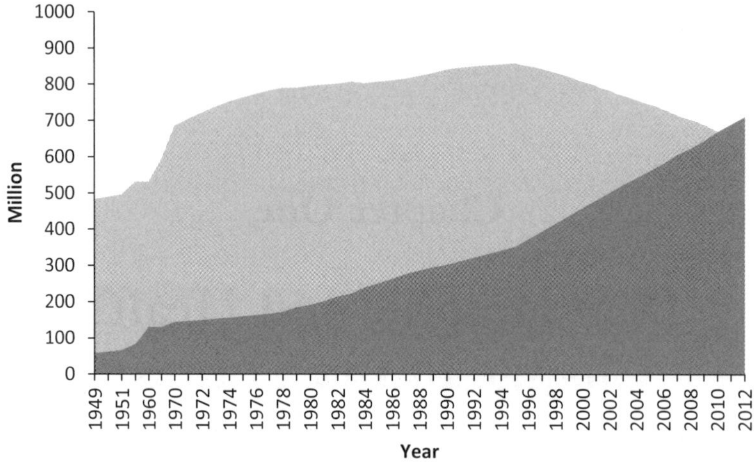

Figure 1.1 Urban and rural population (1949–2012).

***Data source*: National Bureau of Statistics PRC. China Statistical Yearbook 2013. [EB/OL]. Beijing: China Statistics Press, 2013.**

Note: Figures 1981 (inclusive) are from household registrations; for the year 1982, 1990, 2000, and 2010 are the census year estimates; the rest of the data covered in those years have been estimated on the basis of the annual national sample surveys of population.

the spatial manifestation of the economic structural transformation dating from the early stage of industrialization, characterized by a massive shift of labor and other inputs away from agricultural and into non-agricultural activities in the production structure (Chan, 1992).

The urbanization level of China at the end of 2012 was 52.57% of the population. This means that the number of people living in urban areas reached 711.82 million. Demographically, the percentage of the urban population in the total population is usually taken as the indicator by which to evaluate the level of urbanization, that is, the 'urbanization rate' (Zuo *et al.*, 2007). Figure 1.1 shows the change in the proportion of urban and rural populations in China from 1949 to 2012 (National Bureau of Statistics PRC, 2013).

The process of urbanization in China has its own characteristics. In general, the level of urbanization in China was relatively low before the 1980s. It rose slowly from the 1950s to the late 1970s, but

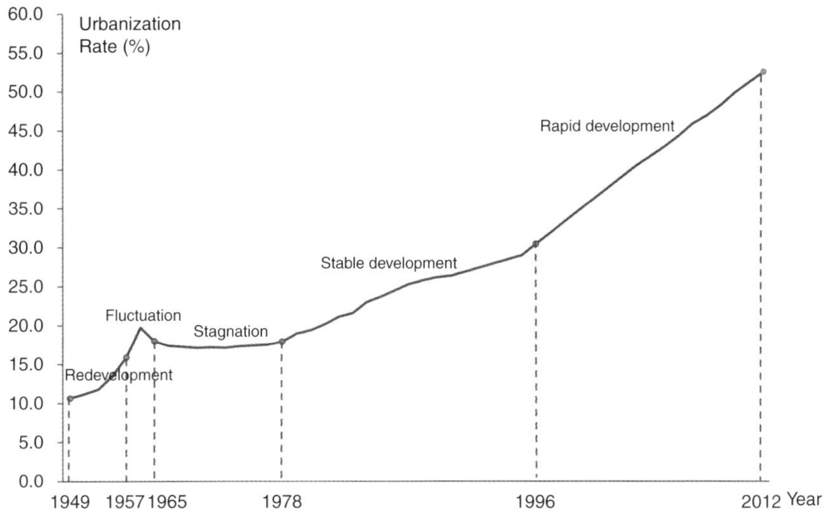

Figure 1.2 The five stages of urbanization in China.

***Data source*: National Bureau of Statistics PRC. China Statistical Yearbook 2013. [EB/OL]. Beijing: China Statistics Press, 2013.**

remained in the under-urbanization[1] stage at the beginning of the 1980s. However, the economic reforms and open-door policy of 1978 have led to the average annual rate of change in urban population increasing significantly.

It is generally agreed among China scholars that the process of urbanization in China since 1949 can be divided into five stages (see Figure 1.2): Redevelopment (1949–1957), Fluctuation (1958–1965), Stagnation (1966–1977), Stable Development (1978–1995), and Rapid Development (1996–2012) (Zuo *et al.*, 2007; Gao *et al.*, 2010; Yang and Tao, 2010; Yang, 2012). Since economic reform and opening up, the number of rural-to-urban migrants has increased significantly, resulting in the so-called 'floating population', that is, people who are not permanently registered in their current place of residence but who have become the majority in an urban population. Although

[1] Under-urbanization is a typical phenomenon of socialist economies and, in the case of China, refers to the achievement of a high industrial growth without a parallel growth in urban population (Zhang and Simon, 2003).

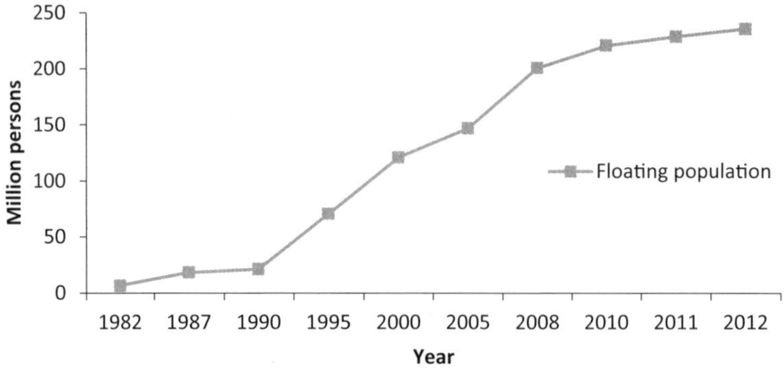

Figure 1.3 The floating population size in China, 1982–2012 (million).

***Data source*: National Bureau of Statistics PRC. China Statistical Yearbook 2013. [EB/OL]. Beijing: China Statistics Press, 2013.**

Note: Data of 1982, 1990, 2000, and 2010 are based on the National Population Census and the rest are estimates based on annual national sample surveys of population.

they are physically living and working in cities, the floating population experiences different social insurance, different services, different rights, and different resources (such as education), compared with local urban residents, that is, people living in the same city. This is called 'semi-urbanization', caused by formal or informal social exclusion at various levels in employment, life, and social interaction (Li, 2010). In 1982, there was a floating population of 6.57 million, and this reached 236 million in 2012 after the rapid increase after the 1990s. The extent of the floating population is shown in Figure 1.3. In terms of the urban population in general, from 1978 to 2012, the urbanization rate increased from 17.92% to 52.57%, one percent per year on average. Between 1996 and 2012, the 'rapid development' period, the average annual rate of change increased up to 1.3%. By comparison, during the rapid urbanization stage in the United States, from 1886 to 1920, the average rate of urbanization increased only 0.5% per year (Zuo *et al.*, 2007).

In recent decades, in the context of rapid urbanization, the size, age structure, and patterns of health of the Chinese population have undergone great transformation. These changes significantly impact on the safety and development of the Chinese population. This chapter discusses demographic and health changes in the context of urbanization in China, focusing on basic demographic variables such as fertility and mortality, and exploring the transition of health patterns related to the cause-of-death structure among the Chinese population.

1.2 Demographic Change in the Context of Urbanization in China

1.2.1 *Birth and fertility*

The demographic transition model, first proposed by Warren Thompson (1929), divides the demographic growth of a country or region into four phases (Berry *et al.*, 1987; De Souza, 1990; Cadwallader, 1996). First is the 'high stationary phase', in which population change is slow, with high levels of both fertility and mortality. In this phase in China, both birth and death rates were high, at nearly 40‰. (This might have varied a little in different counties and regions.) The second phase is the 'early expanding phase', in which the birth rate is high, death rates decrease and the population grows fast. The Chinese birth rate in this phase was up to 35–40‰, but death rates decreased to about 10‰. The third phase is the 'late expanding phase', in which the death rate is low, under 10‰, the birth rate gradually declines from around 35‰ to under 10‰, and the population grows fast. The fourth phase, the 'low stationary phase' is characterized by a low birth rate, a low death rate and slow population change. In China, during this phase, both the birth rate and the death rate were between 5–10‰ (Chen, 2010).

Following this model, the process of demographic change since the foundation of the new China can be divided into the following four stages (Yang, 2012). The first stage spanned 1949–1970, during which the population transition was led by mortality change. This stage was characterized by the death rate decreasing but the birth rate remaining high, except during the natural disaster period (1959–1961) when the birth rate decreased sharply and the death rate

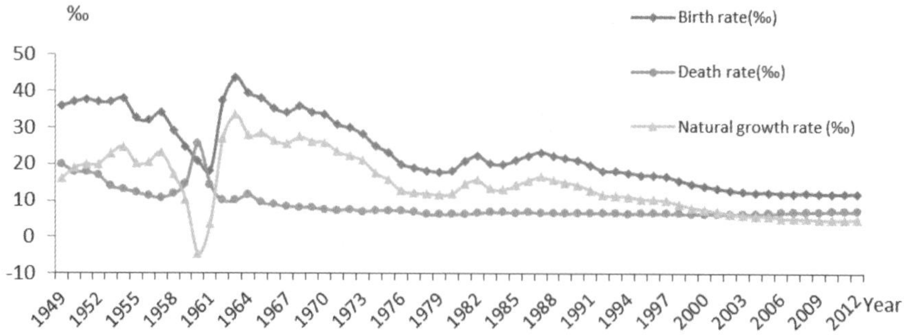

Figure 1.4 The change of birth rate, death rate, and natural growth rate (1949–2012).

Data source: **National Bureau of Statistics of China.**

Note: Figures 1981 (inclusive) are from household registrations; for the year 1982, 1990, 2000, and 2010 are the census year estimates; the rest of the data covered in those years have been estimated on the basis of the annual national sample surveys of population.

increased significantly (Figure 1.4). The total fertility rate[2] was around six children, consistent with the birth rate except during the natural disaster period (Figure 1.5). From the second stage (1971–1980), the birth rate became the most prominent factor in the population transition of China. Throughout the 1970s, the birth rate decreased sharply from 30‰ to less than 20‰ and the total fertility rate decreased from six children to fewer than three children (Figures 1.4 and 1.5). In the third stage (1980–1990), the birth rate showed a downward trend, hovering at just 20‰ or higher in most years. The total fertility rate fluctuated between two and three children, almost to replacement level (Figures 1.4 and 1.5). The fourth stage (since 1990), has manifested in a stable decrease in the birth rate to a relatively low level with the total fertility rate remaining under the replacement level (Figures 1.4 and 1.5).

These declining fertility statistics show that urbanization rates reflect the levels of social and economic development, as these have

[2] Total fertility rate refers to the average number of children a hypothetical cohort of women would have at the end of their reproductive period if they were subject during their whole lives to the fertility rates of a given period and if they were not subject to mortality. It is expressed as children per woman (United Nations, 2013).

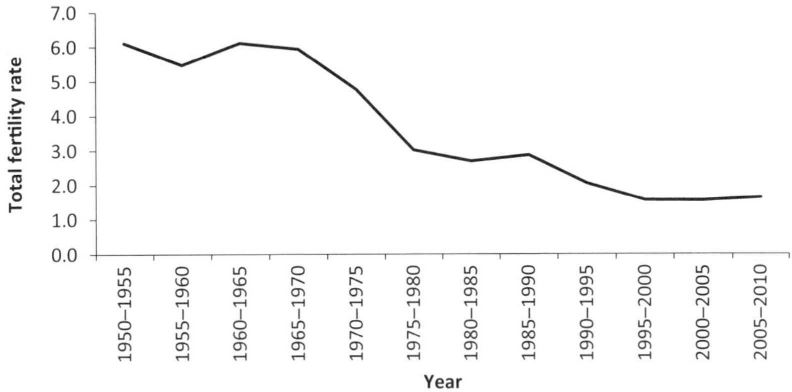

Figure 1.5 The total fertility rate of China.

***Source*: United Nations, Department of Economic and Social Affairs, Population Division (2013). World Population Prospects: The 2012 Revision, DVD Edition.**

Note: For statistical purposes, the data for China do not include Hong Kong and Macao, Special Administrative Regions (SAR) of China, and Taiwan Province of China.

an important impact on fertility (Thompson, 1930; Notestein, 1953). The urbanization rate is one of the variables included in the statistical model used in researching the influence of socio–economic development on fertility, and many studies have demonstrated that urbanization is a key factor in decreasing Chinese fertility levels (Jiang, 1986; Gu, 1989; Li, 2004). Because of urbanization and industrialization, some factors, such as the decline in infant mortality and the rise in the cost of raising children, have changed people's attitudes to fertility, resulting in lower birth rates (Preston, 1986).

In addition, in the 1980s, the Chinese government introduced the family planning policy, commonly known as the 'one child policy', which reduced the birth rate of the Chinese population sharply (Ding and Hesketh, 2006). Significantly, urbanization also played an important role in the implementation of the policy and its effect on the change in fertility. That is to say, urbanization contributed to the broader implementation of the more restrictive family planning policy, which would help reduce birth rates. There were significant disparities in the implementation and enforcement of the one-child policy throughout the country, specifically between the urban and rural areas. In urban areas, the policy was stricter, only allowing a couple to have one child, and the cost of policy violation was higher. In many rural areas, couples were also bound by the one-child limit if the firstborn was a son. However, rural couples whose firstborn was a daughter were allowed a second child, referred to as the 'one-and-a-half child policy' (Sanderson and Tan, 1995).

In the context of urbanization, a population that migrates from rural areas to urban areas, and those people whose residence status changes from 'rural' to 'city' residents because of the adjustment of administrative division, have a major impact on fertility rates. A study by You and Poston (2004) indicates that the relationship between population migration and fertility in China is consistent with migration and fertility theory in the West, that is, fertility levels of rural-to-urban migrants were likely to decline after they migrated from rural to urban areas. Registered rural-to-urban migrants and people whose identities changed from rural to urban because of the adjustment of administrative division[3], have to follow the more strictly enforced urban fertility policy, which allows only one child per couple. This has resulted in the decline in their fertility (Chen, 2006). Therefore, in the process of China's urbanization, the naturally growing urban population, the floating population, the registered migrants and the population that has become urban due to the adjustment of administrative division, have all contributed to the decline in fertility and subsequent population stabilization (Figure 1.6).

1.2.2 *Mortality and life expectancy*

The crude 'death rate' of the Chinese population underwent a sharp decline from 1949 to 1959, fluctuated from 1959 to 1961, and then

[3]The household registration (*hukou*) system in China divides citizens into urban household registration and rural household registration according to biological inheritance and geographic location. This system has aroused more and more controversy and criticism because of the inequality in welfare and rights between urban and rural residents. The Chinese government has been reforming this system since 2005, but the effect of reform is yet to be assessed.

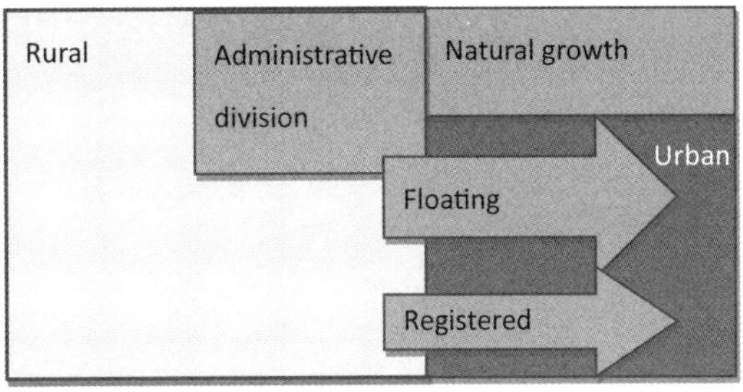

Figure 1.6 The source of urban population growth of China.

stabilized at a low level from then on (see Figure 1.4). It seems that rapid urbanization mainly affects fertility and birth rates, rather than mortality or death rates. However, if the death rates of some specific groups are analyzed, the influence of urbanization on death can also be confirmed. Figure 1.7 shows the neonatal mortality rate, infant mortality rate, mortality rate of children under five years, and the maternal mortality rate in China from 1991 to 2012. Obviously, mortality among all four groups in both the urban and rural populations decreased sharply during those 20 years, and the speed of the decline in rural areas was faster than that in urban areas. The gap between rural and urban areas became smaller, although the levels of mortality in rural areas were still higher.

A study by Fu *et al.* (2011) indicated that urbanization promoted economic development, and economic development raised the level of infrastructure, improved traffic conditions, and increased the incomes of people both in urban and rural areas. The abovementioned factors promoted the utilization of services of maternity and child care and reduced the incidence of malnutrition in children, thus reducing mortality. Similarly, the improvement of medical health technology in maternity and child care in the context of urbanization reduced the risk of puerperal and infant mortality.

In addition, although the crude death rate of the total population remained at a stable low level, the sustained decline of infant mortality resulted in the life expectancy of the Chinese population increasing from 67.77 years in 1982 to 74.83 years in 2010. The life expectancy of women reached 77.37 years in 2010 (Figure 1.8).

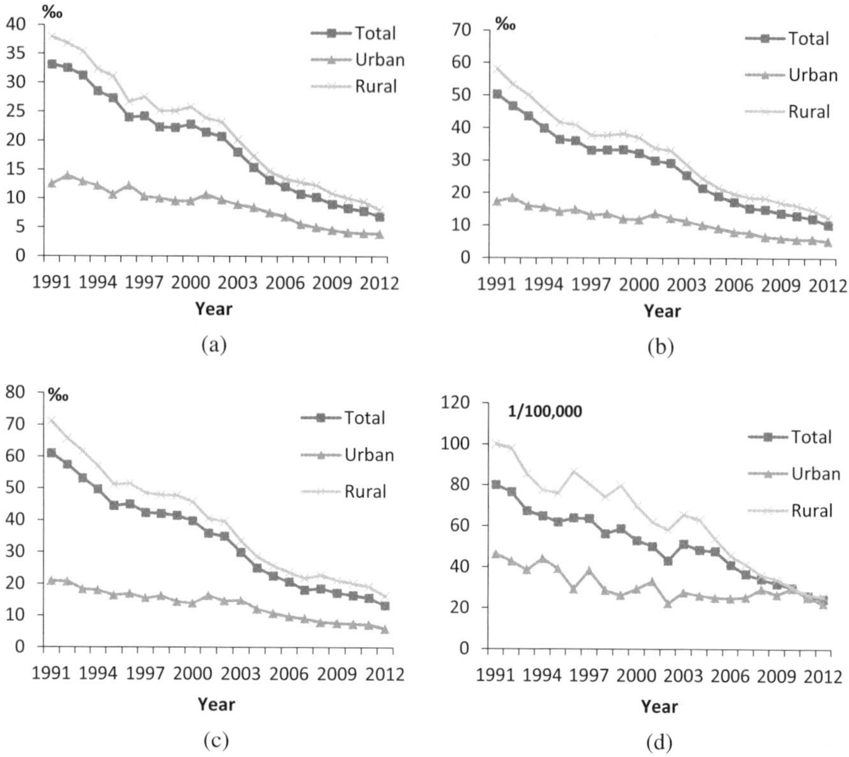

Figure 1.7 (a) Neonatal mortality rate (b) Infant mortality rate (c) Mortality rate of children under 5 (d) Maternal mortality rate.

***Data source*: National Bureau of Statistics PRC. China Statistical Yearbook 2013. [EB/OL]. Beijing: China Statistics Press, 2013.**

1.2.3 *Age structure and aging*

The age structure of the Chinese population in both rural and urban China, has undergone great change during the process of urbanization. The proportion of the age group 0–14 years has decreased gradually while the proportion of the age group over 65 years has gradually increased. Figure 1.9 shows four age–sex pyramids representing the Chinese population in 1982, 1990, 2000, and 2010, based on data from the four most recent censuses in China, conducted by the National Bureau of Statistics PRC. As the pyramids

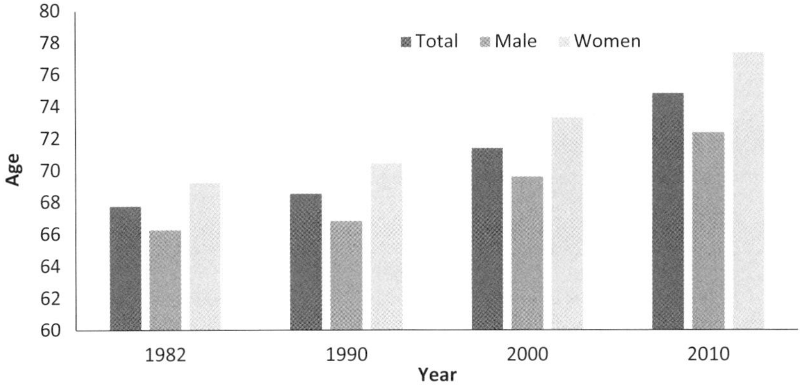

Figure 1.8 Life expectancy of Chinese population.

***Data source*: The census office of the state council. National Bureau of Statistics PRC. Data of the Third/Fourth/Fifth/Sixth Population Census China. [EB/OL]. Beijing: China Statistics Press, 1982/1990/2000/2010.**

suggest, the age structure of China changed from a youth bulge to a bulge in middle and old age. The proportion of people older than 65 years was 4.91% in 1982, 5.57% in 1990, 6.96% in 2000, and 8.87% in 2010. China has one of the world's fastest aging populations (Kinsell and He, 2009). The estimated number of people older than 65 years in China in 2012 was 127 million, accounting for 9.4% of the total population (National Bureau of Statistics PRC, 2013).

Based on the experience of many of the world's developed countries, the interaction between changes in population 'age type' and the various periods of urbanization can be summarized as follows: the 'young bulge' population corresponds with the primary stage of urbanization; the 'adult bulge' population corresponds with the rapid development of urbanization; and the 'old age bulge' corresponds with the ultimate stable stage of urbanization. When the age structure of the population turns from the young to the adult type, the proportion of young people decreases distinctly, as indicated in the olive-shape of the population pyramid, showing people at the labor age forming the main body of the population. This kind of population structure has proven to be of great benefit to the development of society, resulting in the rapid development of urbanization. Moreover,

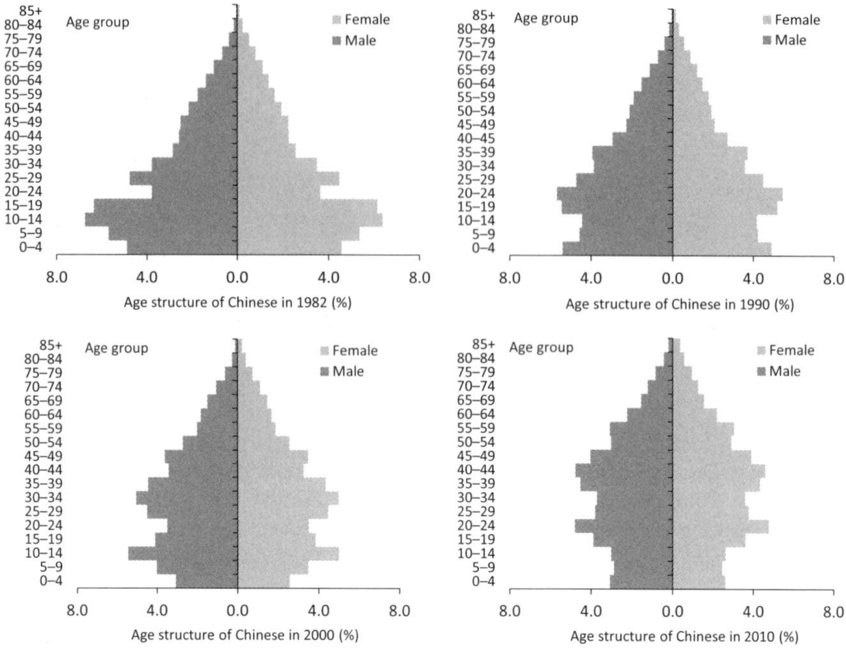

Figure 1.9 Population age–sex pyramids of Chinese population, in 1982, 1990, 2000, 2010.

***Data source*: The census office of the state council. National Bureau of Statistics PRC. Data of the Third/Fourth/Fifth/Sixth Population Census China. [EB/OL]. Beijing: China Statistics Press, 1982/1990/2000/2010.**

the urban areas had particular appeal to the labor force dominant in that period, thus playing a considerable role in the development of urbanization. When the population age structure developed into the aged society, the cycle of population reproduction became longer and the increase of the urban population slowed. Therefore, the urban population tended to increase slowly and the urbanization process went into the stable stage at a relatively high level (Li, 1995).

In China, the population age structure is in the 'old age bulge' now, while urbanization is still developing rapidly. This is because, on the one hand, China came up with the family planning policy in the 1970s, which promoted the sharp decrease in fertility. The rigorous policy as an external force contributed to the fast aging of China's population by reducing the number of births, in addition to increasing the longevity of people (Mu, 2006). So the problem of the dual function of 'aging at the bottom' caused by the decrease in fertility, and 'aging at the top' caused by the increase in life expectancy, led China's population to age faster than the pace of urbanization, while still leaving room for a large rise in the development of urbanization. On the other hand, the large population base of China indicates that there is much potential for the further growth of rural-to-urban migration.

In addition, because the majority of the working population migrates from rural areas to urban areas, the aging in the rural population is greater than in urban areas. According to the sixth population census of China (2010), the proportion of people older than 65 years is 7.8% in urban areas, and 10% in rural areas (National Bureau of Statistics PRC, 2010). The left-behind elderly in rural areas, as well as the left-behind children, have become an important problem for China. Perhaps the key to solving the problem of the left-behind elderly is to balance development between rural and urban areas, as well as to reform the household registration system.

1.3 Transitions in Patterns of Health in the Context of Urbanization in China

1.3.1 *The change in the epidemic pattern of major diseases in China*

Quantity and quality are two complementary aspects of population. Besides demographic changes during the past 60 years, the major diseases that impact the health of the Chinese have also changed a lot. The mortality of infectious diseases, tuberculosis, diseases of the respiratory system and the digestive system significantly declined, while the mortality of malignant tumors, heart diseases, cerebrovascular diseases and external causes of injury and poisoning (such as pesticides and carbon monoxide) rose. There were some differences between rural and urban areas in the mortality of major diseases: the death rates from infectious diseases, diseases of the respiratory and digestive systems and injuries in the rural population were higher than in the urban population; death rates from malignant tumors, heart diseases, and cerebrovascular diseases were higher in urban areas.

The most important transition in health and death patterns has been the decline in the morbidity and mortality of infectious diseases — the main cause of death in the Chinese population before 1949. A survey in Guangxi province between 1939 and 1942 suggested that death caused by infectious diseases represented more than 40% of total deaths (Shao, 2001). Since then, because of active control, various infectious diseases including respiratory system diseases, intestinal diseases, natural-focal disease and insect-borne diseases have decreased more than 80%, contributing greatly to a decrease in death rates among the total population, from around 2,000:100,000 in the early 1950s to 700:100,000 in the 1990s, where it remains today.

The top 10 causes of death in urban and rural areas of China changed significantly from 1949 to 2010. A number of Non-communicable chronic diseases (NCDs) — malignant tumors, heart diseases, and cerebrovascular disease–replaced infectious diseases, parasitic disease, and maternal and child diseases in the top ten. By 2012, the top five causes of death in urban areas were malignant tumor, heart diseases, cerebrovascular disease, diseases of the respiratory system and external causes of injury (such as poisoning); in rural areas within the top five causes of death by 2012, only the ranks of heart diseases and cerebrovascular disease interchanged (National Bureau of Statistics PRC, 2013).

Besides the death rate, there were also changes in the causes of death. In the early 1950s, infectious diseases were the main cause of death, accounting for about 30% of total deaths. By the late 1990s, NCDs became the main cause of death. The number of deaths caused by NCDs represented 90% of overall deaths, with the proportion in rural areas reaching 80%. Also, the combination of the top five causes of death made up a larger percentage of total deaths. In urban areas at the beginning of the health transition, when infectious diseases were the main cause of death, the top five causes accounted for less than 50% of total deaths. However, when NCDs became the main cause of death in the late period of transition, the top five became responsible for almost 80% of total deaths. The trend in rural areas is similar to that in urban areas. It can be said that in China, NCDs have had the most impact on population health and death patterns.

1.3.2. *The characteristics of health patterns in the rapid development period of urbanization*

During the rapid development period of urbanization, the health patterns of Chinese people in urban and rural areas showed some characteristics that reflected the special influence of urbanization on health. In urban areas, from 1990 to 2010, the crude death rates from malignant tumors, heart diseases, and endocrine, nutritional and metabolic diseases showed rising trends. The crude death rates from cerebrovascular disease increased in the first decade, and despite decreasing a little during the next decade, remained at high levels. The death rate from diseases of the respiratory system and diseases of the digestive system each showed a downward trend. The death rates from external causes of injury and poisoning, and infectious disease and parasitic disease were also on a downward trend from 1990 to 2000, but rallied a little in the second decade.

In rural areas, during these 20 years, the death rate from malignant tumors, heart diseases, cerebrovascular disease, and endocrine, nutritional and metabolic diseases showed rising trends. Meanwhile, the death rate from infectious disease and parasitic disease, diseases of the respiratory system, diseases of the digestive system, and external causes of injury and poisoning were still on downward trends (Figures 1.10 and 1.11).

In terms of diseases, during the 20 years between 1990 and 2010, the mortality caused by NCDs such as malignant tumors, heart diseases, and endocrine, nutritional and metabolic diseases kept increasing in both urban and rural areas, and the rates in urban areas were always higher than those in rural areas. Specifically, deaths caused by cerebrovascular disease in urban areas stopped increasing, although it was still at a high level, while its prevalence rate in rural areas continued to increase. In 2010, the death rate for cerebrovascular disease in rural areas, which was lower before 2000, was already higher than that in urban areas. Mortality from infectious diseases, parasitic

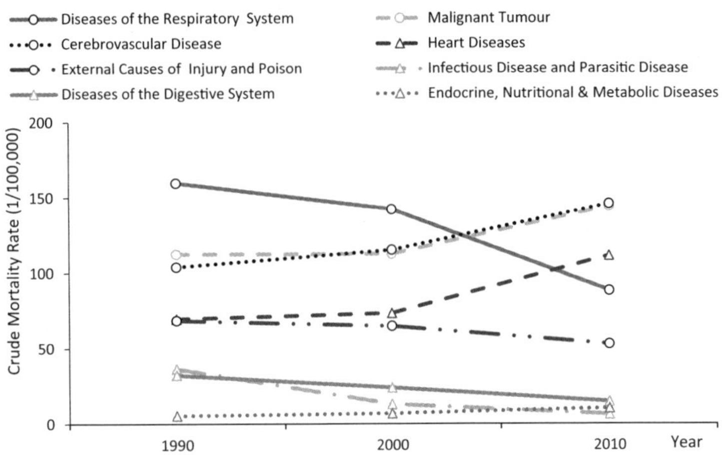

Figure 1.10 The death rate of major diseases in rural areas of China, 1990, 2000, 2010.

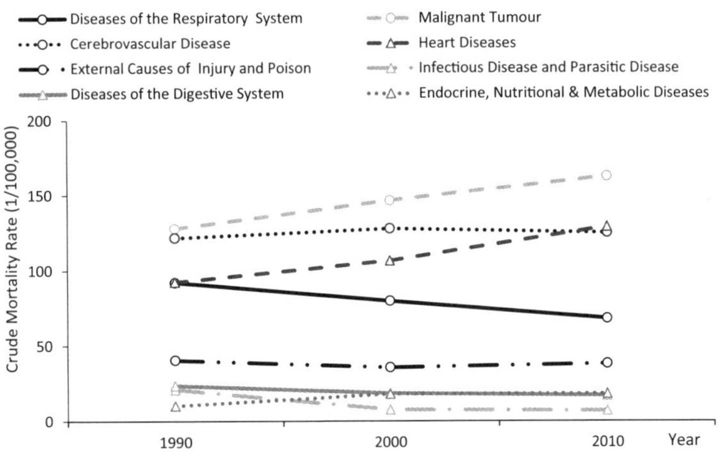

Figure 1.11 The death rate of major diseases in urban areas of China, 1990, 2000, 2010.

disease, diseases of the digestive system, and respiratory system, were declining in both urban and rural areas. While death rates from infectious diseases, parasitic disease, and diseases of the digestive system in rural areas dropped to lower levels than those in urban areas, diseases of the respiratory system in rural areas were still higher, compared with urban areas. Death from external causes of injury and poisoning were the same in both areas (Figures 1.10 and 1.11).

There were not many differences among the ranks of major causes of death in urban areas, except that cerebrovascular disease and heart disease changed places in 2010 and endocrine, nutritional and metabolic diseases rose one rank per decade, from eighth in 1990 to sixth in 2010. In rural areas, the main changes happened with diseases of the respiratory system and cerebrovascular disease. Diseases of the respiratory system were the major cause of death in both 1990 and 2000, but dropped down to fourth in 2010. Conversely, cerebrovascular disease rose one rank per decade, from third in 1990, up to being the main cause of death for rural people in 2010. As a result, the top three causes of death in urban and rural areas included the same three diseases: malignant tumors, heart disease, and cerebrovascular disease, although there was a little difference in the ranks (Table 1.1).

In addition, the three major NCDs, malignant tumors, heart disease, and cerebrovascular disease, together accounted for a larger proportion of deaths per decade in both rural and urban areas, especially during the second decade in rural areas. In 2010, the total proportions of the top three major causes of death in rural and urban areas almost reached the same level, accounting for nearly 70% of total deaths, indicating that NCDs played increasingly important roles in both urban and rural people's health in the context of urbanization (Figure 1.12).

Overall, in rural areas, the NCDs, particularly cerebrovascular disease, developed a stronger momentum, especially after 1990. Rural people became a higher risk population for NCDs than urban people, because of which may be caused by the weaker health service system and poorer medical resources in the rural areas. In addition, prevention and control of external causes of injury and poisoning should still be the key point in rural areas because rapid urbanization means that the rural population — the left-behind elderly, children and women — is the group most vulnerable to injury. In urban areas, in addition to the prevention and control of NCDs, more attention should be paid to preventing the recurrence of infectious disease and

Table 1.1 The rank of death rate of major diseases in urban and rural areas of China, 1990, 2000, 2010

	Urban				Rural		
Cause of death	1990	2000	2010	Cause of death	1990	2000	2010
Malignant tumor	1	1	1	Diseases of the respiratory system	1	1	4
Cerebrovascular disease	2	2	3	Malignant tumour	2	3	2
Heart diseases	3	3	2	Cerebrovascular disease	3	2	1
Diseases of the respiratory system	4	4	4	Heart diseases	4	4	3
External causes of injury and poison	5	5	5	External causes of injury and poison	5	5	5
Diseases of the digestive system	6	6	7	Infectious disease and parasitic disease	6	7	8
Infectious disease and parasitic disease	7	8	8	Diseases of the digestive system	7	6	6
Endocrine, nutritional & metabolic diseases	8	7	6	Endocrine, nutritional & metabolic diseases	8	8	7

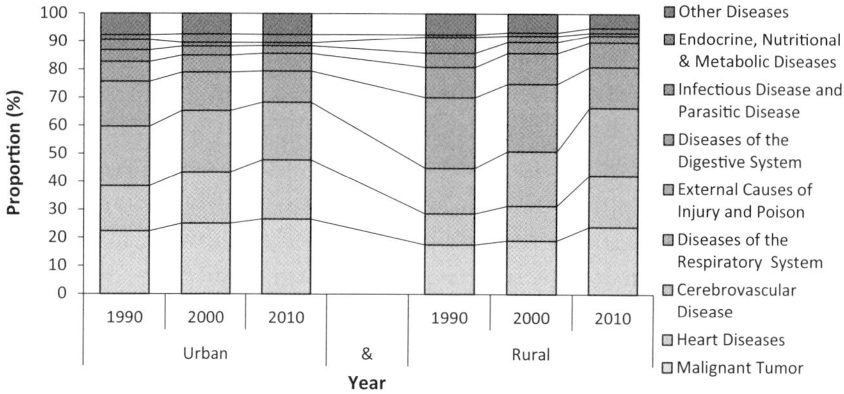

Figure 1.12 The proportions of major causes of death in China, 1990, 2000, 2010.

parasitic disease, as the numbers of migrants and floating people increase with the rapid development of urbanization.

1.4. Conclusion

People play an important role in the process of urbanization, and are impacted by the changes that urbanization causes. Therefore, people should be helped to cope with these demographic and health changes more positively. The most important challenge presented by China's urbanization is to balance the development of rural and urban areas, while improving the equality of policy, resources and services, to tackle the problem of the left-behind elderly, children and women, in the areas of education, social insurance, medical requirements and so on. At the same time, rural and urban areas should focus on different key points, according to the specific needs of each. For example, in addition to the most common cause of death, NCDs, preventing and controlling the external causes of injury and poisoning should still be a key consideration in rural areas where the groups who are most vulnerable to these injuries — again the left-behind elderly, children and women — still live. However, in the urban areas, more attention should be paid to preventing the recurrence of infectious disease and parasitic disease, because of the increasing numbers of migrants and floating people as the rapid development of urbanization continues.

In addition, some population problems occurring with urbanization, such as the current low fertility, suggest that China should take more effective measures to prevent the situation from deteriorating even further. Recently some active measures have been taken. For example, a more generous family planning policy allowing families to have two children if one of the parents is an only child, has been gradually implemented since November 2013. Furthermore, an urbanization plan for 2014–2020 that aims to steer China's urbanization onto a human-centered and environmentally friendly path was unveiled in March 2014 (Xinhuanet, 2014). This suggests that China might have changed its focus from economic development to human development, and is paying more attention to other developmental goals and measures besides GDP. Despite this, more effort is warranted in addressing the challenges brought by the demographic and health changes in the context of urbanization.

References

Berry, B.L.J, Conkling, E. and Ray, D. (1987). *Economic Geography*, Prentice-Hall, New Jersey.

Cadwallader, M.T. (1996). *Urban Geography: An Analytical Approach*, Prentice Hall, New Jersey.

Chan, K.W. (1992). Economic Growth Strategy and Urbanization Policies in China, 1949–1982, *International Journal of Urban and Regional Research* **2**: 275–305.

Chen, Y.G. (2010). The Corresponding Relationships between the Demographic Transition, Urbanization Process, and Industrial Development of China, *Geographical Research* **12**: 2109–2120 (in Chinese).

Chen, Y.H. (2006). The Household Registration System Reform and Family Planning Work, *Population Research* **6**: 82–88 (in Chinese).

De Souza, A.R.A. (1990). *A Geography of World Economy*, Columbus, Ohio.

Ding, Q.J. and Hesketh, T. (2006). Family Size, Fertility Preferences, and Sex Ratio in China in the Era of the One Child Family Policy: Results from National Family Planning and Reproductive Health Survey, *British Medical Journal* **333**: 371–373.

Fu, J.X., Feng, X.L. and Guo, Y. (2011). Effect of Urbanization on Mortality of Children in China, *Maternal & Child Health Care of China* **18**: 2725–2728 (in Chinese).

Gao, X.C., Zhou, Y. and Xu, J. (2010). The History of China's Urbanization Process, *Academic Exchange* **1**: 97–99 (in Chinese).

Gu, B.C. (1989). Analysis on the Role of Social and Economic Development and Family Planning in the Decline of Fertility Rates in China, *Chinese Journal of Population Science* **1**: 2–11 (in Chinese).

Jiang, Z.H. (1986). The Influence of Social and Economic Factors on China's Fertility Rate, *Population Research* **3**: 25–30 (in Chinese).

Kinsell, K. and He, W. (2009). *An Aging World: 2008*, National Institute on Aging, U.S. Census Bureau, Washington DC.

Li, H. (1995). Interaction between Population Age Structure and Urbanization, *Statistics and Decision* **9**: 23–24 (in Chinese).

Li, J.M. (2004). Birth Reason and Reproductive Decision-making and the Transition of the Stable Mechanism for Low Birth Level in China, *Journal of Population Research* **6**: 2–18 (in Chinese).

Li, Q. (2010). *Thirty Years of Reform and Social Changes in China*, Brill Academic Publishers, Boston.

Mu, G.Z. (2006). The Risk Prospect of Demographic Transition in China, *Journal of Zhejiang University (Humanities and Social Sciences)* **6**: 25–34 (in Chinese).

National Bureau of Statistics PRC (2013). *China Statistical Yearbook 2013*, China Statistics Press, Beijing.

National Bureau of Statistics PRC (2010). *Data of the Sixth Population Census China*, China Statistics Press, Beijing.

Notestein, F.W. (1953). *Economic Problems of Population Change*, Oxford University Press, Oxford.

Preston, S.H. (1986). Changing Values and Falling Birth Rates, *Population and Development Review* **12**: 176–195.

Sanderson, W.C. and Tan, J.P. (1995). *Population in Asia*, World Bank, Washington D.C.

Shao, R.T. (2001). China's Disease Transition Model and Countermeasures, *China Medical News* **15**: 2–5 (in Chinese).

Thompson, W.S. (1929). Population, *American Journal of Sociology* **34**: 959–975.

Thompson, W.S. (1930). *Population Problems*, McGraw Hill, New York.

Xinhuanet (2014). *National New Urbanization Plan (2014–2020)*. Available at http://news.xinhuanet.com/politics/2014-03/16/c_119791251.htm [Accessed 15 January 2015].

Yang, F. and Tao, S.W. (2010). The Development Process, Characteristics and Trends of China's Urbanization, *Lanzhou Academic Journal* **6**: 75–78 (in Chinese).

Yang, S. (2012). The Level of China's Urbanization, Based on the Demographic Transition, *China Economic & Trade Herald* **26**: 60–62 (in Chinese).

You, H.X. and Poston, D.L. (2004). Are Floating Migrants in China "Childbearing Guerillas": An Analysis of Floating Migration and Fertility, *Asia and Pacific Migration Journal* **13**: 11–29.

Zhang, L. and Simon, X.Z. (2003). Reinterpretation of China's Under-urbanization: A Systemic Perspective, *Habitat International* **27**: 459–483.

Zhao, Y. and Li, S. (2009). The Relationship between Urbanization and Real Estate Industry: Evidence from Chinese Regions, *International Journal for Housing Science & Its Applications* **4**: 195–206.

Zuo, X.J.,· Zhu, Y. and Wang, G.X. (2007). *Population Urbanization in China and Coordinated Urban–rural Development*, Xuelin Publishing House, Shanghai (in Chinese).

Chapter Two

Population Aging: Social Consequences and Challenges

He Chen and Tuo Hong Zhang

Abstract

Like the rest of the world, China's population is aging. Rapid urbanization attracts young people from the land to large metropolitan centers, exacerbating the aging problem in remote rural areas. There are social consequences and challenges in this situation, such as increasing numbers of 'empty-nest' families whose children have left home, and a corresponding lack of social care and appropriate physical infrastructure. The situation calls for government regulations, governance and the development of civil society. This chapter examines the social consequences and challenges of aging in China on the economy, health service delivery, long-term care and pension systems. Recent government and social developments in tackling Chinese aging issues are also discussed. Population aging does not only present *challenges* to the current society, but could also provide opportunities for building a better one in the future. Whether they are challenges or opportunities largely depends on the ability of Chinese society to deal with the issue of aging. Recommendations are provided where solid evidence exists in the literature.

2.1 Introduction

In the 21st century, population aging and urbanization are two global trends that come together to form a major force, shaping societies, especially in middle and low income countries (WHO, 2007). China[1] is no exception. Since the 1970s, the combination of rising life expectancy and rapidly declining fertility have resulted in a dramatic demographic transition (Flaherty *et al.*, 2007). The percentage of persons aged 60 and over rose from 7.5% in 1950 to 12.4% in 2010 and is predicted to further climb to 32.8% by 2050 (United Nations, 2013), as discussed in more detail in Chapter One, 'Demographic and Health Change in the Context of Urbanization in China'. China experienced a stagnation of the urbanization process in the late 1960s and early 1970s, and a subsequent upturn since the 1980s. The proportion of China's population classed as urban was 11.8% in 1950, 19.4% in 1980 and then quickly increased to 49.2% in 2010 (United Nations Department of Economic and Social Affairs Population Division, 2014a). In 2014, China had the largest urban population (758 million) in the world; Shanghai with 23 million inhabitants and Beijing with 19.52 million inhabitants are among the 10 largest mega-cities in existence (United Nations Department of Economic and Social Affairs Population Division, 2014b).

Similar to the trend of population aging in China, urbanization will continue, and is projected to reach 75.8% in 2050 (United Nations Department of Economic and Social Affairs Population Division, 2014a). In this process of urbanization, population aging will probably bring issues that will negatively affect the sustainability of social development. However, these issues may also significantly drive Chinese society to adapt and develop. This chapter will discuss the challenges presented by population aging on the economy, health service delivery, long-term care, the opportunities for pension reform and the development of age-friendly cities.

---

[1] Without specification, "China" in this chapter refers to "mainland China".

2.2 Economic Implications

2.2.1 *The negative impact of aging on economic development in China*

Workforce and private savings are the main mechanisms through which aging influences economic development. The Chinese 'economic miracle' over the last 30 years has largely depended on high inputs of cheap capital and labor (Jackson *et al.*, 2009). However, as population aging continues, these comparative advantages are gradually diminishing. With all other conditions held constant, aging will theoretically impede economic development in China by reducing workforce supply and lowering saving rates (Banister *et al.*, 2012; Peng, 2008).

It was estimated that the favorable population age structure contributed 15–25% of per-capita GDP growth during 1980 and 2010 in China (Wang, 2012). However, this demographic dividend is being exhausted (Cai and Wang, 2006; Cai, 2010). Between 1950 and 2050, the year 2010 was the turning point for Chinese workforce supply, when the working-age population, whether in absolute number or as a percentage of total population, achieved its apex (Figure 2.1). As a result, persons in the working-age range 15–59 in 2050 are projected to make up only 76.9% of the population in 2010 (United Nations, 2013). Moreover, due to urbanization, especially the migration of the working-age population to the cities, rural China has experienced a faster aging process compared with urban areas (Tong, 2014). When the labor shortage occurs, the cost of the workforce will go up (Eggleston *et al.*, 2013), which tends to increase cost and decrease profit. In addition, an aged workforce may lack the capability to absorb new knowledge and engage effectively with technology, which hinders improvements in productivity (Zhang, 2013).

Saving patterns vary across different age groups. Usually, those aged 30–50 years have the highest saving rate, while the elderly population tends to save less due to decreased net income (Wang, 2012). In China, the percentage of people aged 30–50 years will decrease from 31.07% in 2015 to 23.92% in 2050 (United Nations, 2013), and therefore private savings are expected to drop. Additionally, population

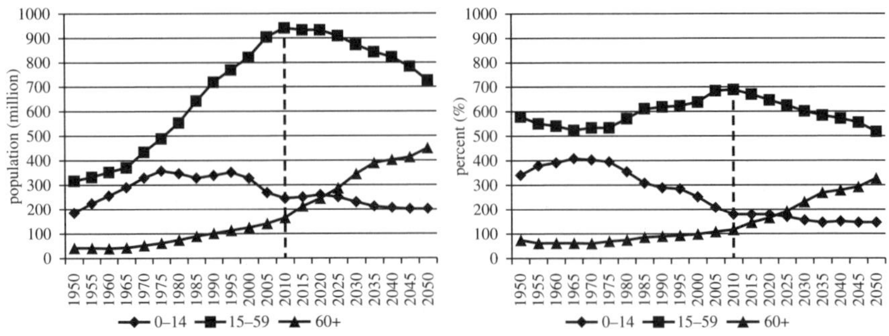

Figure 2.1 The number and percentage of population aged 0–14, 15–59, and 60+ in China between 1950–2050 (million).

Source: United Nations (2013).

aging is likely to further reduce government savings through higher expenditure on pensions, health care and long-term care. The overall savings rate in China is expected to decline, which will impede future economic investment and growth (Banister *et al.*, 2012).

2.2.2. *The factors mitigating the impact of aging on china's economy*

Though the impact of aging on the Chinese economy is a matter of concern, there are ways to mitigate the impact. Firstly, China has the potential to increase the workforce through measures such as encouraging the participation of women. The employment participation of women is lower than that of men in almost all age groups. Even in the age group 25–45, when people are most likely to be in the workforce, around 80% of women had a job in 2010 (Figure 2.2) and the gap between male and female employment has been increasing (Chi and Li, 2014)" into "Even in the age group 25–45, when people are most likely to be in the workforce, around 80% of women had a job in 2010 and the gap between male and female employment has been increasing as displayed in Figure 2.2 (Chi and Li, 2014). At least two factors contribute to the gap: child care and household responsibilities significantly decrease the opportunities for female labor participation (Zhang *et al.*, 2008; Du and Dong, 2013); and the disparity in pay

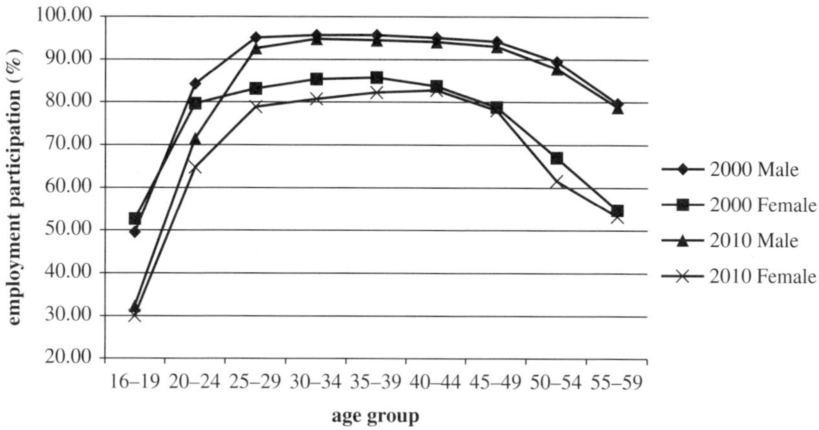

Figure 2.2 Employment participation by sex and age group in China, 2000 and 2010.

***Source*: Population Census Office of China (2002 and 2012).**

forces women out of the labor market, especially women on low wages (Chi and Li, 2014). Measures such as increasing the availability and affordability of child care and housekeeping services, promoting gender equality in wages and providing more part time or flexible time jobs, might encourage more women into the labor market.

Secondly, improvement in agricultural productivity and progress in urbanization may provide more workforces to industry and service sectors in China (Banister *et al.*, 2012). Zhang and Bruemmer (2011) estimated that the total factor productivity of Chinese agriculture had a net cumulated increase of 222% from 1979 to 2008. Chemical fertilizer made the most important contribution to this impressive progress; machinery use also made a positive but lesser contribution (Zhang and Bruemmer, 2011; Li and Zhang, 2013). The level of machinery use in the Chinese agriculture sector is quite low compared to the U.S. and other countries, such as Australia. According to the Food and Agriculture Organization of the United States (2013), in 2007, the value of machinery and equipment stock per economically active person in the agriculture sector in the U.S. was US$100,261,300, which was 500 times higher than that in China (US$195,400). There was also a huge difference in the number of combine harvester-threshers in use per thousand economically active persons in agriculture sector between the U.S. (129.5) and China (1.3) (Food and Agriculture Organization of the United States, 2014). It was estimated that the contribution of machinery to output growth in Chinese agriculture was only 6.25% during 1985 and 2010 (Li and Zhang, 2013). It is reasonable to speculate that more investment in agricultural machinery and the increasing use of this machinery in Chinese agricultural activities will release a surplus workforce from farming. Some researchers suggest that government subsidies of machinery investment and promotion of farmland transfer might facilitate machinery use (Liu *et al.*, 2014; Li, 2014; Cao *et al.*, 2010).

The relationship between urbanization and agricultural productivity improvement is more complicated. On the one hand, improved agricultural productivity will push the surplus workforce to enter non-agricultural sectors, which usually promotes urbanization; on the other hand, if urban areas can provide adequate and highly paid jobs, farmers will leave rural areas, requiring the agricultural sector to improve their productivity (Xia and Liu, 2012). For this to happen, attractive job opportunities in urban areas and the household registration (*Hukou*) system reforms are essential (Banister *et al.*, 2012).

Moreover, productivity improvement in the industrial and service sectors may reduce the need for a growing workforce (Peng, 2008). The China economic miracle largely depends on its comparative advantage embodied in labor-intensive products with low added value (Lin *et al.*, 2003). China has been carrying out industrial transformation and upgrading, which emphasizes total factor productivity improvement (Zhang, 2008; Zhu and Chen, 2011) and, if the upgrading succeeds, workforce needs may decrease (Bloom *et al.*, 2010).

Raising statutory retirement age is one of the most straightforward ways of increasing workforce supply (Jackson *et al.*, 2009). In 2013, the central government announced the progressive raising of the retirement age in order to keep people in the workforce longer and to delay the burden of pension costs (The Central Committee of the Communist Party of China, 2013). This, however, has generated a lot of debate and no clear plans have been released.

The burgeoning 'grey' market also helps to fight against the downside of the aging impact on the economy. More than 200 million

Chinese aged 60 and over form a huge consumer group. They have specific needs in areas such as long-term care, food, real estate and tourism. As described by Jin and Wang (2010), in 2010 spending by the aged was 1.18 trillion RMB, accounting for 9.83% of total national spending, and the figure is predicted to reach 1.73 trillion RMB in 2040, accounting for one fifth of the total national consumption of goods and services. This huge potential market creates enormous business opportunities.

2.3 Health Service Delivery System

2.3.1 *The challenge confronted by the health service delivery system*

Along with demographic transition, China has been undergoing a profound health transition. Chronic and non-communicable diseases (NCDs) have become the predominant disease burden among elderly Chinese (Yang *et al.*, 2013; Yang *et al.*, 2008). Like other aging societies, China is confronted with a huge challenge of how to adapt the health service delivery system to current population health (OECD, 2011). The health system in China consists of community health centers, secondary and tertiary hospitals in the urban areas, village clinics, township health centers, and county hospitals in the rural areas (Yip *et al.*, 2010). Community health centers, village clinics, and township health centers are primary care providers. For now, China needs to control its disease burden related to chronic diseases, which requires primary health facilities to do a better job in disease prevention and management (WHO, 2008). However, such facilities, especially those in rural areas, are disadvantaged by a lack of human resources, equip ment and technologies, and social prestige (Chen, 2009; Fang *et al.*, 2014), which makes them unable to act efficiently as a health gatekeeper. Chinese patients' trust in primary health providers is low, and thus they often seek care at large secondary or tertiary hospitals for simple health problems (Yip *et al.*, 2012; Yip and Hsiao, 2014). Such a hospital-centered model does not match the population's health needs, especially in a time of health transition when chronic and non-communicable diseases are the most common diseases in China.

The integration of health services and long-term care systems is the key to guaranteeing that elderly persons have accessible and continuous health care services. A high proportion of aged care institutions in China, however, do not provide health care services. Enrollees of health insurance schemes must obtain services in designated health facilities in order to be reimbursed (Li *et al.*, 2011). To become designated health facilities for health insurance schemes, facilities need to apply to the Ministry of Human Resources and Social Security. However, only a small proportion of health facilities in the aged care sector have succeeded in such applications, which makes most medical services consumed in aged care institutions non-reimbursable. Due to the lack of national statistics on this issue, we will take Beijing as an example (Liu, 2011). In 2011, there were 387 aged care institutions in Beijing, among which 103 (26.6%) had established their own clinics, 138 (35.7%) had signed contracts with nearby medical facilities and the remaining 145 (37.5%) had neither clinics nor contracts. In those 103 institutions with clinics, 52 (50.5%) had obtained approval from Beijing Municipal Health Bureau (now Beijing Municipal Commission of Health and Family Planning), which made their medical practice legal, and a further 21 (20.4%) had become designated health facilities for health insurance. It is difficult for the sick elderly to gain timely and adequate access to the medical services of those 138 institutions having contracts with health facilities, as these institutions often already have an existing heavy burden of providing health services. Thus, when the elderly become ill, they have to be transferred between home, health and long-term care institutions. More importantly, disabled or partly disabled elderly people cannot access adequate curative or rehabilitation services in aged care institutions (Mu, 2012).

Huang and Meng (2014) identified a number of causes for the segmentation between health and long-term care systems. Firstly, the official requirements for health facilities are high. Considering significant costs (such as investing in premises, medical equipment and human resources) and possible legal issues involved in medical disputes, aged care facilities have no strong incentive to provide medical services. Secondly, the charges in institutions with integrated health and long-term care services are very high, and not many consumers can afford them, which reduces the number of consumers and further limits the development of such institutions. Thirdly, the system involves multiple government ministries. Common aged care facilities are under the management of the Ministry of Civil Affairs, community-based aged care facilities are under the National Committee on Aging, while medical facilities are under the National Health and Planning Commission and health expenditure reimbursement is under the Ministry of Human Resources and Social Security. The spread of administrative functions across these ministries complicates the integration of health and long-term care systems.

2.3.2 *Efforts to improve the health service delivery system*

In order to deal effectively with the demographic and health transition, the health service delivery system needs to transform from the hospital-centered model to a primary-care-centered model, and to shift the service focus from curing to preventing disease. In 2009, the Chinese Government launched a new round of health reform, elaborated on in Chapter Fifteen: 'Urbanization, Population Health and Health Systems'. Some components of the reform will help to fight chronic diseases, and the importance of primary health care is emphasized. In the last five years, the primary health facilities have been built, rebuilt or upgraded, and the health personnel capability in the primary health care facilities has been strengthened through means such as general practitioner training. Furthermore, China, for the first time, set up a National Basic Public Health Service Package in 2009. Governments at various levels are responsible for financing this package, and the minimum contribution from the each government is 30 RMB. Residents are able to receive certain public health services free. The package covers eleven service items (Table 2.1), some of which specifically target elderly persons, for example health management of the elderly promoting healthy aging, health education and the management of such conditions as hypertension and type 2 diabetes. These services are mostly provided by the public primary health centers. To date, the 2009 health reform has achieved some success in

Table 2.1 The service list of Chinese national basic public service packages

Item	Market	Content
Establish health archives	Permanent residents[1]	Establish and maintain health archives
Health education	Residents	Health education materials distribution; health education notice board updates; health counseling services; health education lectures; personalized health education
Planned immunization and vaccination	Children aged 0–6 and other priority population	Manage and implement immunization and vaccination and deal with suspected abnormal cases
Child health management	Children aged 0–6	Newborn visits; health management for children aged 0–6
Maternal care management	Pregnant women	Health management for pregnant women at early, middle or late stages; postnatal visits; checkups after postnatal 42 days
Elderly health management	Permanent residents aged 65+	Lifestyle and health status assessment; annual physical examination; auxiliary medical examination; Health guidance
Health management of hypertension patients	Primary hypertension patients aged 35+	Screening; follow-up assessment and categorized intervention; physical examination
Health management of type 2 diabetes patients	Type 2 diabetes patients aged 35+	Screening; follow-up assessment and categorized intervention; physical examination
Management for patients with major mental illness	Major mental illness patients living in their own home	Information collection and management of these patients; follow-up assessment and categorized intervention; physical examination
Report and deal with infectious disease and sudden public health event	Residents	Risk-manage, discover, register, report and deal with infectious disease and sudden public health event

(*Continued*)

Table 2.1 (*Continued*)

Item	Market	Content
Health management using Chinese medicine	Permanent residents aged 65+ and all the children aged 0–3	Mange the elderly and children health using Chinese medicine
Health supervision and assistant management	Residents	Food safety information report; occupational health consultation and guidance; water sanitation inspection; school health service; illegal medical practice and illegal blood draw and supply information report

Note: [1]Those without local Hukou but living there for more than half a year are also included

Source: The notice on 2013 national basic public health service work issued by National Health and Family Planning Commission, Ministry of Finance, and State Administration of Traditional Chinese Medicine.

expanding health insurance coverage and providing improved equality in public health services. Its influence on the outcomes of chronic disease needs more evaluation (Yip and Hsiao, 2014; Yip *et al.*, 2012).

In order to deliver health services more efficiently to the elderly, China is promoting the integration of medical and long-term care service systems (*Yi-yang-jie-he* in Chinese), a program which shares some features with the Program of All-Inclusive Care (PACE) in the U.S. (Hirth *et al.*, 2009). Cities such as Tianjin, Hefei, Zhengzhou, Changsha, and Qingdao have already set up some aged care facilities that provide both medical and long-term care services (Huang and Meng, 2014). Such an integrated model has two components. Firstly, the medical and long-term care infrastructures are physically located together. The long-term care institutions can choose to build medical facilities, such as clinics, by themselves or contract medical facilities nearby. Secondly, the elderly who consume medical services under the integrated model are able to get reimbursement from health insurance. As medical expenditure in China is high, and over 93% of elderly Chinese are now covered by health insurance (CHARLS Research Team, 2013), the reimbursement from health insurance greatly increases the feasibility of the integrated model. The integrated model is still in its early stage, and more assessment and improvement are needed.

2.4 Long-term Care

2.4.1 *The traditional old age support system is under threat*

In Chinese culture, under the influence of Confucian philosophy, children have the responsibility to support their aged parents (Zhao *et al.*, 2014), which is further enforced by the Law of the People's Republic of China on Protection of the Rights and Interests of the Elderly (2012 Revision). Currently, informal long-term care is still the main resource for the care of older adults (Feng *et al.*, 2011). More than 80% of disabled elderly people are looked after by family members, such as daughters-in-law and spouses (CHARLS Research Team, 2013; Zhang and Zheng, 2010).

In an aging society, the increasingly mobile workforce has posed several challenges for meeting the long-term care needs of some population groups. The Chinese tradition and China's current aged care structure are no longer consistent with the changing lifestyles of younger generations. Today, Chinese people are living longer, with life expectancy increasing from 44.6 years between 1950 and 1955 to 75.2 years between 2010 and 2015 (United Nations, 2013). Without effective disease and disability prevention strategies, prolonged life expectancy will lead to prolonged duration with disability, which requires more long-term care. Liu *et al.* (2009) showed that from 1987 to 2006, the life expectancy of those living with a disability (i.e. the average number of years spent with disability by a person) at age 60, went up in China, especially among the female elderly.

While older people are living longer, many do suffer from disability due to poor health. Children are now less available to care for their elderly parents than in decades before. Since the family planning policy, also known as the 'one-child policy' was adopted in the late 1970s, the total fertility rate in China has dropped from 3.01 between 1975 and 1980 to 1.66 between 2010 and 2015 (United Nations, 2013). The 2010 Chinese census showed that, of households with older adults, 31.8% were 'empty nests'. The proportions in Shandong and Zhejiang provinces even reached about 45% (Zhang, 2012). As the first cohort of parents affected by the one-child policy are now in their 50s, its effects will be felt in the coming two decades (Zhao *et al.*, 2014). Moreover, urbanization has drawn many young people from rural China to cities for greater opportunities. The older rural parents are left physically and socially isolated in remote hometowns, and are less likely to be able to rely upon their children than in the past (Powell, 2012; Li *et al.*, 2013). Zeng *et al.* (2012) estimated that, under the scenario that the one-child policy is unchanged, the average burden of home-based care cost for the disabled elderly (aged 65 and over) per worker (aged 18–64) in 2030 would be at least 3.0–4.1 times as large as that in 2000, and in 2050 it would be at least 6.8–12.6 times as large. It is apparent that the burden is too great to be placed on the shoulders of individuals and families. Therefore, government officials, researchers and other stakeholders alike are calling for the establishment of a national long-term care system.

2.4.2 *Establishing a national long-term care system*

A recent, nationally representative study in China showed 38.1% of the elderly reported having one disability (defined as having any difficulty completing basic daily activities on their own), and 23.8% reported requiring assistance with basic daily activities (CHARLS Research Team, 2013). While family support of elderly members is decreasing, the relevant market and voluntary services have not been fully developed (Glass *et al.*, 2013). Effort from the Chinese government is especially needed to fill the gap between long-term care need and supply. In those countries where the population aging process started earlier than in China, public finance plays an important role in providing long-term care. For example, in France, the public long-term care spending accounts for 1.7% of GDP, and in Japan the figure is 1.4% (Colombo *et al.*, 2011). The Chinese government is gradually taking on its responsibility in supporting the aged members of society. It aims to set up a long-term care system with home-based care as the basis, community-based long-term care as the support and institutionalized long-term care as the supplement (General Office of the State Council of the PRC, 2006; State Council of the PRC, 2013). A series of policies has also been implemented, such as The Notice on the Construction of Social Aged Care Service System (2011–2015) (General Office of the State Council of the PRC, 2011), which sets goals and steps for building an improved social aged care service system between 2011 and 2015, and the Starlight Project (Ministry of Civil Affairs of PRC, 2001), which specifically targets building community-based aged care facilities and senior citizen centers.

Since 2011, the Chinese government has made great efforts to build aged care institutions and to train professional long-term care workers. Policies also encourage private capital to enter the long-term care market. Table 2.2 shows the subsidies to each bed in aged care

Table 2.2 The construction subsidies to each bed in aged care institutions in 31 province-level administration units in mainland China

Provinces	Implementation year	Subsidy per bed (RMB)	Provinces	Implementation year	Subsidy per bed (RMB)
Beijing	2011	8000–16,000	Henan	2011	1500–3000
Tianjin	2011	10,000	Hubei	2012	500–1000
Hebei	2010	3000	Hunan	2011	3000
Shanxi	2012	1000	Guangdong	2011	2000–3000
Neimeng	2011	5000–9000	Guangxi	2012	1000–3000
Liaoning	2012	6000–7000	Hainan	2012	2500
Jilin	2011	2000	Chongqing	2012	2000–4000
Heilongjiang	2011	1000	Sichuan	2011	10000
Shanghai	2011	10000	Yunnan	2011	1000
Jiangsu	2012	3000–1000	Shaanxi	2011	2000–3000
Zhejiang	2011	1000–6000	Gansu	2012	5000
Anhui	2012	1200–5000	Qinghai	2010	5000
Fujian	2012	2500–5000	Ningxia	2012	5000
Jiangxi	2011	2000	Xinjiang	2011	1000
Shandong	2011	2000–5000			

Source: Wang L. (2013).

institutions in 31 provincial administrations in China (Wang, 2013). Nationally, the overall number of beds per 1000 elderly persons has increased by 21% from 2010 (17.8 per 1,000 elderly persons) to 2012 (21.5 per 1,000 elderly persons). In the meantime, the Ministry of Human Resources and Social Security has developed national occupational skill standards for caregivers of older adults, and aims to train more qualified caregivers. The number of certified caregivers for older adults has increased significantly in recent years (Ministry of Civil Affairs of China, 2013). Despite the increase, the number of qualified caregivers is still extremely low, considering that there were 44 million Chinese elderly needing assistance with their basic daily activities in 2011 (CHARLS Research Team, 2013). In addition, in China, some paid caregivers without certification are a vital part of the long-term care workforce (Mu, 2012). Huang *et al.* (2012) found that in Liaoning Province, only 7% of long-term care providers in aged care institutions had obtained a certificate for nursing or caregiving for older adults. However, there are no national statistics on the actual number of these non-certified caregivers.

There are significant disparities between urban and rural China in the long-term care system. On average, the rural elderly have more beds in residential care facilities than their urban counterparts. Statistics from the Ministry of Civil Affairs of China (2013) showed that in 2012, there were 10 beds per 1000 elderly in urban areas, which was much lower than that in rural areas, with 26.3 beds per 1000 elderly. At least two factors may contribute to such urban–rural difference: welfare policies and economic development. As required by central government policies, local governments need to build homes for the aged for *Wubao* elders[2] in rural areas and welfare institutes for *Sanwu*

[2] According to Regulations on the Work of Providing Five Guarantees, *Wubao* elders refer to aged residents in rural China who have no ability to work, no source of income, and no statutory obligors to provide for them or support them, or whose statutory obligors have no ability to provide for them or support them. They shall enjoy the five guarantees in rural areas, including food, clothing, housing, medical care, and burial expenses.

elders[3] in urban areas (Wu *et al.*, 2008). These facilities are sponsored by public finance and collective economy. In the last three decades, the income of older people in urban areas was significantly elevated, which has largely reduced the number of *Sanwu* elders — thus the need for residential care facilities is reduced. However, the income of older persons in rural areas has not increased as much as in urban areas. In 2012, 99,000 urban residents were eligible for *Sanwu* while 5.46 million rural residents were still classified as *Wubao*, which largely explains why rural areas have considerable advantages in the number of subsidized aged care beds.

Urban and rural long-term care services may have a different structure and quality. Firstly, in recent years, more private funds have been invested in establishing aged care institutions in urban areas than in rural areas, and the beds in such private-run facilities have become an important complementary resource (Li *et al.*, 2013). Second, the quality of the workforce in urban aged care facilities is generally higher. For example, in 2012, there were 77 registered social workers per 1000 residential aged-care facilities in urban areas, but only 12 in rural areas (Ministry of Civil Affairs of China, 2013). In addition to poor availability of informal long-term care, rural residents are less capable of purchasing formal long-term care services due to lower income (Li *et al.*, 2013; Sicular *et al.*, 2007). These factors combined put the rural population at a significant disadvantage for adequate aged care. This further perpetuates inequality in the chronic disease burden and inequity in aged care between the urban and rural elderly.

The Chinese government has allocated some limited financial support for long-term care. This support is provided through multiple systems, instead of a single one: first, medical insurance covering some long-term care expenditure in health facilities such as hospitals or nursing homes; second, medical aids that help to relieve the long-term

[3] According to Interim Measures for Social Assistance, *Sanwu* elders refer to aged residents in urban China who have no ability to work, no source of income, and no statutory obligors to provide for them or support them, or whose statutory obligors have no ability to provide for them or support them. They are eligible to receive the following support: cash or in kind to guarantee basic living standard, long-term care if disabled, medical care, and burial expenses.

care expenditure burden of elderly persons with extremely low income; third, an elderly welfare system providing an advanced-age allowance and vouchers for buying home-based aged care service; fourth, elderly aids supply money (cash or in kind) and aged care services to *Wubao* or *Sanwu* elderly, who have no ability to work, no source of income, and no alive or capable statutory obligors to support them." However, these financial supports are scattered across multiple social security systems, which makes it difficult for elderly persons to understand and use them. Currently, the long-term care finance model in China is somewhere between the OECD finance models of mixed systems and means tested safety net schemes (Colombo *et al.*, 2011). Some scholars such as Dai (2012) advocate that China should establish a nationwide long-term care insurance like those in Japan and Germany, which would require more public finance investment from government. Several cities such as Qingdao have piloted such insurance, but the nationwide long-term care insurance still has a long way to go.

2.5 Pension System

2.5.1 *Chinese pension system under pressure from aging population*

The central government has implemented three types of pension schemes in China in the past decade; all three schemes covered roughly 788.23 million people in 2012, accounting for 70% of Chinese aged 16 years and over (National Bureau of Statistics of China, 2013). Significant institutional fragmentation exists among these schemes (Wang *et al.*, 2014a; Wu, 2013):

- *Basic Old-age Insurance System for Enterprise Employees Scheme.* This scheme covers enterprise staff, self-employed persons and individuals in flexible employment. Participation in 2012 was 282.72 million (National Bureau of Statistics of China, 2013). This scheme is financed by employers, employees, and government. It currently mainly runs under the pay-as-you-go model, which is more sensitive to population age structure (Williamson *et al.*,

2012; Cai and Cheng, 2014; Yang, 2013). From 1989 to 2012, the elderly dependency ratio within this scheme[4] dropped from 5.39 to 3.09 (Ministry of Civil Affairs of China, 2013). Thus, current working employees have to contribute more compared with two decades ago in order for the system to generate enough money to pay for the already retired people.

- *Basic Old-age Insurance System for Civil Servants Scheme.* This scheme includes all the civil servants and most public institution employees. Participation in 2012 was 21.55 million (National Bureau of Statistics of China, 2013). Public finance contributes to this scheme. After years of piloting, at the beginning of 2015, the Chinese government announced the decision to reform this scheme, aiming to reduce the pension inequality among different workforce segments and to adopt a co-contribution model, requiring public institution employees to pay part of the insurance contribution.
- *Basic Old-age Insurance System for Urban and Rural Residents Scheme.* This scheme was established in 2014, and combines the previous old-age insurance system for urban residents and rural social endowment insurance, which together covered 483.97 million in 2012 (National Bureau of Statistics of China, 2013). All residents who are 16 years old and over (excluding students) and have not participated in the above two pension schemes are eligible for this new scheme. This scheme is financed by local and central governments, collective enterprise, individuals and other sponsors.

As in other societies with aging populations, the Chinese pension system is facing huge pressure from the sheer number of aging people (Zeng, 2011; Sikken *et al.*, 2008; Williamson *et al.*, 2012). The Basic Old-age Insurance System for Enterprise Employees Scheme is confronted with the low retirement age issue. Currently, the statutory retirement age in China is 60 for males, 55 for female civil servants and 50 for female employees (Wang *et al.*, 2014b). This was determined in the 1950s when Chinese life expectancy was about 45 years,

[4] In the Basic Old-age Insurance System for Enterprise Employees, elderly dependency ratio is computed as the ratio of the number of employees and the number of retirees.

but now life expectancy has reached about 75 years (United Nations, 2013). Furthermore, because of problems such as diseases and disabilities, the average actual retirement age is even lower, only 53.3 years (Yang, 2013). Considering the heavier burden on the current workforce and prolonged life expectancy, it seems reasonable and necessary to raise the statutory retirement age.

2.5.2 *The emerging consequences and measures taken by the government*

The negative impact of aging on the Basic Old-age Insurance System for Enterprise Employees has gradually emerged in recent years. Government subsidies to this scheme continue to escalate. For example, in 2012, the subsidies were 264.8 billion RMB, which accounted for 2.26% of total public finance in that year, and represented an increase of 37.6 billion over the year before. Excluding the central government subsidies, among the 32 mainland province level administrations (including Xinjiang Production and Construction Corps), only 12 provinces had total insurance premiums higher than insurance expenditure, and the scheme deficit in Liaoning and Heilongjiang provinces actually reached over 20 billion RMB (Zheng, 2013). Moreover, in the same year, the average contribution rate[5] was 16.88% and the replacement rate was only 49.23%, which indicates that working people had to pay a high percentage of their wages towards this pension scheme and retired people had to lower their living standards compared with their pre-retirement time (Zheng, 2013).

In order to increase the sustainability of its pension systems, the Chinese government has implemented some measures in recent years. Firstly, several provinces such as Heilongjiang have been selected as pilots to reform the Basic Old-age Insurance System for Enterprise Employees Scheme, aimed at improving the defined contribution. Secondly, part of the central government's deepening reform is to

[5] In the Basic Old-age Insurance System for Enterprise Employees, contribution rate = average premium per month/average wage per month; replacement rate = average pension per month/average wage per month.

develop a policy for progressively raising the retirement age (The Central Committee of the Communist Party of China, 2013). In the same document, the central government announced that the family planning policy, that is the one-child policy, is to be relaxed so that couples in which at least one partner is a single child can have two children. This policy is expected to increase fertility rates and help to balance the pension system (Zeng, 2011). However, the sustainability issue of Chinese pension systems, for now, is far from being solved.

2.6 Age-Friendly Cities

2.6.1 *Urbanization and the need for age-friendly cities*

Along with urbanization, the proportion of the elderly population in urban areas has also increased. In 2000, 9.68% of permanent residents in urban China were aged 60 and over, and in 2010, the proportion climbed to 11.69% (Population Census Office of China, 2002; Population Census Office of China, 2012). In the mega-cities, that is, cities with 10 million inhabitants or more, the proportion of persons aged 60 and over is even higher (for example, in Shanghai it is 14.78%). The figures have very likely been understated as a result of urbanization, which brings large numbers of working age migrants to mega-cities (Tong, 2014). Due to physical and social changes associated with aging, elderly people particularly need supportive and enabling living environments, but there are still many barriers to this in China. For example, bus decks are too high for the elderly to get on and off easily (Zhao *et al.*, 2013); public vehicles lack the space for wheelchairs (Jia *et al.*, 2014); technical or skill barriers hinder older persons from accessing government or other websites (Guo, 2012; Zhao, 2013).

Age-friendly cities are helpful in guaranteeing the wellbeing of elderly persons and encouraging them to contribute to social development: "In practical terms, an age friendly city adapts its structures and services to be accessible to and inclusive of older people with varying needs and capacities" (WHO, 2007). In addition, age-friendly cities promote active aging by optimizing opportunities for good health,

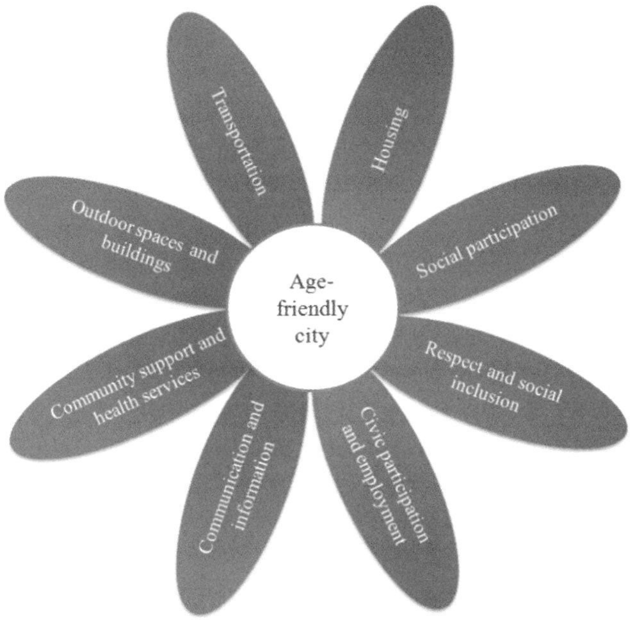

Figure 2.3 Age-friendly city topic areas.
Source: WHO (2007).

active social participation and security that enhance quality of life as people age (WHO, 2002). Figure 2.3 illustrates the eight key elements of an age-friendly city: housing, social participation, respect and social inclusion, civic participation and employment, communication and information, community support and health services, outdoor spaces and buildings, and transportation.

2.6.2 *The progress of age-friendly cities in china*

In China, the construction of age-friendly cities, accompanied by livable communities, officially started in 2009. From then until 2013, there were 14 pilot sites in total (Table 2.3). In 2011, the city of Qiqihaer in Heilongjiang Province was admitted as a member to the WHO Global Network of Age-friendly Cities and Communities. It is the only Chinese city in this Network (Hu and Shen, 2014). Further pilot cities have been developed and customized to the framework of age-friendly

Table 2.3 Pilots of age-friendly cities and livable communities conducted during 2009 and 2012 in China

Time	Pilots
2009 (9 pilots)	Qiqihaer City in Heilongjiang Province, Jianhua District in Qiqihaer City, Bayuquan District in Yingkou City, Qingdao City in Shandong Province, Xuanwu District in Nanjing City, Huangpu District in Shanghai City, Yangpu District in Shanghai City, Changning District in Shanghai City, Huzhou City in Zhejiang Province
2010 (3 pilots)	Pudong District in Shanghai City, Gulou District in Nanjing city, Jinchang District in Suzhou City
2011 (1 pilot)	Taizhou City in Shandong Province
2012 (1 pilot)	Yunxi City in Yunnan Province

Source: WHO (2007).

cities in the Chinese context. Shanghai can be used as an example (Shanghai Committee on Aging, 2013) to demonstrate the key features of a Chinese age-friendly city. The Shanghai Municipality age-friendly framework contains eight components, including outdoor spaces and buildings, transportation, housing, social security and assistance, social and health service, education and physical exercise, social participation and contribution, respect and preferential treatment. Compared with the WHO guideline for age-friendly cities (WHO, 2007), the Shanghai model focuses on issues such as the development of a policy of preferential treatment of elderly persons and promotion of senior citizen association, rather than on the aspects which are less relevant in the Chinese urban environment, such as employment. No official or academic assessment has yet been conducted or published on the progress of these pilot projects. For the civil-society-led projects to be effective, it will need strong government support and coordination of all relevant sectors and the establishment of a monitoring and evaluation system so the effects of the projects can be evaluated properly.

2.7 Conclusion

Population aging is a result of social stability, economic growth and improved health in China. However, it brings multiple challenges to sustainable development. The economy, health service delivery, long-term care and pension systems and whole cities are facing great challenges due to such dramatic demographic changes. More importantly, the aging-related problems are further complicated by urbanization, which, for example, accelerates the pace of an aging rural workforce and reduces the provision of informal long-term care for rural elderly persons.

However, aging should not mean that senior citizens in the society have to live miserable lives. This largely depends on how the Chinese government and civil society respond. The Chinese government has taken some action which may have some effect on mitigating the negative impact of population aging. Population aging can also have positive influences. Many older people still contribute to society by engaging in formal jobs or providing informal care for their families. There are lessons that China can learn from other countries in tackling population aging problems more effectively.

References

Banister, J., Bloom, D.E. and Rosenberg, L. (2012). Population Aging and Economic Growth in China, in Aoki, M. and Wu, J. (eds.), *The Chinese Economy: A New Transition*, 114–149, Palgrave Macmillan, New York.

Bloom, D.E., Canning, D. and Fink, G. (2010). Implications of Population Ageing for Economic Growth, *Oxford Review of Economic Policy* **26**: 583–612.

Cai, F. (2010). Debating the Lewis Turning Point in China, *China Economic Journal* **3**: 107–119.

Cai, F. and Wang, M. (2006). Challenge Facing China's Economic Growth in its Aging but Not Affluent Era, *China & World Economy* **14**: 20–31.

Cai, Y. and Cheng, Y. (2014). Pension Reform in China: Challenges and Opportunities, *Journal of Economic Surveys* **28**: 636–651.

Cao, G., Zhou, L., Yi, Z. *et al.* (2010). The Influence of Agricultrual Machinery Subsidy on Purchasing Behavior of Farmers, *Chinese Rural Economy* **6**: 38–48 (in Chinese).

CHARLS Research Team (2013). Challenges of Population Aging in China, *National Baseline Survey of the China Health and Retirement Longitudinal Study* (*CHARLS*).

Chen, Z. (2009). Launch of the Health-care Reform Plan in China, *The Lancet* **373**: 1322–1324.

Chi, W. and Li, B. (2014). Trends in China's Gender Employment and Pay Gap: Estimating Gender Pay Gaps with Employment Selection, *Journal of Comparative Economics* **42**: 708–725.

Colombo, F., Llena-Noza, I.A., Mercier, J. *et al.* (2011). Help Wanted? Providing and Paying for Long-term Care, *OECD Health Policy Studies.* Available at http://www.oecd.org/els/health-systems/47836116.pdf [Accessed 20 February 2015].

Dai, W. (2012). *The Construction of Long-term Care Insurance System in China*, People's Publishing House, Beijing (in Chinese).

Du, F. and Dong, X-y. (2013). Women's Employment and Child Care Choices in Urban China During The Economic Transition, *Economic Development and Cultural Change* **62**: 131–155.

Eggleston, K. Oi, J.C., Rozelle, S. *et al.* (2013). Will Demographic Change Slow China's rise? *Journal of Asian Studies* **72**: 505–518.

Fang, P., Zou, X. and Sun, Y. (2014). Key Points of the Hierarchical Medical System Research in China, *Chinese Hospital Management* **34**: 1–3 (in Chinese).

Feng, Z.L., Zhan, H.J., Feng, X.T. *et al.* (2011). An Industry in the Making: The Emergence of Institutional Elder Care in Urban China, *Journal of the American Geriatrics Society* **59**: 738–744.

Flaherty, J.H., Liu, M.L., Ding, L. *et al.* (2007). China: The Aging Giant, *Journal of the American Geriatrics Society* **55**: 1295–1300.

Food and Agriculture Organization of the United States (2013). *FAO Statistical Yearbook 2013.* Rome: World Food and Agriculture.

Food and Agriculture Organization of the United States (2014). FAOSTAT. Available at http://faostat.fao.org/ [Accessed 20 January 2015].

General Office of the State Council of the PRC (2006). *The Notice on Accelerating the Development of Aged Care Industry Issued by Office of National Aging Work Commission and National Development and Reform Commission and Forwarded by General Office of the State Council of the PRC*, Beijing: PRC (in Chinese).

General Office of the State Council of the PRC. (2011). *The Notice on the Construction of Social Aged Care Service System (2011–2015)* Issued by General Office of the State Council of the PRC, Beijing: PRC (in Chinese).

Glass, A.P., Gao, Y. and Luo, J. (2013). China: Facing a Long-term Care Challenge on an Unprecedented Scale, *Global Public Health* **8**: 725–738.

Guo, J. (2012). On the Accessibility of Provincial Government Websites in China, *Journal of Intelligence* **31**: 165–169 (in Chinese).

Hirth, V., Baskins, J. and Dever-Bumba, M. (2009). Program of All-inclusive Care (PACE): Past, Present, and Future, *Journal of the American Medical Directors Association* **10**: 155–160.

Hu, T. and Shen, S. (2014). Research Progress and Construction Practice of Age-friendly City, *Modern Urban Research* **9**: 14–20 (in Chinese).

Huang, F., Zhang, H. and Yin, J. (2012). The Status and Need of Professional Training of Long-term Care Providers in Aged Care Institutions in Liaoning Province, *Chinese Journal of Gerontology* **32**: 570–573 (in Chinese).

Huang, J. and Meng, F. (2014). Integrating Pension Service with Medical Service for the Elderly: Necessity Dilemmas and Solutions, *Chinese Journal of Health Policy* 7: 63–68 (in Chinese).

Jackson, R., Nakashima, K. and Howe, N. (2009). *China's Long March to Retirement Reform: The Graying of the Middle Kingdom Revisited*, Washington: CSIS and Prudential Foundation Programs.

Jia, Z., Yang, J. and Shen, L. (2014). Status and Countermeasures of Barrier-free Facilities at Urban Rail Transit Stations, *Urban Mass Transit* **9**: 62–66 (in Chinese).

Jin, X. and Wang, H. (2010). The Influence of Old-age Consumption on Economic Development in China and Relevant Policy Implications, *Consumer Economics* **26**: 74–78 (in Chinese).

Li, C., Yu, X., Butler, J.R.G. *et al.* (2011). Moving Towards Universal Health Insurance in China: Performance, Issues and Lessons From Thailand, *Social Science & Medicine Journal* **73**: 359–366.

Li, M., Zhang, Y., Zhang, Z., *et al.* (2013). Rural urban Differences in the Long-term Care of the Disabled Elderly in China, *PLOS One* **8**(11): e79955.

Li, Y. (2014). Institutional Predicament and Reform Ways of China's Agricultural Mechanization, *Journal of Chinese Agricultural Mechanization* **35**: 312–315 (in Chinese).

Li, Z. and Zhang, H-p. (2013). Productivity Growth in China's Agriculture During 1985–2010, *Journal of Integrative Agriculture* **12**: 1896–1904.

Lin, J.Y., Cai, F. and L,i Z. (2003). *The China Miracle: Development Strategy and Economic Reform*, Chinese University Press, Hong Kong.

Liu, J.F., Chen, G., Song, X.M. *et al.* (2009). Trends in Disability-free Life Expectancy Among Chinese Older Adults, *Journal of Aging and Health* **21**: 266–285.

Liu, M. (2011). Solve the Problem in Providing Medical Services in Aged Care Institutions, *Beijing Observation* **6**: 20–21 (in Chinese).

Liu, X., Han, X. and Dou, M. (2014). Analysis of the Behavior County Agricultural Mechanization Based on SPSS, *Journal of Chinese Agricultural Mechanization* **35**: 22–35 (in Chinese).

Ministry of Civil Affairs of China (2013). *China Civil Affairs' Statistical Yearbook (2013)*, China Statistics Press, Beijing (in Chinese).

Ministry of Civil Affairs of PRC (2001). *The Implementation Plan on "Community Aged Welfare Service Starlight Project"* Beijing: PRC (in Chinese).

Mu, G. (2012). The Dilemma and Countmeasures in Developing Aged Care Institutions in China, *Journal of Huazhong Normal University (Humanities and Social Sciences)* **51**: 31–38 (in Chinese).

National Bureau of Statistics of China. (2013). *Labour Statistical Yearbook of China*, China Statistics Press, Beijing.

OECD (2011). *Health Reform: Meeting the Challenge of Aging and Multiple Morbidities.* Available at http://www.oecd.org/els/health-systems/49151107.pdf [Accessed 15 January 2015].

Peng, X. (2008). Demographic Shift, Population Ageing and Economic Growth in China: A Computable General Equilibrium Analysis, *Pacific Economic Review* **13**: 680–697.

Population Census Office of China (2002). *Tabulation on the 2000 Population Census of the People's Republic of China*, China Statistics Press, Beijing (in Chinese).

Population Census Office of China (2012). *Tabulation on the 2010 Population Census of the People's Republic of China*, China Statistics Press, Beijing (in Chinese).

Powell, J.L. (2012). China and the Bio-medicalization of Aging: Implications and Possibilities, in Chen, S. and Powell, J.L. (eds.), *Aging in China: Implications to Social Policy of a Changing Economic State*, New York: Springer.

Shanghai Committee on Aging (2013). *Notice on Age-friendly City Construction Guideline (Trial) Issued by Shanghai Committee on Aging* Beijing: PRC (in Chinese).

Sicular, T., Ximing, Y., Gustafsson, B., *et al.* (2007). The Urban–rural Income Gap and Inequality in China. *Review of Income and Wealth* **53**: 93–126.

Sikken, B.J., Davis, N., Hayashi, C., *et al.* (2008). *The Future of Pensions and Healthcare in a Rapidly Ageing World: Scenarios to 2030*, Geneva: World Economic Forum.

State Council of the PRC (2013). *Several Opinions of the State Council on Accelerating the Development of Elderly Services* PRC: Beijing (in Chinese).

The Central Committee of the Communist Party of China (2013). *Decision of the Central Committee of the Communist Party of China on Some Major Issues Concerning Comprehensively Deepening the Reform* PRC: Beijing (in Chinese).

Tong, Y. (2014). Changes and Challenges of Labour Supply in China in the Context of Population Ageing, *Journal of Population Research* **38**: 52–60 (in Chinese).

United Nations (2013). *World Population Prospects: The 2012 Revision*, UN: New York.

United Nations Department of Economic and Social Affairs Population Division. (2014a) *World Urbanization Prospects: The 2014 Revision*, UN: New York.

United Nations Department of Economic and Social Affairs Population Division. (2014b) *World Urbanization Prospects: The 2014 Revision, Highlights*, (ST/ESA/SER.A/352). UN: New York.

Wang, F. (2012). Racing Towards the Precipice, *China Economic Quarterly* **June**: 17–21.

Wang, L. (2013). Develop Service and Relevant Industries of the Elderly with Great Effort as a National Strategy, in Wu, Y. (ed.) *China Report of the Development on Aging Cause* (2013), 140–167, Social Science Academic Press, Beijing (in Chinese).

Wang, L., Beland, D. and Zhang, S. (2014a). Pension Fairness in China, *China Economic Review* **28**: 25–36.

Wang, L., Beland, D. and Zhang, S. (2014b). Pension Financing in China: Is There a Looming Crisis? *China Economic Review* **30**: 143–154.

WHO (2002). Active Ageing: A Policy Framwork, Available at http://www.who.int/ageing/publications/active_ageing/en/ [Accessed 20 Feburary 2015].

WHO (2007). Global Age-friendly Cities: A Guide, Available at http://www.who.int/ageing/age_friendly_cities_guide/en/ [Accessed 20 Feburary 2015].

WHO (2008). Primary Health Care: Now More Than Ever. Available at http://www.who.int/whr/2008/en/ [Accessed 20 February 2015].

Williamson, J.B., Price, M. and Shen, C. (2012). Pension Policy in China, Singapore, and South Korea: An Assessment of the Potential Value of the Notional Defined Contribution Model, *Journal of Aging Studies* **26**: 79–89.

Wu, B., Mao, Z. and Xu, Q. (2008). Institutional Care for Elders in Rural China, *Journal of Aging & Social Policy* **20**: 218–239.

Wu, L. (2013). Inequality of Pension Arrangements Among Different Segments of the Labor Force In China, *Journal of Aging & Social Policy* **25**: 181–196.

Xia, C. and Liu, W. (2012). The Empirical Study on the Relationship Between Agricultural Modernity, Urbanization and Industrialization, *Journal of Agrotechnical Economics* **5**:79–85 (in Chinese).

Yang, G.H., Kong, L.Z., Zhao, W.H. *et al.* (2008). Emergence of Chronic Non-communicable Diseases in China, *The Lancet* **372**: 1697–1705.

Yang, G.H., Wang, Y., Zeng, Y.X. *et al.* (2013). Rapid Health Transition in China, 1990–2010: Findings from the Global Burden of Disease Study 2010, *The Lancet* **381**: 1987–2015.

Yang, X. (2013.) Breakthrough in China's System of Security for the Elderly in Wu, Y. (ed.), *China Report of the Development on Aging Cause* (2013), 73–93, Social Science Academic Press, Beijing (in Chinese).

Yip, W. and Hsiao, W. (2014). Harnessing the Privatisation of China's Fragmented Health-care Delivery, *The Lancet* **384**: 805–818.

Yip, W.C.M., Hsiao, W., Meng, Q.Y. *et al.* (2010). Realignment of Incentives for Health-care Providers in China, *The Lancet* **375**: 1120–1130.

Yip, W.C.M., Hsiao, W.C., Chen, W., *et al.* (2012). Early Appraisal of China's Huge and Complex Health-care Reforms, *The Lancet* **379**: 833–842.

Zeng, Y. (2011). Effects of Demographic and Retirement-age Policies on Future Pension Deficits, With an Application to China, *Population and Development Review* **37**: 553–569.

Zeng, Y., Chen, H. and Wang, Z. (2012). Analysis on Trends of Future Home-Based Care Needs and Cost for Elderly in China, *Economic Research Journal* China **47**(1): 134–149 (in Chinese).

Zhang, J. (2013). Population Aging, Change of Labor Market and Social Security for the Old Age: How to Improve the Basic Pension Insurance System for Urban Workers, *Scientific Research on Aging* **1**: 11–19 (in Chinese).

Zhang, J. and Zheng, X.Y. (2010). Research on Health Status and Health Care of the Elderly in China (in Chinese), *Population & Development* **16**: 60–66.

Zhang, Q. (2008). Evolution of Comparative Advantage and Path of Industry Upgrading, *China Industrial Economics* **2008–2009**: 58–68 (in Chinese).

Zhang, Y. (2012). The Trend of Small Family, Core Family, Empty-Nest Family in China, *Studies on Socialism with Chinese Characteristics* 87–94 (in Chinese).

Zhang, Y. and Bruemmer, B. (2011). Productivity Change and the Effects of Policy Reform in China's Agriculture Since 1979, *Asian-Pacific Economic Literature* **25**: 131–150.

Zhang, Y., Hannum, E. and Wang, M. (2008). Gender-based Employment and Income Differences in Urban China: Considering the Contributions of Marriage and Parenthood, *Social Forces* **86**: 1529–1560.

Zhao, F. (2013.) Survey on the Government Website Accessibility Status in China, *Archives Science Study* 66–70 (in Chinese).

Zhao, L., He, P., Xu, Z. *et al.* (2013). Study on Barrier-free Environment of Public Vehicles in Urban China *Urban Problems* 42–46 (in Chinese).

Zhao, Y., Smith, J.P. and Strauss, J. (2014). Can China Age Healthily? *The Lancet* **384**: 723–724.

Zheng, B. (2013). *China Pension Report 2013*, Economic & Management Publishing House, Beijing (in Chinese).

Zhu, W. and Chen, L. (2011). The Study on the Components and Models of Industrial Upgrading: Take the Industrial Upgrading in Guangdong Province as an Example, *The Economist* **1843**: 60–66 (in Chinese).

Chapter Three

Surveillance of Non-Communicable Disease Risk Factors

Ji Xiang Ma, Jian Hong Li, Zeng Ge
and Yang Feng Wu

Abstract

Non-communicable chronic diseases (NCDs) are the leading cause of death in China, accounting for close to 70% of the disease burden and over 80% of the total mortality. The four main NCDs in China are cardiovascular diseases (CVDs), diabetes, cancer, and chronic obstructive pulmonary diseases (COPDs). Over 50% of the NCD burden is preventable by modifying health factors such as tobacco use, harmful alcohol use, poor diet, particularly high consumption of fast foods that are rich in fat and salt and sugar-rich soft drinks, and physical inactivity.

China's urban population endures a high prevalence of overweight individuals, obesity, hypertension, and diabetes. This chapter describes major NCD trends and their risk factors in urban areas of China. An analysis of mortality will demonstrate current major causes of death, the burden of disease and 'disabilities adjusted life years' (DALYs) in urban populations, and changes in the mortality and disease burden during the past decades. Risk-factor analysis will show the prevalence of and trends in behavioral risk factors such as smoking, harmful alcohol use, unhealthy diet, physical inactivity as well as pre-NCD conditions such as obesity, hypertension, and diabetes. These analyses will provide strong suggestions for policy makers and public healthcare providers in shaping future policies and programs which address these risk factors.

3.1 Introduction

Non-communicable chronic diseases (NCDs) are chronic conditions not caused by infections. Therefore, they are not 'contagious' or 'communicable'. These conditions often have multiple and complex risk factors, over prolonged courses, which could result in major disability and thus poor quality of life. Of the 57 million deaths that occurred globally in 2008, 36 million — almost two thirds — were due to NCDs, mainly cardiovascular diseases, cancers, diabetes, and chronic lung diseases (Alwan *et al.*, 2010). Although the causes of NCDs are very complex, there are, largely, four common risk factors: tobacco use, unhealthy diet, insufficient physical activity, and the harmful use of alcohol — pervasive aspects of economic transition, rapid urbanization and, 21st century lifestyles. The World Health Organization (WHO) has prioritized these four as the key modifiable behavioral risk factors for prevention and control of NCDs (WHO, 2010). Elimination of these modifiable risk factors would prevent 80% of premature heart disease, 80% of premature stroke, 80% of type 2 diabetes and 40% of cancer (WHO, 2009a).

The rapid development of urbanization in China, has resulted in the urban population more than tripling in the past 30 years (Yeh *et al.*, 2011; NBSC, 2010). Although urbanization offers opportunities for improvements in population health in China (such as access to improved health care and basic infrastructure), it can also lead to substantial health risks, including ambient air pollution, occupational and traffic hazards, poor diet and reduced physical activity. These are the main factors of the increasing disease burden and death rate from chronic diseases.

NCDs are now the leading causes of death in China, accounting for close to 70% of the disease burden and over 80% of total mortality

(WHO, 2009b; Wang *et al.*, 2005). The most prevalent NCDs in China are cardio- and cerebrovascular diseases, diabetes, cancer, and chronic obstructive pulmonary diseases (COPDs) (Yu, 2012). This chapter focuses on risk factor analysis, showing the prevalence and trend of major behavioral risk factors, including smoking, harmful alcohol use, unhealthy diet, physical inactivity; and pre-NCD metabolic conditions such as hypertension, elevated cholesterol levels, diabetes, and overweight individuals and obesity, based on data from the China National Chronic Disease Surveillance System (established in 2005), and other relevant nationally representative survey results. The National Chronic Disease Surveillance System is set to collect data by multi-stage randomized cluster sampling every three years from 145 monitoring points covering 31 provinces, with the sample size of about 71 million people in each wave.

It is hoped a major reduction in the burden of NCDs will come from population-wide interventions, targeting the key modifiable risk factors. These interventions are cost effective and may even be revenue-generating, as is the case, for instance, with increases in tobacco and alcohol tax. The analysis of the major risk factors presented in this chapter provides strong suggestions for policymakers and public health-care providers to consider when shaping policies and programs. This is particularly relevant to the promotion of healthy lifestyles, including healthy eating and physical activity, and the reduction of smoking and alcohol consumption.

3.2 Modifiable Behavioral Risk Factors for NCDs

3.2.1 *Smoking and tobacco use*

Smoking has been established as the leading cause of preventable death worldwide (WHO, 2013). According to the WHO report, smoking was responsible for approximately 5.4 million deaths globally in 2004, and that number is projected to rise to more than 8.3 million deaths per year by 2030, at which point it will represent almost 10% of all causes of death globally (WHO, 2004). In China, there were an estimated 301 million smokers in 2010 (approximately 28% of persons aged 15 years and over), making the country the world's largest consumer of cigarettes, and contributing considerably to the global burden of smoking-related death (Li, *et al.*, 2011).

According to findings from the National Tobacco Surveys, the prevalence of smoking had significantly decreased from 31.8% in 1996 to 25.0% in 2002, but rose again to 26.1% in 2010 (Yang, *et al.*, 2005). The prevalence of smoking among men slightly decreased, but still remained at a high level. In urban areas of China, the prevalence of smoking among adults has significantly decreased over the last two decades. Although the prevalence of smoking in men was lower in urban areas than in rural areas, the survey showed the opposite for women. This could be partially attributed to public health programs. In 2003, China signed the Framework Convention on Tobacco Control. This came into force in 2006 and its implementation has started to gain momentum in recent years. Tobacco control has now received significant attention and support from the Chinese governments and Chinese residents. Several large-scale programs for tobacco control, mainly in urban areas, have been undertaken, such as smoking bans in hospitals, government buildings and other public places. These programs have achieved some results under the guidance of Monitor, Protect, Offer, Warn, Enforce, and Raise (MPOWER) strategy (Yang and Hu 2011).

3.2.2 *Alcohol consumption*

Alcohol abuse is a major global risk factor for premature deaths and disabilities. With urbanization come lifestyle changes, such as the adoption of a more Western-style diet, high in fat, sugar and salt; less physical activity; greater alcohol consumption; and weight gain. Every year, alcohol abuse is responsible for 2.5 million deaths worldwide (WHO, 2014). It is the eighth leading risk factor for deaths globally, and alcohol abuse accounted for almost 4% of all deaths in the world in 2004 (WHO, 2014). The average volume of consumption, as well as drinking patterns, are linked to many long-term and acute health and social consequences, and result in a huge disease burden (WHO, 2009c; Rehm *et al.*, 2003). Deaths from liver cancer secondary to alcohol use in China in 2010 was 67,500, up from 44,000 in 1990, whereas deaths from cirrhosis of the liver secondary to alcohol use decreased from 35,000 to 25,000 from 1990 to 2010 (Yang *et al.*, 2013).

The National Chronic Disease Risk Factors Surveillance data shows that in China, in 2010, the per capita intake of alcohol in adults aged 18 years and over was 20.3 grams, while the stratified consumptions by gender, age, and urban or rural living showed 24.1 grams and 4.8 grams among males and females respectively; 17.4 grams, 22.8 grams and 25.6 grams in people aged 18–44, 4–59, and over 60 years old respectively; and an overall 17.9 grams and 21.6 grams in urban and rural areas respectively. For both genders, the consumption of alcohol was higher for drinkers living in rural areas than for those living in urban areas. The rate of harmful drinking, defined as per capita consumption of pure alcohol equal to or greater than 61.0 grams for males and 41.0 grams for females, was 9.3% in Chinese adults aged 18 years and over. With rapid social and economic development people now have higher disposable incomes, and this, coupled with increasing alcohol production and alcoholic beverage advertisements in the mass media, has probably contributed to the rapid increase in alcohol consumption (Ma *et al.*, 2005; Cochrane *et al.*, 2003).

3.2.3 *Unhealthy diet: high fat intake*

Dietary fat is important for maintaining energy balance in the human body. Due to different dietary structures, the proportion of diet fat to fatty-acid intake varies. High dietary fat intake can contribute to chronic diseases, such as coronary heart disease, diabetes, and certain cancers. A study looking into fat consumption in urban and rural settings shows that between 1991 and 1997, the intake of dietary fats, the mean percentage of energy from total fat, and the intake of cholesterol increased in people who lived in urban, suburban, and town environments. The increased consumption of animal food (especially meat and meat products), and vegetable oil were the main causes of the increase in dietary fat intake. This means the percentage of energy from saturated, monounsaturated and polyunsaturated fatty acids increased, whereas the fat consumption had not changed very much (Wang, *et al.*, 2003).

3.2.4 *Unhealthy diet: high salt intake*

Excess dietary sodium is a major contributor to hypertension (high blood pressure). Reduction in sodium intake has been shown to lower blood pressure significantly, in both normotensive and hypertensive people (He *et al.*, 2013). In a 2002 meta-analysis, He and MacGregor found that a reduction of 100 mmol/day in sodium intake could result in a 3.6 mmHg reduction in systolic and 1.7 mmHg in diastolic blood pressure among normotensive persons, and a 7.1 mmHg fall in systolic and 3.9 mmHg fall in diastolic blood pressure among hypertensive persons (He *et al.*, 2002).

Traditionally, dietary salt intake has been high in Chinese people. People living in rural areas, in particular, have always had higher salt consumption than those living in urban areas. Based on findings from the China Chronic Disease Risk Factors Surveillances, and the National Health and Nutrition Examination Surveys which have been conducted every 10 years since 1982, the average dietary salt intake decreased from 13.0 grams per day in 1982 to 12.0 grams per day in 2002, and further to 10.6 grams per day in 2010. That is, between 1982 and 2010 the average dietary salt intake had decreased by about 18.5% (2.4g) in Chinese adults (He *et al.*, 2005; Wang, 2005; NCNCD, 2010). However, there is a long way to go for China to reach the global target of 30% relative reduction intake (WHO, 2014) in the mean population's salt/sodium.

Most dietary sodium in developed countries comes from sodium added to foods before purchase, whereas only 5–6% is added at home during cooking and 5–6% at the table (Institute of Medicine of the National Academies, 2011). However, in China, most dietary sodium consumed comes from home cooking. This may be one of the reasons dietary sodium intake among the Chinese is higher than in other developed countries. Although the salt intakes for both urban and rural populations have been decreasing during the last 30 years (as shown in Figure 3.1), the daily dietary salt intake values are still twice the Adequate Intake (AI) (5.0 grams per day) recommended by the WHO (Joint WHO/FAO Expert Consultation, 2003). Over 80% of families still had dietary salt intake above five grams per person in 2010 (NCNCD, 2010).

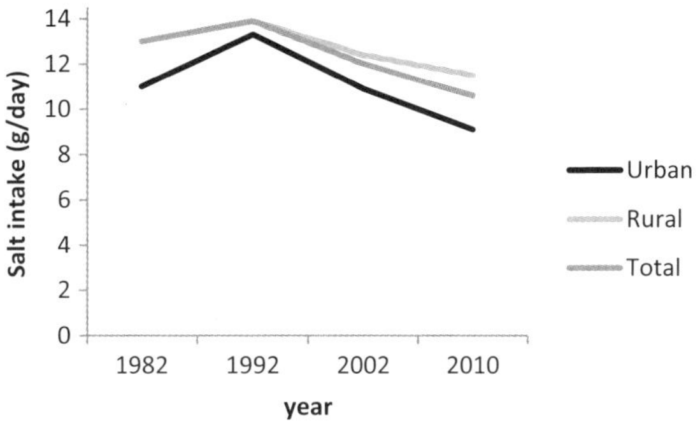

Figure 3.1 The trend comparison of dietary salt intake from 1992 to 2010.

Source: National Nutrition and Health Survey in China in 1982, 1992 and 2002, and Chronic disease risk factor surveillance in China in 2010, Chinese Centre for Disease Control and Prevention.

3.2.5 *Physical inactivity*

Insufficient physical activity (PA) is one of the leading risk factors for mortality. Worldwide, approximately 3.2 million deaths and 32.1 million 'disabilities adjusted life years' DALYs (representing about 2.1% of global DALYs) each year are attributable to insufficient physical activity (WHO, 2014). Regular physical activity is critical to overall health and fitness. People who are physically active generally live longer and have a lower risk of heart disease, stroke, type 2 diabetes, depression, some cancers, and premature mortality. Physical activity can also help control weight (WHO, 2014). The National Chronic Disease Risk Factor Surveillance used the global physical activity questionnaire (GPAQ) to evaluate the physical activity of Chinese adults (WHO, n.d). Results revealed that only 11.9% of Chinese adults 18 years and over regularly engaged in physical exercise in 2010. The prevalence of regular leisure-time physical activity (casual activities of at least 10 minutes at a time, at least three times per week) was higher in males (13.1%) than in females (10.6%), and higher for people living in urban areas (19.9%) than for those living in rural (8.2%) (NCNCD, 2010).

Further, the prevalence of regular leisure-time physical activity was increasing among people living in urban areas as they aged, while decreasing among their rural counterparts (Figure 3.2). For example, the prevalence of regular leisure-time physical activity in the population

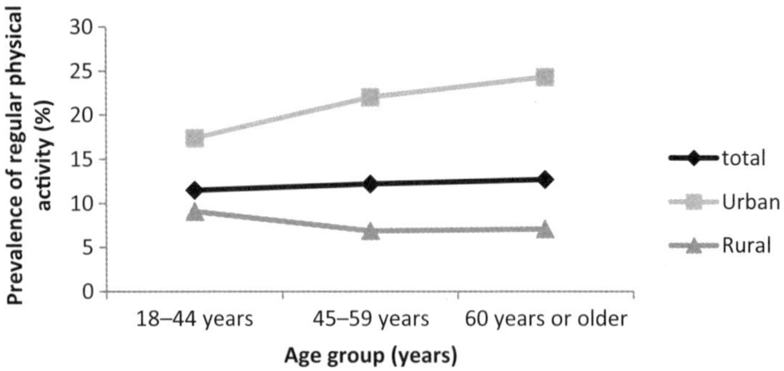

Figure 3.2 The prevalence of regular physical activity by age group in Chinese adults in 2010.

***Source*: Chronic disease risk factor surveillance in China in 2010, Chinese Centre for Disease Control and Prevention.**

aged 60 years and over was 24.3% among participants living in urban areas versus 7.1% among participants living in rural areas (NCNCD, 2010). Though the proportions of regular physical activity are still small, surveys indicate that from 2002 to 2010, the prevalence of regular leisure-time physical activity increased 23.2% among women overall (from 15.1% to 18.6%) and 42.3% among men (from 14.9% to 21.2%) in the urban population (NCNCD, 2010; Wang, 2005). It can be speculated that inequity in health promotion — particularly relevant to NCD prevention — and in the availability of facilities between urban and rural areas plays a part. It should be noted that this survey only measures the leisure-time physical activity, rather than all forms of physical activities (NCNCD, 2010; Wang, 2005). The different levels of participation in physical activity between urban and rural adult populations as they get older also reflects the fact that urban residents have more free time to participate in leisure-time physical activity after retirement, while poor physical health and aging prevent rural residents from participating in any form of physical activity.

Meanwhile, the National Chronic Disease Risk Factor Surveillance results reveal that in Chinese adults about 2.7 hours per day was spent in sedentary behaviors, such as watching television, reading, using computers or playing games. Those aged 18–24 years spent most time, on average 3.8 hours per day, in sedentary behaviors, and the time reduced with age. More time on sedentary behaviors was spent by males (2.9 hours per day) than by females (2.6 hours per day), and more hours were spent on sedentary activities in urban populations (3.3 hours per day) than in rural populations (2.9 hours per day) (Chen, *et al.*, 2012).

3.3 Pre-NCD Metabolic Conditions

Certain lifestyle choices and behaviors can lead to changes in physiological or biological markers and influence the outcome of some pre-NCD conditions. Preventing these conditions or achieving a better control can significantly reduce the risk of individuals developing NCDs.

3.3.1 *Hypertension*

Changes in diet and lifestyle associated with urbanization contribute to raised blood pressure (hypertension), defined as systolic and/or diastolic blood pressure ≥140/90 mmHg, in adults aged 18 years and over. In 2014, the global prevalence of raised blood pressure was about 22% (WHO, 2014). It was estimated that hypertension had caused 9.4 million deaths and represented 7% of the disease burden in terms of disabilities adjusted life year (DALY) worldwide in 2010 (Lim *et al.*, 2012). Hypertension is not only a serious condition by itself, but it is also a risk factor for heart attacks, strokes, and kidney failure.

In urban China, the prevalence of hypertension among adults has significantly increased over the last two decades. Findings from the National Hypertension Survey in 1991, the 2002 National Health and Nutrition Examination Survey, and the 2010 China National Chronic Disease Risk Factors Surveillance show an upward trend in the prevalence of hypertension, from 12.8% (14.4% in men and 11.4% in women) in 1991 to 19.3% in 2002, and 34.7% (37.6% in men and 31.8% in women) in 2010 (Wang, 2005; NCNCD, 2010; Wu *et al.*, 1995). The surveys all used national representative samples and the results were weighted. The prevalence of awareness; treatment; and control of hypertension, on the other hand, increased significantly from 35.6%; 17.1%; and 4.1% in 1991, to 41.1%; 35.1%; and 9.7% in 2002, respectively (Wang, 2005; Wu *et al.*, 1995). Additionally, the 2007 and 2010

China National Chronic Disease Risk Factor Surveillance data demonstrated that the proportion of participants who were aware of their hypertensive status and were being treated with antihypertensive medications increased from 72.5% in 2007 to 80.1% in 2010. The percentage of participants with hypertension who had their hypertension controlled was 22.9% (NCNCD, 2010; CDC of China, 2010).

3.3.2 *Cholesterol*

Raised cholesterol levels increase the risk of heart disease and stroke (Wu, *et al.*, 2001). Globally, a third of ischaemic heart disease is attributable to high cholesterol (WHO, 2010). Raised total cholesterol is a major cause of disease burden in both the developed and developing worlds, as a risk factor for ischaemic heart disease and stroke.

In 2010, the levels of serum total cholesterol among Chinese adults aged 18 years and over was 4.04 mmol/L overall. When looking at the data by age, gender, and urban or rural living segregations, the levels were 3.86, 4.29, and 4.33 mmol/L for 18–44, 45–59, and over 60 years old, respectively. There was little difference between male and female, being 4.06 mmol/L and 4.03 mmol/L, respectively; and the levels were 4.08 mmol/L and 4.03 mmol/L in urban and rural residents, respectively. The mean total cholesterol increased 0.12 mmol/L from 2002 to 2010, and it showed the same increasing levels by age group, gender and location, that is urban or rural settings (Wang, 2005; NCNCD, 2010) (Figure 3.3).

According to the National Chronic Disease Risk Factor Surveillance in China in 2010, the elevated cholesterol level in adults was 3.3%. The prevalence by age, gender, and urban or rural living location was 3.0%, 4.5%, and 2.9% in the age groups of 18–44, 45–59, and 60 years old or over, respectively; 3.4% and 3.2% in males and females, respectively, and 4.2% and 2.9% in urban and rural residents, respectively. The prevalence of hypercholesterolemia in urban residents was significantly higher than that of people from rural areas. The prevalence of hypercholesterolemia in Chinese adults increased from 1.3% in 2002 to 3.3% in 2010, which is 153.8% increase in less than 10 years. What is particularly concerning is that the increase in the

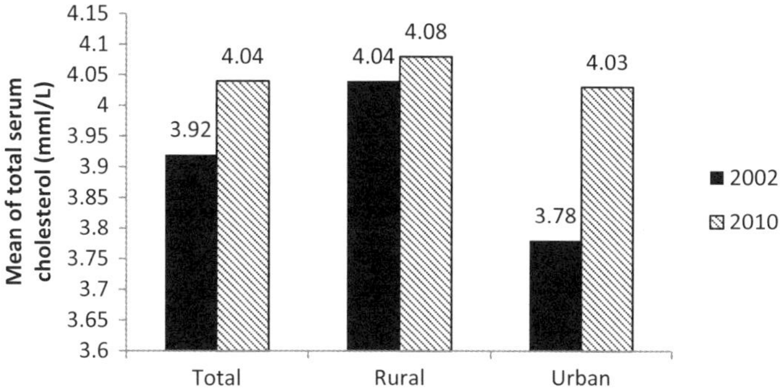

Figure 3.3 Comparison of mean total serum cholesterol between 2002 and 2010.

Source: Chronic disease risk factor surveillance in China in 2010, Chinese Centre for Disease Control and Prevention; National surveys on nutrition in China in 2002.

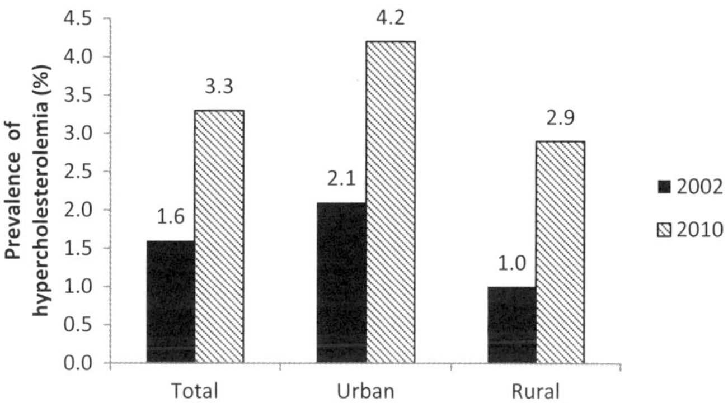

Figure 3.4 Comparison of prevalence of hypercholesterolemia between 2002 and 2010.

Source: Chronic disease risk factor surveillance in China in 2010, Chinese Centre for Disease Control and Prevention; National Nutrition and Health Survey in China in 2002.

prevalence of hypercholesterolemia was higher in younger male participants, 18–29 years, living in rural areas (Figure 3.4).

3.4 Diabetes

Type 2 diabetes mellitus is a serious public health problem worldwide because of its high prevalence and concomitant risks of all-cause mortality, and has the largest absolute disease burden of diabetes in the world. The prevalence of diabetes was estimated to be 8.3% worldwide in 2012, meaning a total of 371 million people living with diabetes (Xu, *et al.*, 2013). The prevalence of diabetes in Asian populations has increased rapidly in recent decades with a disproportionate representation among young- and middle-aged individuals. For instance, it was estimated that the national prevalence of diabetes was 9.0% in India (International Diabetes Federation, 2012).

A comparison of results from the 1980, 1986, and 1994 diabetes censuses with the 2002 National Health and Nutrition Examination Survey, indicates that the prevalence of diabetes in China has significantly increased, and the rates of increase show no signs of slowing. Even more alarmingly, China has replaced India as the country with the largest population of diabetic patients.

According to a national cross-sectional study involving 46,239 adults selected from 14 provinces and municipalities from June 2007 to May 2008, in urban areas of China, the prevalence of diabetes was 12.0% (12.8% in men and 10.1% in women) and of pre-diabetes 13.6% (15.5% in men and 14.3% in women) (Yang, *et al.*, 2010). The 2010 China National Chronic Disease Risk Factor Surveillance reported that the overall prevalence of diabetes was 9.7% in Chinese adults 18 years and over and it was 12.3% in urban areas and 8.4% in rural areas (NCNCD, 2010). It is possible that the difference in diabetes prevalence between urban and rural residents is due to differences in lifestyle in the two settings. The estimated prevalence of diabetes in the Chinese population is similar to the United States population (11.3%) even though being overweight and obesity, the main risk factors for diabetes, are much more common in the United States (Centers for Disease Control and Prevention, 2011; Flegal *et al.*, 2012).

3.5 Being Overweight and Obesity

China is undergoing rapid urbanization, accompanied by the adoption of a Western-style diet (Zhai *et al.*, 2009). Along with these changes, both being overweight and obesity have become more prevalent in China. The prevalence of overweight (BMI 24–28 kg/m^2) and obese (BMI >28 kg/m^2) Chinese adults aged 18 years and over in urban areas in 2002, using the cut-offs for Asian populations (WHO Expert

Consultation, 2004), was estimated at 22.6% and 8.2%, respectively (WHO, 2013).[1]

The prevalence of obesity (BMI ≥28 kg/m^2) in Chinese adults aged 18 years and over increased from 9.8% in 2002 to 14.2% in 2010 in the urban population, and from 6.0% to 10.9% in the rural population (Wang, 2005; NCNCD, 2010). The 2004, 2007, and 2010 China Chronic Disease Risk Factors Surveillances also demonstrated the trend (NCNCD, 2010). The prevalence is higher in females (increased from 8.5% in 2004 to 9.1% in 2007, and to 10.2% in 2010) than in males (increased from 6.5% in 2004 to 7.0% in 2007, to 10.6% in 2010); and higher among people living in urban areas (increased from 8.3% in 2004 to 8.7% in 2007, to 11.1% in 2010) than participants living in rural areas (increased from 6.7% in 2004 to 7.4% in 2007, to 9.4% in 2010) (NCNDC, 2010; He *et al.*, 2005; NCNCD, 2009, and CDC of China, 2009) (Figure 3.5). Chapter Six in this volume discusses the rising incidence of childhood obesity in China.

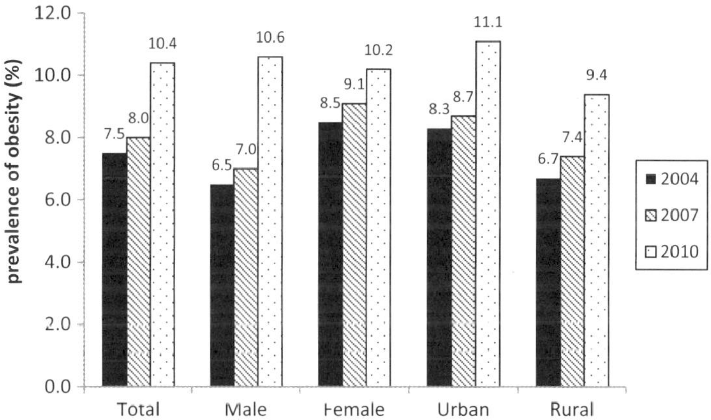

Figure 3.5 The trend comparison of prevalence of obesity from 2004 to 2010.
***Source*: Chronic disease risk factor surveillance in China in 2004, 2007, and 2010, Chinese Centre for Disease Control and Prevention.**

[1] BMI cut-off values were defined according to the association between epidemiology of obesity and risk of related diseases. The WHO standard was seen as unsuitable for Asian populations, including the Chinese. Therefore, The Working Group China Obesity put forward new BMI cut-off values for the Chinese population based on the analysis of 13 large sample epidemiological investigations of China.

3.6 Conclusion

The prevalence of NCDs is closely linked to a range of issues, such as socio–economic conditions, ecological environment, culture and lifestyle, and other factors. Along with population aging, as demonstrated by the data presented here, the number of Chinese living with NCDs has been increasing dramatically. At the same time, the extraordinary pace of urbanization in China has exacerbated this trend. NCDs have become the leading causes of death in China. The proportion of NCDs attributable to individual behavior and practices is steadily rising. The most important of these behaviors include unhealthy diet, smoking, excessive alcohol consumption, and physical inactivity. Therefore, public health policies should be formulated to help curb this chronic disease epidemic.

The Chinese government has increasingly paid attention to chronic and non-communicable disease control and prevention. The China National Plan for NCD Prevention and Treatment (2012–2015) was developed jointly by the Ministry of Health and 14 other ministries and state administrations on 8 May 2012 (CDC of China, 2012). The plan has laid down some basic principles for Chronic Disease Prevention and Treatment, including, firstly, government leadership, inter-sector cooperation and social participation; secondly, a focus on priorities, classified guidance based on various conditions, and results-oriented principles; and thirdly, prevention-first, integrating prevention with treatment, and emphasizing primary healthcare. The current health reforms will also have significant implications for the implementation of this plan.

As the data presented in the chapter has shown, many NCDs risk factor patterns are different among different age groups, and vary between the urban and rural settings (although the gaps are shrinking). This should provide the evidence for developing specific policies and prevention or intervention programs targeting the right population groups. This is not only important for achieving desirable health outcomes and reaching the nine global targets for the prevention and control of non-communicable diseases, it is also important in promoting population health and investing in human capital, which will bring enormous benefits to future economic and socially sustainable development.

References

Alwan, A., MacLean, D.R., Riley, L.M., *et al.* (2010). Monitoring and Surveillance of Chronic Non-communicable Diseases: Progress and Capacity in High-Burden Countries, *The Lancet* **376**: 1861–1868.

Centers for Disease Control and Prevention (2011). *National Diabetes Fact Sheet: National Estimates and General Information on Diabetes and Prediabetes in the United States, 2011*, Centers for Disease Control and Prevention, Atlanta, GA.

Chen, Xiaorong, Yong Jiang, Limin Wang, *et al.* (2012). Leisure-Time Physical Activity and Sedentary Behaviors Among Chinese Adults in 2010, *Chinese Journal of Preventive Medicine Med* **46**: 399–403 (in Chinese).

CDC of China (Center for Disease Control and Prevention) (2012). *China National Plan for NCD Prevention and Treatment (2012–2015).* Available at http://www.chinacdc.cn/en/ne/201207/t20120725_64430.html [Accessed 20 January 2015].

CDC of China (Center for Disease Control and Prevention) (2010). *Report on Chronic Disease Risk Factor Surveillance in China, 2007.* People's Medical Publishing Press, Beijing (in Chinese).

Cochrane, J., Chen, H., Conigrave, K.M., *et al.* (2003). Alcohol Use in China, *Alcohol* **38**: 537–542.

Flegal, K.M., Carroll, M.D., Kit, B.K., *et al.* (2012). Prevalence of Obesity and Trends in the Distribution of Body Mass Index Among US Adults, 1999–2010, *JAMA* **307**: 491–497.

He, F.J., Li, J. and MacGregor, G.A. (2013). Effect of Longer-term Modest Salt Reduction on Blood Pressure. *Cochrane Database of Systematic Reviews.* DOI: 10.1002/14651858.CD004937.pub2.

He, F.J. and MacGregor, G.A. (2002). Effect of Modest Salt Reduction on Blood Pressure: A Meta-Analysis of Randomized Trials. Implications for Public Health, *Journal of Human Hypertension* **16**: 761–770.

He, Y., Ma, G., Li, Y., *et al.* (2005). Study on the Current Status and Trend of Food Consumption Among Chinese Population, *Zhonghua Liu Xing Bing XueZaZhi* **26**: 485–488 (in Chinese).

Institute of Medicine of the National Academies (2010). *Strategies to reduce sodium intake in the United States.* Available at http://www.iom.edu/reports/2010/strategies-toreduce-sodium-intake-in-the-united-states.aspx [Accessed 5 December 2011].

International Diabetes Federation (2012). *Diabetes Atlas: 5th ed.* Available at http://www.idf.org/sites/default/files/attachments/5E_IDFAtlas Poster_2012_EN.pdf [Accessed 28 December 2012].

Joint WHO/FAO Expert Consultation (2003). WHO Technical Report Series: Diet, nutrition and the prevention of chronic disease. WHO, Geneva.

Li, Q., Hsia, J. and Yang, G. (2011). Prevalence of Smoking in China in 2010, *The New England Journal of Medicine* **364**: 2469–2470.

Lim, S.S., Vos, T., Flaxman, A.D., *et al.* (2012). A Comparative Risk Assessment of Burden of Disease and Injury Attributable to 67 Risk Factors and Risk Factor Clusters in 21 Regions, 1990–2010: A Systematic Analysis For The Global Burden Of Disease Study 2010, *The Lancet* **380**: 2224–2260.

Ma, G.S., Zhu, D.H., Hu, X.Q., *et al.* (2005). The Drinking Practice of People in China, *ActaNutr Sin* **27**: 16–19 (in Chinese).

NCNCD (National Center for Chronic and Non-communicable Disease Control and Prevention), Chinese Center for Disease Control and Prevention (2010). *Report on chronic disease risk factor surveillance in China, 2010.* Military Medical Science Press, Beijing (in Chinese).

NCNCD (National Center for Chronic and Non-communicable Disease Control and Prevention), Chinese Center for Disease Control and Prevention (2009). *Report on Chronic Disease Risk Factor Surveillance in China, 2004.* Peking Union Medical College Press, Beijing (in Chinese).

National Bureau of Statistics of China (2011). National statistics yearbook. National Bureau of Statistics of China, Beijing.

Rehm, J., Room, R., Graham, K., *et al.* (2003). The Relationship of Average Volume of Alcohol Consumption and Patterns of Drinking to Burden of Disease: An Overview, *Addiction* **98**: 1209–1228.

Wang, Huijun, Fengying, Zhai and Shufa, Du, *et al.* (2003). The Changing Trend of Dietary Fat Intake of Chinese Population: An Eight Provinces Case Study in China, *Ying Yang Xue Bao* **25**(3): 230–234.

Wang, Longde (2005) *Report on 2002 National Nutrition and Health Survey.* Beijing: People Health Publishing House (in Chinese).

Wang, Longde, Kong Lingzhi, Wu Fan, *et al.* (2005). Preventing Chronic Diseases in China, *The Lancet* **366**: 1821–24.

WHO (n.d). Global Physical Activity Questionnaire (GPAQ) Analysis Guide. Available at http://www.who.int/chp/steps/resources/GPAQ_Analysis_Guide.pdf [Accessed 10 February, 2015].

WHO (2004). *The Global Burden of Disease, 2004 update.* WHO, Geneva.

WHO (2009a). *Global Health Risks. Comparative Risk Assessment Project.* WHO, Geneva.

WHO (2009b). *Interventions on Diet and Physical Activity: What Works, Summary Report.* WHO, Geneva.

WHO (2009c). *Global Health Risks: Mortality and Burden of Disease Attributable to Selected Major Risks.* WHO, Geneva.

WHO (2010). *Global Status Report on Non-Communicable Diseases, 2010.* WHO, Geneva.

WHO (2013). WHO report on the Global Tobacco Epidemic, 2013. WHO, Geneva.

WHO (2014). Global Status Report on Non-Communicable Diseases. WHO, Geneva.

WHO Expert Consultation (2004). Appropriate Body-mass Index for Asian populations and its Implications for Policy and Intervention Strategies, *The Lancet* **363**: 157–163.

Wu, X., Duan, X., Gu, D. *et al.* (1995). Prevalence of Hypertension and its Trends in Chinese Populations, *International Journal of Cardiology* **52**, 39–44.

Wu, Z., Yao C., Zhao, D., *et al.* (2001). Sino-MONICA Project: A Collaborative Study on Trends and Determinants in Cardiovascular Disease in China, Part I: Morbidity and Mortality Monitoring, *Circulation* **103**, 462–468.

Xu, Y., Wang, Limin, He, Jiang, *et al.* (2013). Prevalence and Control of Diabetes in Chinese Adults, *JAMA* **301**: 948–958.

Yang, G.H. and Hu Angang. (2011). *Tobacco Control and China Future — The Evaluation Report on Tobacco Use and Control from Chinese and Foreign Experts.* Economic Daily Press, Beijing.

Yang, G.H., Ma, J.M., Liu, N., *et al.* (2005). Smoking and Passive Smoking in Chinese, 2002, *Zhonghua liu xing bing xue za zhi* **26**: 77–83 (in Chinese).

Yang, W., Lu, J. and Weng, J., *et al.* (2010). Prevalence of Diabetes Among Men and Women in China, *New England Journal of Medicine* **362**: 1090–1101.

Yeh, A.G.O., Xu, J. and Liu, K. (2011). China' s Post-Reform Urbanization: Retrospect, Policies and Trends. United Nations Population Fund (UNFPA) and International Institute for Environment and Development (IIED), New York.

Yu, W. (2012). National Disease Surveillance Points System-Death cause surveillance 2010. Military Medical Science Press, Beijing (in Chinese).

Zhai F, Wang H, Du, S., *et al.* (2009). Prospective Study on Nutrition Transition in China, *Nutrition Review* **67**, S56–S61.

Chapter Four

Urbanization and Road Traffic Injury in China

Li Ping Li

Abstract

As urbanization continues to expand in China, capacity cannot meet the daily transport demands of people's social and economic lives, despite record construction of the road network. At the same time, the structure of most urban transport systems is unbalanced, and the transport resource utilization and design of the traffic system are inefficient and unreasonable. As a consequence, China has one of the highest numbers of road traffic accidents resulting in mortality and injury in the world. Road traffic safety has become a major public health concern. There is an urgent need to establish a road safety and life protection system to improve the prevention and reduction of road traffic accidents.

4.1 Introduction

Urbanization is the process of population migration from rural to urban areas; the transformation of production, lifestyle and community structure; and the accumulation of population, wealth, technology and services (Lu *et al.*, 2006). China has been experiencing dynamic urbanization and motorization due to rapid economic growth. From

Table 4.1. Changes in economics, population, urbanization and motorization between 1980 and 2013

Year	GDP (billion US$)	Population (10,000 persons)			Per capita GDP S$/ person)	Motor vehicle ownership (10,000 units)	Motor vehicle drivers (10,000 persons)
		Total	Urban	%			
1980	58	98,705	19,140	19	59	178	245
1985	115	105,851	25,094	24	108	321	462
1990	237	114,333	30,195	26	207	551	791
1995	773	121,121	35,174	29	638	1040	1673
2000	1261	126,743	45,906	36	995	1609	3747
2005	2326	130,756	56,212	43	1,779	3160	8018
2010	5927	134,091	66,978	50	4,394	7802	15,130
2013	9185	136,072	73,111	54	6,767	12,670	21,743
2013/ 1980	158.36	1.4	3.8	2.8	114.7	71.2	88.7

Source: China Statistical Yearbook 2014.

1980 to 2013, the overall Gross Domestic Product (GDP) increased by approximately 158 times, the urban population increased close to four times, while the total population increased by 40%. During the same period, the numbers of motor vehicles and drivers increased approximately 71 times and 89 times, respectively (Table 4.1).

As urbanization progresses, the quality of the environment, including air and water pollution, nutrition and lifestyle choices and access to health care services contribute to the disease burden both in urban and rural areas. Traffic-related accidents also pose a major public health threat, as the country becomes increasingly motorized (Gong *et al.*, 2012). The central government has made transport policy reform and implementation one of the priorities of its national economic development strategy, aiming at the construction of an integrated transport infrastructure (General Office of the State Council, 2011).

This has been particularly important since the 1997 Asian Economic Crisis. The Chinese government introduced proactive fiscal policies and strengthened investment in infrastructure development. For example, investment in highway construction reached around 3% of total GDP. Investment in transportation infrastructure has directly contributed to national economic growth, as well as greatly improving transport systems.

Due to its widespread accessibility, adaptability and flexibility, road transport has been developing rapidly in China. A road network has been created, consisting of complex systems with major hubs that include the national capital Beijing, the municipalities directly under the central government, namely Shanghai, Tianjin and Chongqing, and provincial capital cities. Routes radiate from each of the economic zones and major highways connect the east coastal areas, the hinterland and the vast rural areas in the west. By the end of 2013, the total distance covered by highways in China reached 4.356 million kilometers (excluding Hong Kong, Macao and Taiwan), and the total length of expressways reached 104,438 kilometers, a remarkable record by any standards.

Thus, as a result of rapid urbanization and dynamic economic change, motorization has increased and road transport infrastructure has been developed. However, road traffic mortality has become an unintentional result and thus, road traffic accidents have emerged as a serious public health problem in China. According to the annual report of the China Road Traffic Accidents Statistics, the number of people who died in road traffic accidents in 2012 was 59,997. Although since 2004 the number of deaths from road traffic accidents is declining (Table 4.2), the total number of fatalities is expected to grow, due to the rapidly increasing number of vehicles and novice drivers on the roads. Mortality from traffic-related injury is ranked first among all types of injuries, followed by drowning and falls. The Potentially Productive Years of Life Lost (PPYLL) from road traffic injuries was 33.6% of all injuries during 2002–2006, and the proportion of road traffic-related mortality among all injury deaths was 32.35% (Wang *et al.*, 2008). This chapter examines how, driven by economic development and urbanization, increased demand on transport capacities has led to transportation mode changes in China.

Table 4.2 Traffic accident data, 1980–2012

Year	Number of accidents	Number of deaths	Number of injuries	Number of deaths per 10,000 vehicles[1]	Number of deaths per 10,0000 people
1980	116,692	21,818	80,824	104.47	2.21
1981	114,679	22,499	79,546	95.85	2.25
1982	103,777	22,164	71,385	85.32	2.81
1983	107,758	23,944	73,957	84.35	2.33
1984	118,886	25,251	79,685	42.99	2,43
1985	202,136	40,906	136,829	62.39	3.89
1986	295,136	50,063	185,785	61.12	4.70
1987	298,147	53,439	187,399	50.37	4.94
1988	276,071	54,814	170,598	46.05	5.00
1989	258,030	50.441	159,002	38.26	4.54
1990	250,297	49.271	155,072	33.38	4.31
1991	264,817	53.292	162.019	32.15	4.60
1992	228,278	58,729	144,264	30.19	5.00
1993	242,343	63,508	142,251	27.24	5.36
1994	253,537	66,362	148,817	24.26	5.54
1995	271,843	71,494	159,308	22.48	5.90
1996	287,685	73,655	174,447	20.41	6.02
1997	304,217	73,861	190,128	17.50	5.97
1998	346,129	78,067	222,721	17.30	6.25
1999	412,860	83,529	286,080	15.45	6.82
2000	616,971	93,853	418,721	15.60	7.27
2001	754,919	105,930	546,485	15.46	8.51
2002	773,137	109,381	562,074	13.71	8.79
2003	667,507	104,372	494,174	10.81	8.08
2004	517,889	107,077	480,864	9.93	8.24
2005	450,254	98,738	469,911	7.57	7.60
2006	378,781	89,455	431,139	6.16	6.84
2007	327,209	81,649	380,442	5.10	6.21
2008	265,204	73,484	304,919	4.33	5.56

(Continued)

Table 4.2 (*Continued*)

Year	Number of accidents	Number of deaths	Number of injuries	Number of deaths per 10,000 vehicles[1]	Number of deaths per 10,0000 people
2009	238,351	67,759	275,125	3.63	5.10
2010	219,521	65,225	254,075	3.15	4.89
2011	210,812	62,387	237,421	2.78	4.65
2012	204,196	59,997	224,327	2.50	4.45

Source: China Road Traffic Accidents Statistics 2012.

[1]Two-wheel motorcycles and some tractors are included.

4.2 Changes in Modes of Transportation

An improved economic position has raised the people's consumption levels across the country. This has required increased spending on travel and transportation. Further, as the urban areas continue to expand, and urban housing costs increase, more and more people are committed to long distance commuting each day. This is coupled with the underdevelopment of the public transport system. Because of the demand, motor vehicle production in China has tripled since the early 1990s (Zhou *et al.*, 2003). These factors contribute to the number of vehicles in many major Chinese cities skyrocketing, reaching saturation point. The increase in the number of vehicles in the last 30 years has unavoidably put a lot of pressure on the existing roads, resulting in road accidents. Changes in modes of transport, housing and lifestyle have contributed to new patterns of accidents and injuries. It is not surprising, therefore, that a large and increasing proportion of China's injury-related mortality and morbidity is due to traffic-related injuries. Globally, over the past few decades, the process of rapid and unplanned urbanization has resulted in an unprecedented revolution in the ownership of motor vehicles and the alarming increase in morbidity and mortality from road traffic injury (Fk *et al.*, 2003).

In the 20 years between 1985 and 2005, the number of automobiles in China increased nine-fold, and the number of motorcycles and other vehicles increased 54-fold. The public health impact of this phenomenal increase is not limited to deaths and injuries but includes harder-to-measure air pollution, the effects of reduced exercise, and other inevitable changes. During this period, reported road traffic mortality in China increased by 95%.

It is clear that rapid urbanization has played a key role in driving the trends of traffic-related and occupational accidents and injuries (Hu *et al.*, 2008). In urban areas, increasingly crowded roadways are shared by a mix of pedestrians and motorized and non-motorized vehicles, competing for road space. In the absence of separate rights of way, pedestrians and cyclists are put at a heightened risk of accidents and injuries, especially at intersections (Pucher *et al.*, 2007). Ironically, slowing of traffic because of the rising number of vehicles on the road which causes congestion in urban areas could have played a part in the stabilization or even reduction in traffic death rates (Hu *et al.*, 2008). However traffic-related accidents and injuries remain the country's leading cause of injury-related deaths (Wang *et al.*, 2008). Cyclists and pedestrians make up 60% of traffic-related deaths.

Despite the fact that motor vehicles have taken over the roadways, non-motorized transport modes are still used for as many as 40–55% of total trips taken in big cities such as Beijing and Shanghai, and a much higher proportion of journeys than those in smaller cities (Pucher *et al.*, 2007). The urban poor — especially rural-to-urban migrants — are most reliant on these non-motorized transport modes in their everyday life, and therefore bear a larger share of the burden of road traffic injuries (Pucher *et al.*, 2007).

Even though urbanization promotes industrialization, encourages economic growth, supports population flow and brings many other significant benefits, it also leads to many problems, such as that of road traffic safety. As a city proceeds to expand and develop, road traffic safety presents significant challenges and pressures, as discussed below.

4.3 Increased Demand on Road Network Capacity

The progress of global economic integration and urbanization promotes the development of countries and cities around the world. In one generation, more than half the world's population, and a quarter of the poor population in developing countries, will live in cities (Xu *et al.*, 2014). Expanding cities create larger demands on roads and transport. Any further expansion of urban population will perpetuate the situation, and worsen it. This is the scenario in China, where the road network capacity cannot meet the demand of rapid urbanization. Residents require a sustainable, safe and healthy traffic environment. This is a huge challenge for the current struggling traffic system.

Ideally, during the process of urban development and rural-to-urban migration, city governments should consider offering employment opportunities to newcomers, with reasonable incomes that meet their daily needs. Cities should also be able to offer them housing or enable them to rent or buy a house, so that they have shelter. Further, cities should provide conditions that encourage newcomers to integrate fully into the city in terms of lifestyle and *suzhi* (personal qualities) (Yu, 2013). Currently, cities are not able to meet these basic needs. The reality is that in cities houses are expensive and employment opportunities are limited, so people spend a lot of time and effort traveling. With the expansion of city space, the distance traveled and time spent traveling increase. In order to save travel time, people choose the car as their preferred means of transport. The great number of cars on city roads has become a necessary part of people's everyday lives in areas undergoing urbanization. As a result, the number of overall road users has increased dramatically — two to three times higher than population growth. Increased traveling inevitably raises the risks of traffic accidents. While cars are convenient, the rapid increase in the number of motor vehicles on the road has also contributed to deterioration in traffic safety (Yu, 2013). Admittedly, the majority of people fail to obey traffic rules. The ownership of cars is continuously climbing. All of these factors pose threats to traffic safety.

The conflict between the increasing transport demands and the unsatisfactory road infrastructure brings about road traffic insecurity. The expansion of the population, the agglomeration of city functions and the rapid increase in the number of motor vehicles are together continually adding more pressure to road traffic facilities, which are incapable of handling the pressure. The problem is several-fold: firstly the current growth rate in numbers of motor vehicles is far greater than the growth rate of road infrastructure; secondly low road infrastructure capacity does not reflect the high demand; thirdly motor vehicles, non-motor vehicles and pedestrians have to share the roads. All these issues are factors in the high frequency of road accidents. Even though the Department of Urban Development has invested heavily in widening roads, building new roads and increasing the proportion of urban development, the finance allocated to the construction of traffic infrastructure, and the available land for such infrastructure development are both limited. This means that the conflict between the demand for more transport capacity and the government's ability to deliver it will become more urgent. Thus, the factors currently causing unsafe road traffic conditions will continue to present a huge challenge to the management of road traffic safety.

Injuries and disabilities caused by accidents are responsible for economic losses not only to the people concerned and their families, but also to the government. Governments of cities should consider investing more in developing and improving the public transport system (such as buses and trains). At the same time, governments should also invest in strengthening the construction of the bicycle and pedestrian network to provide safer traveling conditions. These measures have been shown to reduce urban traffic pollution and traffic injuries, as well as to reduce the costs of mobility to poor populations who are mostly reliant on these means of transport. Commuter research in Shanghai shows that the mortality rate among those who ride a bike to work is 30% lower than among those who travel to work using other means of transport (WHO, 2011).

4.4 Need to Improve the Structure and Utilization of the Urban Transport System

Urbanization in China has entered a critical period with rapid development and serious consequences emerging. The ecological and environmental problems, which occurred in developed countries around the world over the last 100 years in their different developmental stages, have been intensely concentrated in China over the last 20 years. Apart from air and water pollution, the most outstanding transportation problems are traffic jams, parking difficulties, high frequency of traffic accidents, motor vehicle exhaust and noise pollution. Some cities are showing an increasing trend of traffic congestion, with a traffic speed of only 20 km/h in the city center, severely restricting the economic and social development of the cities (Shen, 2008).

The problems are caused, to a large extent, by the unbalanced urban traffic structure, incapable of accommodating the mixed modes of transport in most cities. There is a lack of effective policy, guidance and strategic planning for managing the urban traffic structure. In addition, the designs of urban road systems are not reasonable: that is they are not taking the needs of various road users into consideration. As a result, the utilization of limited road resources is ineffective. The conflict between supply and demand for urban parking facilities is also a manifestation of poor planning. In developed countries, each car usually has on average 1.2–1.5 parking spaces. However, in China on average, a hundred cars share less than 35 parking spaces (Yu, 2007). As a consequence, many cars are parked along roads, further occupying the limited space and exacerbating the situation.

Furthermore, public transport, such as the urban rail network, has lagged behind the pace of urban development. Most cities depend entirely on road-using motor vehicles and these are unable to meet the growing transport demands. In addition, urban land resources are limited. There is a shortage of land available for road traffic infrastructure expansion. As the high-intensity and high-density urban development continues, the conflict between demand and supply of effective transport will persist if no alternatives are put in place. There is an urgent need to develop public transport, and to speed up the construction of rail transport in cities. In addition, the government should consider the logical use of underground space and enhancing the land utilization rate, for example, building underground car parking, and developing the underground transport system. This would help to manage the crowds of people and traffic on the roads, and hence reduce traffic accident rates. The subsequent increase in road traffic speed would alleviate traffic congestion and reduce harmful emissions.

It is evident that in many cities there are some people or businesses who use the limited land resources for the purpose of building big roads, commercial properties or malls for profit, without considering an overall urban development plan (Yu, 2007). To ensure sustainability the government should, therefore, take into account the population, resources, and environmental capacity and condition in urban planning. More importantly, the urban development should adapt to the socio–economic situation, and adopt an appropriate developmental speed guided by scientific evidence.

4.5 Need to Establish a Road Safety System

According to the "Global Status Report on Road Safety" published by WHO in 2013, there are approximately 124 million road traffic fatalities each year worldwide. Since 2007, the death rate has barely changed (WHO, 2013). It is significant that the number of registered cars has increased by 15% around the world in the same period. This suggests that interventions designed to reduce road traffic mortality have been effective.

China is a country with a high incidence of road traffic accidents. However, national road traffic statistics data released by the Traffic Management Department reveal fewer incidents than those reported by the WHO. For example, in 2009, it was reported that 70,000 people died in traffic accidents, and a further 300,000 were injured. The WHO report revealed that every day 600 people died in traffic accidents, and 45,000 were injured. This means that the total number of deaths and injury was 219,000 and 16,425,000 respectively every year. The WHO's data are more objective compared to the official report in China (Wang, 2013). Additionally, during the period 2002–2007, the rate of death from road traffic injuries based on death registration data was about twice as high as the rate reported by the police. Linear regression analysis showed a significant decrease of 27% (95% confidence interval, CI: 35–19) in the death rate over the period according to police sources but no significant change according to death registration data (Hu *et al.*, 2011). In other words, the police-reported data did not reflect the true situation. The quality of the data obtained from police reports that inform decision-making by the Government of China and international organizations needs to be improved. Accurate records of the number of road traffic fatalities is essential for planning effective policies aimed at reducing these deaths.

Road traffic injury was ranked third in 2013 for years of life lost in China (GBD, 2013; Mortality and Causes of Death Collaborators, 2014). Obviously, the road traffic safety problem has become one of China's top public health problems. According to the result of a six year National Injury Surveillance System in China, from 2006 to 2011, the annual number of recorded injuries increased from 340,000 to 630,000, the majority being male (65%), and over 80% aged 15–64 years (Duan, 2015). The Chinese Center for Disease Prevention and Control Disease Surveillance Points (DSP) data support this; there were a total of 15,012 road traffic deaths in 2008. Among them 11,603 were male (77%), and 3876 deaths (26%) occurred in urban areas. The highest incidence of road traffic deaths occurred among young male adults aged 20–45 (Ma, 2012). Thus it can be said that road traffic injury mainly affects the labor force population. For China, therefore, there are significant social and economic implications that require urgent measures to reduce road accidents.

By November 27, 2014, the number of registered vehicles in China reached 264 million with 154 million cars, accounting for 58.9% of all motor vehicles, a 33.3% increase from ten years ago. The number of motor vehicle drivers has surpassed 300 million. The number of drivers and the vehicle growth rate is now ranked first in the world. The traffic structure has also undergone a fundamental change (Wang *et al.*, 2014). However the capabilities of management, the safety facilities, and the traffic control abilities are underdeveloped and urgently need to be strengthened and improved.

With the rapid development of China's economy and increased household income, the affordability of cars has improved markedly. Currently, one in every three adults drives a motor vehicle. Now many new drivers, particularly young drivers, are on the roads. Studies have confirmed that young people are putting themselves and other road users at risk, as motor vehicle crashes involving new drivers are the leading cause of death. (Weiss *et al.*, 2014) In other words, new drivers are the hidden danger to road safety. There are approximately

27.4 million young drivers under 25 years old. In terms of driving experience, about 29.3 million drivers have been driving for less than one year, which is about 10% of all drivers (Jia, 2014).

The road traffic safety problem is of concern in China. Compared with more mature motorized countries or societies, China has a higher incidence of traffic accidents and mortality. China is one of the 10 countries most seriously affected by traffic deaths globally (Hyder and Bisahi, 2012). Research on the prevention of urban traffic accidents has shown that there is a relationship between the number of vehicles on the road and the number of deaths (Wang, 2011). However, an increase in the number of vehicles does not necessarily have to lead to an increase. In the process of fast-paced motorization, phenomena including violations of traffic regulations and abusive driving styles are very common. One of the key issues is to improve the education and safety training of drivers.

It is worth noting that deaths from car accidents are closely related to the level of economic development, the management of road traffic safety and the capacity to rescue and treat the injured effectively. Vehicles in developed countries account for 70% of the total motor vehicles worldwide, but only contribute 15% of traffic fatalities. In recent decades, many developed countries such as the United States of America, Japan and some of the Western European countries have adopted effective preventive measures. Their experience in strengthening road traffic management, and enhancing the capacity to rescue the injured have made road traffic safer by significantly reducing the number of fatalities. Thus, powerful and effective measures for traffic management should be taken seriously as a matter of priority, and should include prevention of traffic accidents and timely rescue and treatment of the injured. To achieve these outcomes, the establishment of a system of road traffic safety and life support adapted from international experience to the Chinese situation needs to be accelerated. Even though road traffic accidents may not be entirely avoidable, many casualties can be prevented before they happen, or managed effectively after they have occurred to minimize the loss of human life. Through the establishment of an efficient and effective system, the safety of road traffic can be substantially increased, despite the continuously increasing number of motor vehicles (Wang, 2011).

Cities in China are facing high traffic accident mortality exceeding the total number of deaths from natural disasters, seriously affecting economic and social development and directly affecting many Chinese people and their families. Governments at all levels have paid great attention to this problem. They call for the establishment of a road safety and life protection system, which means the development of strategies for the prevention and reduction of the impact of road traffic accidents. The traffic safety and life protection system needs to be comprehensive, involving social considerations and technological requirements, all in specific practical detail. The system needs to take people, vehicles, roads, environment and management into consideration. There is also a need to set up a specific institution with a mandate to prevent road traffic accidents, responsible for developing and implementing road safety and life protection strategies. This institution should collaborate with departments of police, transport, education, health and social development. It is also important to establish a road accident prevention governance body. It should follow the principles of 'solving the problem from its roots', 'managing systematically', 'managing comprehensively' and 'managing according to the law'.

Preventive measures should mainly focus on the following:

- Improving the management planning, policies and regulations, and institutional system of road traffic safety.
- Increasing the investment in road transport infrastructure, technology, equipment and management.
- Improving the management system of road traffic safety. The responsibility for preventing road traffic accidents should be undertaken by all levels of government and transport enterprises. There is a need for cooperation in building and developing intra-departmental working systems, to form a coordinated, efficient working mechanism with clear responsibilities.
- Targeting the drivers to prevent and reduce road traffic accidents According to the three main factors that matter to drivers (their physical ability, driving capability and the complex traffic

environment) preventive measures should be developed in these three aspects: a driver suitability test, safe driver training, and the comprehensive management of the traffic environment using modern technology. This approach would help to shape a safer driving environment and achieve the aim of preventing road traffic accidents.

To achieve sustainable national economic development and urbanization, and for the beneficial purpose of developing a healthy, safe and harmonious society, the central government, local departments of traffic management and all road users need to work together towards road traffic safety.

References

Duan, L., Xiao, D., Yuan, W., *et al.* (2015). The National Injury Surveillance System in China: A Six-year Review, *Injury.* Available at http://dx.doi.org/10.1016/j.injury.2014.12.013 [Accessed 18 December 2014].

Afukaar, F.K., Antwi, P. and Ofosu-Amaah, S. (2003). Pattern of Road Traffic Injuries in Ghana: Implications for Control, *International Journal of Injury Control and Safety Promotion* **10**: 69–76.

GBD 2013 Mortality and Causes of Death Collaborators (2014). Global, regional, and national age-sex specific all-cause and cause-specific mortality for 240 causes of death, 1990–2013: a systematic analysis for the Global Burden of Disease Study 2013. Available at http://dx.doi.org/10.1016/S0140-6736(14)61682-2 [Accessed 18 December 2014].

General Office of the State Council (2011). Several opinions of promoting the sustainable healthy development of the common road on further perfecting the investment and financing policy. Available at http://www.gov.cn/zwgk/2011-04/27/content_1853587.htm [Accessed 18 December 2014].

Gong, P., Song, L. and Carlton, E.J., *et al.* (2012). Urbanisation and Health in China, *The Lancet* **379**: 843–852.

Hu, G., Wen, M. and Baker, T.D., *et al.* (2008). Road-Traffic Deaths in China, 1985–2005: Threat and Opportunity, *Injury Prevention* **14**: 149–153.

Hu, G., Baker,T. and Baker, S.P. (2011). Comparing Road Traffic Mortality Rates from Police-Reported Data and Death Registration Data in China, *Bulletin of the World Health Organization* **89**: 41.

Hyder, A.A. and Bishai, D. (2012). Road Safety in 10 Countries: A Global Opportunity, *Traffic Injury Prevention* **13**: 1–2. DOI: 10.1080/15389588.2011.650023.

Jia, S. (2014). China's motor vehicle drivers amount exceed 300 million. *The Beijing News*, 27 November. Available at http://news.sina.com.cn/c/2014-11-27/205831213615.shtml [Accessed 30 December 2014].

Lu, D. and Liu, H. (2006). Urbanization and environmental issues in China, in Wang, W., Krafft, T. and Kraas, F. (eds.), *Global Change Urbanization and Health*, China Meteorological Press, Beijing.

Ma, S., Qingfeng, L., Zhou, M., *et al.* (2014). Road traffic injury in China: A Review of National Data Sources, *Traffic Injury Prevention* **13**(S1): 57–63.

National Bureau of Statistics of China (2014). *China Statistical Yearbook*, China Statistics Press, Beijing.

National Statistics Bureau of China (2014). *China Statistical Yearbook of Communication & Transportation 2014*, China Statistics Press, Beijing.

Pucher, J., Peng, Z.R., Mittal, N., Zhu, Y. and Korattyswaroopam, N. (2007). Urban Transport Trends and Policies in China and India: Impacts of Rapid Economic Growth, *Transport Reviews* **27**: 379–410.

Shen, Y. (2008). Urban road traffic evaluation method and the development of evaluation system. Unpublished master's thesis, Beijing Jiaotong University.

Traffic Administration Bureau of the Ministry of Public Security (2013). *China Road Traffic Accidents Statistics* 2012. China Statistics Press, Beijing.

Wang, S.Y., Li, Y.H., Chi, G.B., *et al.* (2008). Injury-related Fatalities in China: An Under-recognised Public-health Problem, *The Lancet* **372**: 1765–1773.

Wang, Zhengguo (2011). *Modern Traffic Medicine*, Chongqing Publishing Group, Chongqing.

Wang, Zhengguo (2013). Road Traffic Safety, *Medical Journal of Communications* **27**(2): 107–109.

Wang, Zihan and Chen, Xiang (2014). Seven kinds of the traffic law violator behavior, Overspeed is the first killer, *Chongqing Morning News* 2 December. Available at http://news.sina.com.cn/o/2014-12-02/061931231555.shtml [Accessed 30 December 2014].

Weiss, H.B., Kaplan, S. and Prato, C.G. (2014). Analysis of Factors Associated with Injury Severity in Crashes Involving Young New Zealand Drivers, *Accident Analysis and Prevention* **65**: 142–155.

WHO (2011). *Health in the Green Economy: Health Co-benefits of Climate Change Mitigation-transport Sector*, World Health Organization, Geneva.

WHO (2013). *Global Status Report on Road Safety: Supporting a Decade of Action*, World Health Organization, Geneva.

Xu, Anning and Yuan, Hua (2014). Advice on the Road Transportation Safety Management Policy in Developing Cities, *Transport Forum* 19–22.

Xu, Haofeng *et al.* (2005). Qualitative investigation about traffic attitude in Guangzhou residents, *South China Journal of Preventive Medicine*, **31**(2): 29–31.

Yu, Guotai (2007). The Environmental Problems in China's Urbanization Road, *Xinhua Abstract* 13.

Yu, Guotai, (2007). Environmental Issues in Chinese Urbanisation, *Science* **59**(2): 36–38.

Yu, Zhiqing (2013). Effect and Countermeasure of Urbanization on Road Traffic Safety, *Journal of Henan Science and Technology* **11**: 158–159.

Zhou, Y., Baker, T.D., Rao, K. and Li, G. (2003). Productivity Losses from Injury in China, *Injury Prevention* **9**: 124–127.

Chapter Five

Infectious Diseases and Urbanization

Jia Zheng Wang, Qiang Zheng Sun, Zhu Jun Shao,
Xiang Feng Dou, Quan Yi Wang, Bu Yun Cui,
Biao Kan, and Jian Guo Xu

Abstract

Urbanization in China is being strongly promoted by the government to sustain economic development. The urbanization trend thus relies on the new politics. The main changes to risk factors for the transmission of infectious disease in the era of urbanization include high population density in cities, lower health protection awareness and habits in rural-to-urban migrants, changes to the processing of food and its supply, and pollution. Some changes due to urbanization such as housing improvement, higher income, and safe water supplies might be beneficial to the control of some infectious diseases. However, these changes also present new challenges to the prevention and control of infectious diseases. In this chapter, the changes in disease morbidity including in the important diseases of respiratory tract infection, diarrhea, and zoonosis are analyzed, as are the corresponding influences of urbanization. Changes in social behavior and the resulting changes in infectious disease are also discussed.

5.1 Introduction

As the level of infrastructure and public services in urban areas are constantly improving with urbanization, urban culture, and lifestyle have become popular, particularly among young people, and are rapidly spreading to rural areas. The National Bureau of Statistics of the People's Republic of China confirmed that by the end of 2011, over half the Chinese population were living in cities, and the proportion has kept growing. Since 1978, urbanization in China has been steadily and rapidly developing. Because urbanization has improved living standards and enhanced sanitation awareness, the spectrum of infectious diseases has undergone some tremendous changes. The disease surveillance data from the China Centre for Disease Prevention and Control (CDC) shows that on the one hand, the incidence of the two class A (plague and cholera) and 26 class B (SARS, AIDS, viral hepatitis, poliomyelitis and so on) infectious diseases reported and managed under the Infectious Diseases Prevention and Control Act of the People's Republic of China)[1] have decreased significantly. A number of infectious diseases that had high incidence previously have been significantly reduced or even eliminated. For example, the smallpox virus was eliminated in 1980, and the polio virus has been almost eliminated. The incidences of cholera and plague are much lower than before. On the other hand, urbanization has also brought new trends in traditional and emergent infectious diseases. As a result, both research and prevention and control of infectious diseases are facing new challenges.

In this chapter we discuss morbidity changes in some common infectious diseases and explore their links to urbanization.

5.2 Changes in the Incidence of Common Infectious Diseases

In China, infectious diseases (such as bacillary dysentery, meningitis, influenza, hemorrhagic fever with renal syndrome) are jointly

---

[1] Infectious Diseases Prevention and Control Act of the People's Republic of China, passed by the People's Congress in 1989, with amendments passed in 2004 and referred to in the chapter as the Infectious Disease Prevention Act.

monitored, reported and controlled by public health administration departments, disease control institutions, and medical institutions. The Chinese infectious disease surveillance and reporting system was established in 1950. After an infectious disease case is admitted to a health facility, the clinician makes a clinical diagnosis or laboratory confirmation. If a case of a notifiable disease (stipulated by the Infectious Disease Prevention Act) is confirmed or suspected, the doctor must complete the infectious disease reporting record card and information will be collected, checked, corrected and filed by the relevant CDC. There is a disease surveillance network, including county, prefecture, provincial, and national level CDCs. Through this surveillance system, the information on changing trends of reported infectious diseases in China can be monitored and accessed.

5.2.1 *Diarrheal diseases*

Diarrhea diseases are a group of diseases caused by multi-factors and multi-pathogens. Those diarrheal diseases specified by the Infectious Disease Prevention Act include cholera and bacillary dysentery, other infectious diarrhea excluding cholera and bacillary dysentery, and diarrhea caused by typhoid or paratyphoid salmonella infections. China's Patriotic Hygiene Campaign (*ai guo wei sheng yun dong*) began in 1949 at the beginning of the People's Republic of China, and continued simultaneously with the early urbanization process. Its purpose is to improve national hygiene standards and people's health (Xiao, 2003). Under the banner of the Patriotic Hygiene Campaign, diarrheal disease prevention and control programs have been implemented throughout the country. The ecological and environmental conditions in China, especially in cities, have significantly improved since 1949. As a result, the incidence of diarrheal disease has been significantly reduced. However, diarrheal diseases today show some concerning new epidemic characteristics.

As a worldwide public health problem, the morbidity and mortality of bacillary dysentery ranks first among all infectious diarrheas. Bacillary dysentery is an intestinal infectious disease caused by various strains of shigella. Among them, *S. flexnery* and *S. sonnei* are the two main species causing diarrhea in China. Bacillary dysentery is a sporadic disease throughout the year, but has a relatively higher incidence in summer and autumn. Disease surveillance data from the CDC shows that in China in the 1950s to 1980s, the incidence of bacillary dysentery varied between 46.4/100,000 and 1018.9/100,000. From 1981 to 2012, the incidence of bacillary dysentery gradually decreased, and the ranking dropped from the first of the statutory infectious diseases to the third. Particularly, between 1999 and 2012, the reported number of bacillary dysentery cases fell from about 600,000 cases a year to 206,000 cases a year, a two-thirds reduction; and the incidence fell from about 50/100,000 to 15.3/100,000 (Figure 5.1). For example, in 2012, there were 205,972 cases identified, and only 13 deaths from bacillary dysentery were reported nationally. The threat of bacillary dysentery to the health of Chinese people has been significantly reduced. However, its incidence is still significantly higher than in developed countries. Because of poor sanitary conditions, the incidence rate still remains high, and there have been sporadic outbreaks due to water and food contaminations.

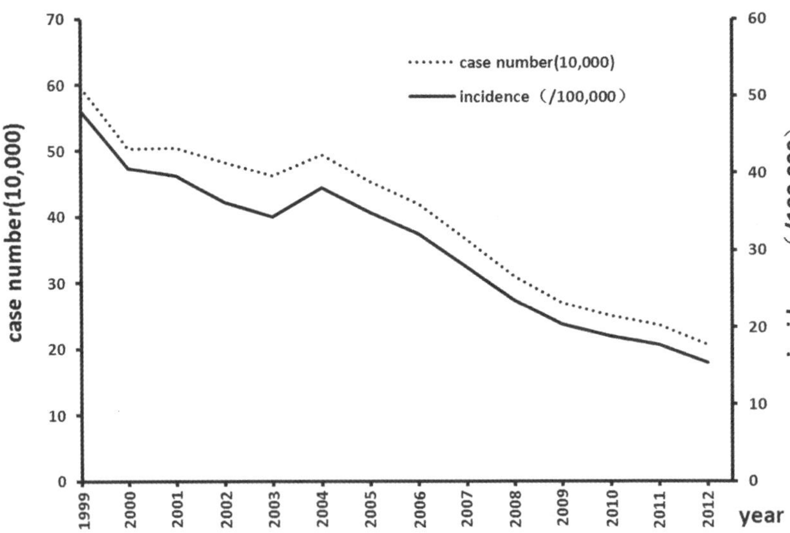

Figure 5.1. Number of cases and incidence rate of bacillary dysentery in 1999–2012 in China.

In urban areas, the disease is especially concentrated in areas, such as places where migrant workers gather.

S. flexneri has long been the dominant pathogenic species of shigella infection in China. The monitoring data from 1999 to 2012 shows that *S. flexneri* accounted for over 60% of all shigella infections. However, the infection rate of *S. sonnei* has been on the rise in recent years. In order to monitor the changes in species and possible associated disease patterns, 20 national monitoring sites were set up in 2012. *S. sonnei* infections are as high as 30%, and have now become the predominant species in some provinces. Meanwhile, a new species of *S. flexneri* has been identified. In essence the pathogen species are evolving but the reasons for these changes are not well understood yet. Of even greater concern is the increasing drug resistance of shigella infections. Traditional antibiotics, such as sulfonamides, tetracyclines, and ampicillin, are no longer effective as the recommended drugs for the treatment of bacillary dysentery. Over-prescribing and misuse of antibiotics and the change of species of the pathogen may have contributed to this.

Although the incidence of dysentery is declining, the emerging specific populations susceptible to bacillary dysentery deserve special attention. As diarrheal diseases are often transmitted by the fecal-oral route, the most vulnerable groups are migrant workers in cities due to their poor hygiene awareness and living conditions. Children who often buy street snack foods are also at higher risk, while AIDS patients are particularly susceptible to dysentery due to their sexual behaviors and compromised immunity.

5.2.2 *Bacterial respiratory infections*

Bacterial respiratory infections are mainly community-acquired pneumonia, meningitis, and other non-invasive infections. Since the comprehensive planned immunization program in China in the 1980s, the incidence of infectious respiratory diseases has been drastically reduced. For example, diphtheria, cerebrospinal meningitis, pertussis and other respiratory diseases have been well controlled (Zhang *et al.*, 2000a and 2000b; Hu, 2004). However, there are new trends of respiratory diseases that demand new prevention and disease control strategies.

Epidemic cerebrospinal meningitis (ECM) is a respiratory infectious disease caused by the *Neisseria meningitidis* infection. Humans are its only host. *N. meningitidis* is spread as coughing and sneezing — patients and carriers project droplets into the air. *N. meningitidis* tends to spread with high efficiency in crowded places, especially among children in childcare and in primary and middle schools. The disease manifests as cerebrospinal meningitis and bacteremia, and it can be fatal. Epidemic flora of ECM in China is undergoing changes and causing disease outbreaks, bringing new challenges to its prevention and treatment.

As a notifiable infectious disease in China, ECM has a relatively high incidence rate and the most prevalent serogroups are serogroup A and serogroup C. For example, national pandemics caused by serogroup A occurred in 1959, 1967 and 1977, with the incidence rate reaching 55.6/100,000, 403/100,000, and 60.1/100,000, respectively (Hu, 2004). Since the 1960s, serogroup A has gone through at least three changes. Serogroup C ECM is known to be mostly responsible for causing sporadic cases. Since the introduction of serogroup A meningococcal vaccine to children 6–18 months old in the 1980s, the disease surveillance data from the China CDC has shown that the incidence rate of ECM has drastically decreased (Figure 5.2). However, in 2003 there was an ECM outbreak in Anhui Province caused by serogroup C (Shao *et al.*, 2010). This outbreak caused an epidemic in 21 provinces, municipalities and autonomous regions, and became the dominant epidemic strain in some provinces in central and eastern China. In response to the epidemic, in 2007 the *N. meningitidis* vaccines of serogroup A+C for people over the age of two were included in the Expanded Program on Immunization in China, leading to the decline of serogroup C ECM. Recently serogroup B ECM, also traditionally known for causing sporadic infections, has shown a growing trend.

In addition, new ECM serogroups that cause epidemic respiratory infections have also been identified. For example, serogroup W135 ECM first appeared in Fujian Province in 2006 and spread to 11 provinces, gradually becoming an epidemic (Shao *et al.*, 2010;

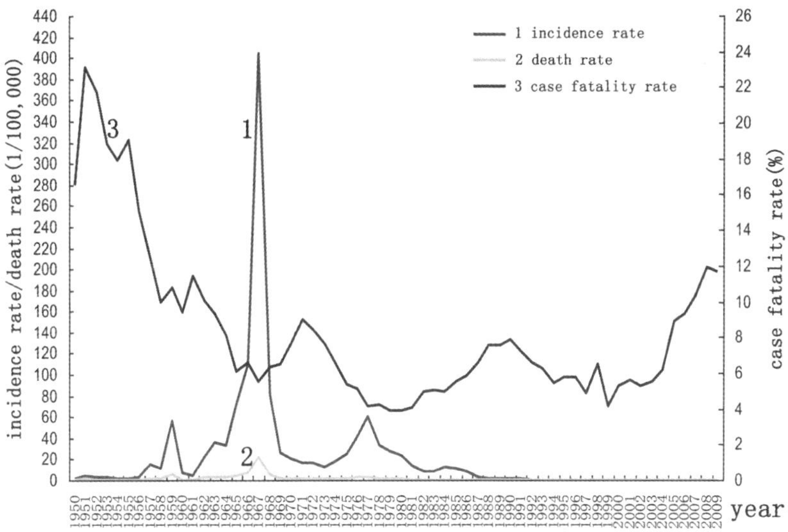

Figure 5.2. Incidence rate, death rate and case fatality rate of ECM in China (1950–2009).

Gao *et al.*, 2013). Serogroup X ECM cases appeared in Beijing in 2007 and in Zhejiang Province in 2013 (Chen *et al.*, 2008). Urbanization and issues that come with it, such as high population density in cities and air pollution have contributed to the increase in bacterial respiratory infectious diseases.

5.2.3 *Viral respiratory infectious diseases*

Viral respiratory infectious disease refers to infectious diseases caused by viruses, such as influenza, measles, mumps and rubella. In the 20th century, there were three major influenza pandemics, two of which started in China. In 1957, the Asian flu (H2N2) first broke out in Guizhou Province and swept the globe rapidly, killing at least one million people, with the incidence rate as high as 15–30% (Cox and Subbarao, 2000; Kilbourne, 2006). In 1968 the Hong Kong flu (H3N2) spread to 55 countries and regions, leading to 1.5–2 million deaths (Chang, 1969; Chu *et al.*, 1957; Shao *et al.*, 2010).

Avian influenza is caused by the Influenza A virus. This highly pathogenic virus can be transmitted to humans, and so has attracted widespread attention both in China and internationally. In 1997 and 1998, several H5N1 and H9N2 AI virus sporadic cases were found in Hong Kong and adjacent Guangdong Province (Yuanji, 2002; Cauthen *et al.*, 2000), which further confirmed the potential risk of the AI virus directly infecting humans. As a pioneering region for the development of urbanization, Guangdong Province has the highest urban development level in China. However, with the development of its live poultry market, Guangdong has always been considered the most likely place for influenza to originate, and is even considered the center of a potential influenza pandemic in Asia and the world (Shortridge, 1997). Guangdong is where the first infections of different AI virus subtypes in humans have appeared (Claas *et al.*, 1998; Gao *et al.*, 2013). It has also been the location of sporadic cases (Chen *et al.*, 2014; Liu *et al.*, 2014; Lu *et al.*, 2014; Xiao *et al.*, 2014; Wang and Lobstein, 2006) as well as where the emergence of new types of AI virus were reported (Lu *et al.*, 2014).

5.3 Zoonoses

Some pathogens can spread between people and animals without relying on humans and animals as the reservoir of infection. The development of urbanization reduces people's contact with wild animals, especially rodents. As a result of this, the incidence of zoonotic diseases in China has showed a downward trend. However, because of the expansion of city borders through urban development, the changes in people's diet, including the consumption of wildlife, the improvement in transport for moving livestock to different areas, and the increased number of domestic pets, diseases caused by zoonosis are not only re-emerging but expressing new epidemic characterizations.

5.3.1 *Hemorrhagic fever with renal syndrome*

Hemorrhagic fever with renal syndrome (HFRS) is a zoonosis caused by hantavirus with small rodents as the vector. China was most affected by hantavirus in the 1970s and 1980s, but the number of HFRS cases started to decline in the 1990s. As a result of rapid urbanization, enhanced immunization programs and rodent control the downward trend continues, particularly in urban areas (Zhang *et al.*, 2004; Guo *et al.*, 2010; Wang *et al.*, 2010). For example, between 2007 and 2012, the incidence of HFRS in Beijing remained at a low level, with fewer than 100 cases each year, below the national average (Table 5.1). However, because of the imbalanced planning and development among different districts of the city, HFRS in Beijing shows a distinctive geographical aggregation pattern. The northern ecological conservation area, the rural–urban fringe of Haidian District in the northwest and the old residential areas in the southern districts of Beijing city have become the three 'hot spots' for HFRS; these are all areas with relatively poor sanitation (Figure 5.3).

5.3.2 *Brucellosis*

Brucellosis is a zoonotic infectious-allergic disease caused by brucella, an infection that mainly affects animals. If transmitted to humans it often becomes chronic and difficult to cure. Brucellosis is listed as a Class B animal epidemic disease by the World Health Organization (WHO) and a class B notifiable disease in China.

Table 5.1 Incidence of HFRS in Beijing during 2007–2012

	Beijing			Nationwide	
Year	Cases	Incidence (/10,0000)	Case fatality rate (%)	Incidence	Case fatality
2007	25	0.16	4.0	0.84	1.31
2008	17	0.11	0	0.68	1.14
2009	12	0.08	0	0.66	1.19
2010	15	0.10	0	0.71	1.24
2011	20	0.10	0	0.80	1.10
2012	18	0.09	0	—	—

Data Source: Beijing Annual Report of Annual Infectious Diseases; Annual Monitoring Report of Key Infectious Diseases and Vectors in China; - No access to relevant data.

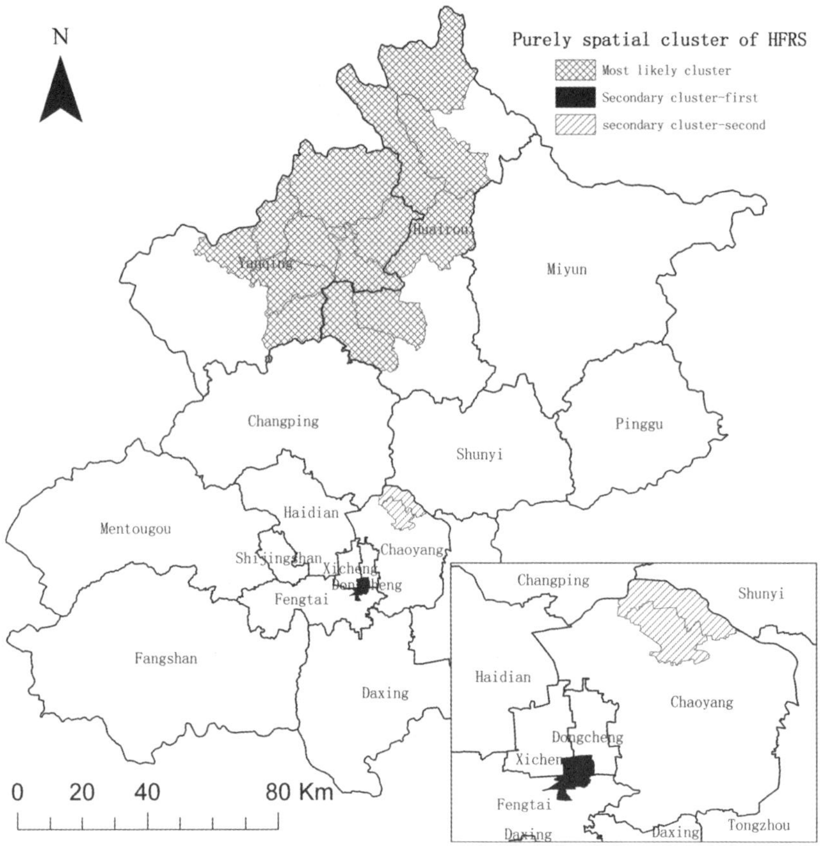

Figure 5.3. Pure spatial scanning analysis of HFRS in Beijing during 2007–2012.

In the 1980s, although brucellosis was found in other provinces, the major epidemiological characteristics of a brucellosis epidemic in China were concentrated in the five pastoral areas of Xinjiang, Tibet, Inner Mongolia Autonomous Regions, and Ningxia and Qinghai Provinces. These areas each had strong animal husbandry sectors. Since the 1990s, the brucellosis endemic has shown sustained growth. It has intensified and transferred to farming–pastoral areas, agricultural areas, cities and small towns (Cui, 2007). The disease surveillance data from the China CDC shows that in 2004 the incidence of brucellosis increased by 87% over the previous year. In 2013, 44,877

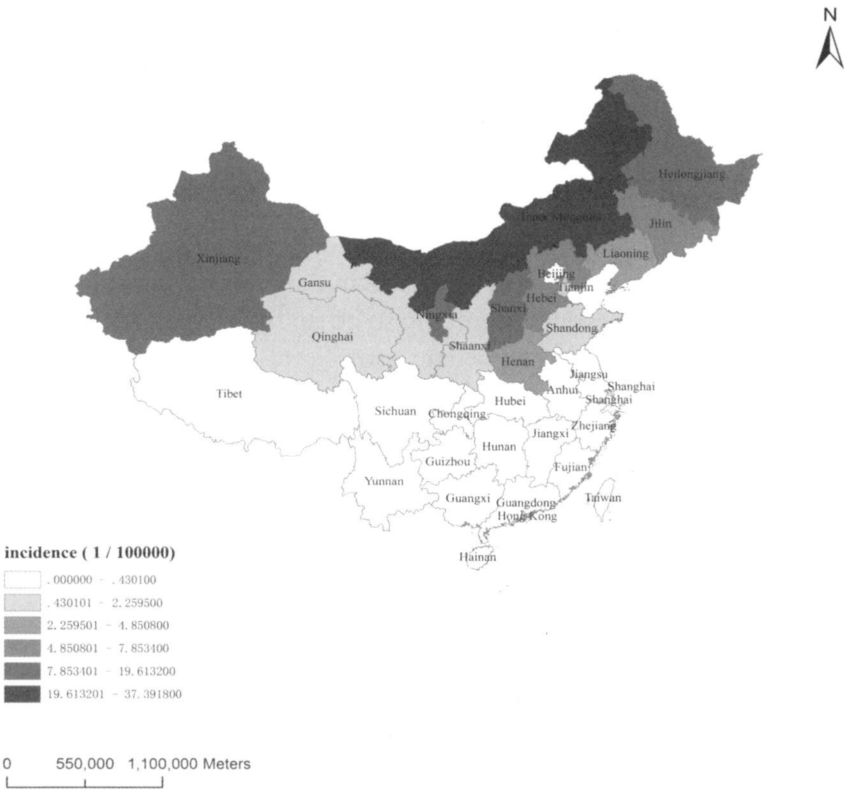

Figure 5.4. Spatial distribution of incidence of brucellosis in China in 2013.

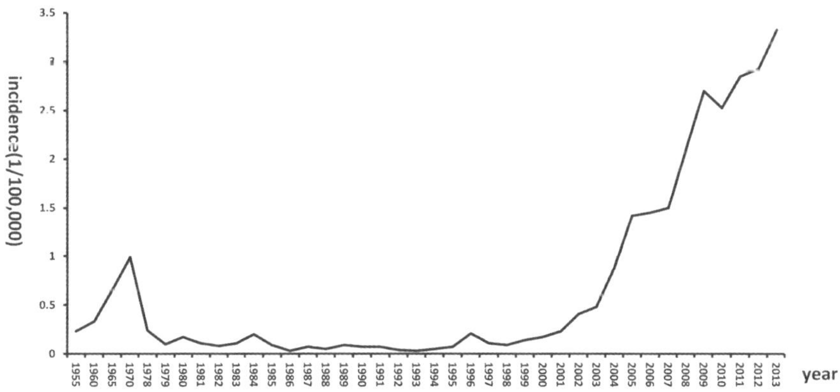

Figure 5.5. Incidence rate of brucellosis in China during 1950–2013.

new cases of brucellosis were reported in China, an increase of 9.5%, compared to the 40,994 cases in 2012. New cases have been reported in all provinces, and distributed across 1412 counties (Figures 5.4 and 5.5). It is estimated that about 10% of cases occurred among people living in urban areas. Cases were mainly spread over 25 provinces. Some of these provinces, such as Yunnan, Jiangsu, Zhejiang and Guangdong that had rarely had cattle and sheep breeding industries before urbanization, are now experiencing significant change in the epidemic and the trend is continuing to go up by the year. Meanwhile, other provinces have also reported various levels of the epidemic. The spread of brucellosis in China is gradually expanding.

5.4 The Relationship Between Chinese Urbanization and the Changing Epidemic of Infectious Diseases

During the urbanization process, with the improvement of socio–economic conditions, the enhancement of environmental sanitary conditions, and strengthened infectious disease prevention and control, the incidence of most infectious diseases has significantly decreased. However, problems generated in this process have also brought about new changes to the incidence rate of certain infectious diseases and endowed them with new features. Urbanization may have influenced these changes in the following aspects.

5.4.1 *Environmental factors*

In the process of urbanization, changes in the environment are inevitable. While improving the quality of life, environmental changes have also dramatically changed the survival and dwelling conditions of pathogenic organisms. Therefore, environmental changes are inextricably linked to changes in the incidence of infectious diseases.

Taking the epidemic changes in hemorrhagic fever with renal syndrome in Beijing presented here as an example, the progress of urbanization and the transformation of agricultural farmlands into industrial and residential areas have drastically reduced biodiversity. Secondly, the ecological environment has undergone a tremendous change and many pathogens have lost their reservoir hosts and living environment. Coupled with improved sanitation and living conditions, the overall incidence of HFRS in Beijing was at a low level between 2007 and 2012. However, the disease is concentrated in a few distinctive 'hot spots'. This localization of the disease distribution is caused by a set of complex environmental and human factors. Firstly, the different urban planning and environmental management in different districts means there are different standards and practices across the city. Secondly, due to the strengthening of ecological protection, the vegetation has being further enriched, and the number of small rodents is also increasing gradually. This provides favorable conditions for the preservation and dissemination of zoonotic pathogens such as hantavirus. Thirdly, the combination of relatively poor living conditions and health status in rural–urban fringe and 'urban villages' (rural villages engulfed by expansion of urban development), and poor health awareness of rural-to-urban migrants who live in these underserviced and overcrowded locations. Finally, during the reconstruction and restoration, many of the old residential districts in the southern part of Beijing were retained, meaning the habitat of rodents has not been eliminated.

Climate change and rising temperatures from heat islands in cities caused by urbanization and population concentration, improper disposal of waste and the poor waste management system have all led to an increasing incidence of mosquito-borne diseases such as dengue fever (Fan *et al.*, 2014). Drinking water contamination in old towns and rural–urban fringe areas has caused *E. coli* and other infectious diarrheal diseases (Wu *et al.*, 2006). Densely populated places such as office buildings and schools contribute to the spread of influenza, pneumonia and other respiratory diseases due to their enclosed environment and poor ventilation (Yan *et al.*, 2012). All these changes in the infectious disease spectrum are closely linked to the environmental changes that urbanization has brought about.

5.4.2 *Economic factors*

Urbanization and economic development have greatly improved not only the living standards of people, but also promoted more diverse lifestyles. A good example of the interaction between urbanization and infectious disease transmission is the live poultry industry and avian influenza. Driven by economic interests and consumer demand, live poultry markets are flourishing in many cities. Some are located in densely populated urban areas, which increases the risk of the transmission and spread of avian influenza to humans. Guangdong Province in Southern China has become the major origin of avian influenza and the expansion of its live poultry markets plays a very important role. Guangzhou Center for Disease Control and Prevention recently conducted monitoring of the human avian influenza virus and investigated the awareness and protection measures of stall owners and employees in live poultry markets. The results revealed that most live poultry stalls fail to implement the 'three separate areas' principles, that is, to separate selling, slaughtering and storing areas. Employees who handle live poultry were found to have poor occupational protection awareness, and failed to apply good hygiene practices. Among people exposed to live poultry handling, latent infection and cross-infection was found (Yuan *et al.*, 2013; Chen *et al.*, 2013, Liu *et al.*, 2014). To investigate the transmission paths, Jiangsu Center for Disease Control and Prevention collected samples from chickens in secondary live poultry wholesale markets, from live poultry retail markets and from human avian influenza patients, and found that the influenza virus was most likely to spread from the secondary wholesale market to live poultry markets, and was then ultimately transmitted to the patients (Bao *et al.*, 2013). The existence of this poultry-to-human transmission path is further supported by the finding that after the live poultry markets were shut down, following the outbreak of avian influenza in Shanghai, Hangzhou, Huzhou and Nanjing in 2013, the infected human population in Shanghai and Hangzhou decreased by 99% and by 97% in Huzhou and Nanjing (Yu *et al.*, 2014). Meanwhile, investigations found that the aggregation of live poultry from different regions in markets provided opportunities for gene recombination of the influenza virus (Lu *et al.*, 2014). This indicates unequivocally that large-scale live poultry markets in major cities are a major infection source of the avian influenza virus and key to its transmission to humans.

The number of reported cases of legionnaires, disease is on the rise, and this may be related to the widespread use of heating systems and heaters, and central air conditioners in particular (Wang and Zhou, 2002). Studies have reported that in major hotels in Beijing, the percentage of air conditioning cooling towers that tested positive for legionella was 55.3% (Peng *et al.*, 2000). In Shanghai, it was discovered that the percentage of central air conditioning systems, surface water and shower facilities in hotels, hospitals, subway stations, department stores and so on that tested positive for legionella was 31.2% (Chen *et al.*, 2000). These studies demonstrate that while improving people's living standards, urbanization and economic development have created favorable conditions for the breeding of pathogens that were once rare in China.

5.4.3 *Medical factors*

New medical technologies, new drugs and vaccines are now readily available to consumers, particularly in urban areas. These advancements have saved many lives, and contribute to the prevention and control of infectious diseases. However, infectious diseases can also arise from improvements in medical care and in medical technologies. For example, advances in medical technologies and services can trigger changes in pathogen behavior, such as their becoming drug resistant, which in turn can affect the effectiveness of infectious disease treatments and controls. Overprescribing and overuse of antibiotics are widespread problems in China. They can lead to disturbances in the normal flora in the human body and can increase the risk of infections of opportunistic pathogens. Even more concerning is that it can cause pathogenic bacteria to evolve and become drug resistant. The implementation of planned immunization has also changed the pathogen spectrum and prevalence trends of some infectious diseases.

Monitoring of drug-resistant shigella dysenteries has found that in recent years the bacteria has developed resistance to the commonly used antibacterial drugs (Zhang *et al.*, 2014). The primary resistance to anti-tuberculosis drugs is an important cause of the recent high incidence of tuberculosis. In addition, the emergence of multi-drug resistant bacteria, such as the methicillin-resistant *Staphylococcus aureus* and extended-spectrum-beta-lactamase producing bacteria, has also created great difficulties for the prevention and control of infectious diseases.

Multi-pathogen infections can be acquired during medical procedures through use of the devices that have not been properly sterilized or through the operators not following disinfection protocols in invasive treatment or procedures, such as in the use of catheters, gastric tubes and endoscopies. HIV and hepatitis virus infections can also be acquired from blood transfusion if the blood donors have not been screened appropriately.

5.4.4 *Social behavior*

While improving people's living standards, the development of urbanization has changed people's behavioral patterns, and thus raised new challenges for infectious disease prevention and control. For example, the incidence of brucellosis has shown a noteworthy upward trend in the recent decade and has spread to many parts of the country. People's behavioral changes in the process of urbanization have played an important role in this new phenomenon. More and more families in urban areas are now keeping dogs as pets. Brucella has been detected in pet dogs, suggesting pet dogs could serve as a vector.

Secondly, the change in eating habits is another reason for the expansion of brucellosis in China. Under the planned economy, poor transport conditions and limited capacity made it difficult to transport beef and mutton produced in northern pastoral areas to other parts of this vast country. Beef and mutton production and consumption were mainly concentrated in a few provinces in the north where there was high incidence of brucellosis. However, with urbanization and the rapid development of a market economy and improvements in transport, beef and mutton have now become an important part of people's diets. The availability of animal meat and the consumption of meat products have increased since the early 1980s (Popkin and Du 2003). Concurrently, brucellosis has spread from five pastoral areas to 25 other provinces.

Furthermore, with urbanization there is a sharp rise in the incidence of some behavior-related infections, including AIDS and sexually transmitted infections, such as gonorrhea and syphilis (Gong *et al.*, 2002). Hepatitis B and hepatitis C cases caused by drug taking and sharing syringes have also increased (Roy, 2000). Further, with increased population movements, transmission of dengue and malaria are also on the rise (Xie *et al.*, 2005).

5.5 Conclusion

In conclusion, the development of urbanization and the incidence of infectious diseases are closely related. Urbanization has provided better sanitation, more favorable living conditions and a more robust monitoring system for prevention and control of infectious diseases. Thus, the overall incidence of most infectious diseases, especially in urban areas, has dropped significantly. However, local environmental changes, changes in food supply patterns, high population density in the cities, hospital-acquired infections and unhealthy lifestyles accompanying urban development have brought with them changes to, and new features of, the incidence of infectious diseases in the cities. In the meantime, many other infectious diseases are continuing to threaten people's lives. Prevention and control of infectious diseases in the 21st century should, therefore, continue to be a top priority on the national public health agenda.

References

Bao, C.J., Cui, L.B., Zhou, M.H., *et al.* (2013). Live-animal Markets and Influenza A (H7N9) Virus Infection, *New England Journal of Medicine* **368**(24): 2337–2339.

Cauthen, A.N., Swayne, D.E., Schultz-Cherry, S., *et al.* (2000). Continued Circulation in China Of Highly Pathogenic Avian Influenza Viruses Encoding The Hemagglutinin Gene Associated with the 1997 H5N1

Outbreak in Poultry and Humans, *Journal of Virology* **74**(14): 6592–6599.

Chang, W. K. (1969). National Influenza Experience in Hong Kong, 1968, *Bulletin of the World Health Organization* **41**(3–4–5): 349.

Chen, C., Zhang, T.G., He, J.G., *et al.* (2008). A First Meningococcal Meningitis Case Caused by Serogroup X Neisseria Meningitidis Strains in China, *Chinese Medical Journal-Beijing-English Edition* **121**(7): 664.

Chen, Y., Shen, J.M., He, Z.C. and Jiang, H. (2000). Investigation on the Status of Clinical Infection and Environmental Contamination by Legionalla in Shanghai [J]. *Shanghai Journal of Preventive Medicine* **12**(7): 305–306.

Chen, Z., Liu, H., Lu, J, *et al.* (2014). Asymptomatic, Mild, and Severe Influenza a (h7n9) Virus Infection in Humans, Guangzhou, China, *Age* **5**: 4–17.

Chen, Z.Q., Lu, J.Y., Xiao, X.C., *et al.* (2013). Evaluation on the Risks of H5, H7 and H9 Avian Influenza Infections in Guangzhou: Using Data from the 2006–2012 Avian Influenza Surveillance Program, *Chinese Journal of Epidemiology* **34**(9): 900–905.

Chu, C.M., Shao, C. and Hou, C.C. (1957). Studies of Strains of *Influenza* Viruses Isolated During the Epidemic in 1957 in Changchun, *Voprosy virusologii* **2**(5): 278.

Claas, E.C., Osterhaus, A.D., van Beek, R., *et al.* (1998). Human *influenza* A H5N1 Virus Related to a Highly Pathogenic Avian *Influenza* Virus, *The Lancet* **351** (9101): 472–477.

Cox, N.J., and Subbarao, K. (2000). Global Epidemiology of *Influenza*: Past and Present, *Annual Review of Medicine* **51**(1): 407–421.

Cui, B. (2007). Epidemic Surveilance and Control of Brucellosis in China, *Disease Surveillance* **22**(10): 649–651.

Fan, J., Wei, W., Bai, Z., *et al.* (2014). A Systematic Review and Meta-analysis of Dengue Risk with Temperature Change, *International journal of environmental research and public health* **12**(1): 1–15.

Gao, R., Cao, B., Hu, Y., *et al.* (2013). Human Infection with a Novel Avian-origin *Influenza* A (H7N9) Virus, *New England Journal of Medicine* **368**(20): 1888–1897.

Gong, X., Ye, S., Zhang, J., *et al.* (2002). Epidemiological Situation of Sexually Transmitted Diseases in China: From 1991 to 2001, *Chinese Journal of Dermatology* **35**(3): 178–182.

Guo, H.Q., Ding, H.L., Bo, Q. and Sun, G. (2010). Epidemic Information of Hemorrhagic Fever with Renal Syndrome in China from 2004 to 2009 in ARIMA Model, *Chinese Journal of Zoonoses* **26**(12): 1137–1140.

Hu, X. (2004). Epidemiological Surveillance and Prevention of Epidemic Cerebrospinal Meningitis, *Chinese Journal of Public Health* **20**(5): 638–640.

Kilbourne, E.D. (2006). *Influenza* Pandemics of the 20th Century, *Emerging Infectious Diseases* **12**(1): 9.

Liu, Y.H., Liu, J.P., Liu, Y., *et al.* (2014). Knowledge, Attitudes and Practices Status About Avian *influenza* A (H7N9) Among People with Occupation Exposure to Wild Birds in Guangzhou. *Disease Surveillance* **29**(1): 21–24.

Lu, J., Wu, J., Zeng, X., *et al.* (2014). Continuing Reassortment Leads to the Genetic Diversity of *Influenza* H7N9 In Guangdong China, *Journal of Virology* JVI-00630.

Peng, X., Pei, H., Li, X., He, X., Yang, A., Tang, Y. and Cao, R. (2000). Studies on Legionella-Contamination to the Air-Conditioning Cooling Towers in Big Hotels and on its Seroprevalence in The Related Populations in Beijing, *Chinese Journal of Epidemiology* **21**(4): 289–291.

Popkin, B.M. and Du, S. (2003) Dynamics of the Nutrition Transition Toward the Animal Foods Sector in China and its Implications: A Worried Perspective, *Journal of Nutrition* **133**: 3898S–3906S.

Roy, R.B. (2000). My Choice: History Repeats Itself. The Prevention of Syringe Transmitted Hepatitis, *Sexually Transmitted Infections* **76**: S10.

Shao, Z., Li, W., Ren, J., *et al.* (2006). Identification of a New Neisseria Meningitidis Serogroup C Clone from Anhui Province, China, *The Lancet* **367**(9508): 419–423.

Shao, Z., Zhou, H., Gao, Y., *et al.* (2010). Neisseria Meningitidis Serogroup W135, China, *Emerging Infectious Diseases* **16**(2): 348–349.

Shortridge, K.F. (1997). Is China an *Influenza* Epicentre? *Chinese Medical Journal* **110**(8), 637–641.

Wang, Y. and Lobstein, T. (2006). Worldwide Trends in Childhood Overweight and Obesity, *International Journal of Pediatric Obesity* **1**: 11–25.

Wang, Q., Zhou, H., Han, Y.H., *et al.* (2010). Epidemiology and Surveillance Programs on Hemorrhagic Fever with Renal Syndrome in Mainland China, 2005–2008, *Chinese Journal of Epidemiology* **31**(6): 675–680.

Wang, S. and Zhou, Y. (2002). Contamination of the Environment by Legionella from Air-Conditioning System and its Control Measures. *Shanghai Journal of Preventive Medicine* **14**(2): 85–86.

Wu, J.G., Zhu, H.B. and Fang, D.C. (2006). Analysis on the Investigation and Control of an Epidemic Outbreak of Infectious Diarrhea, *Disease Surveillance* **21**(6): 304–306.

Xiao, A. (2003). Review of Patriotic Hygiene Campaign from 1949 to 1959. *Contemporary China History Study* **10**(1): 97–102.

Xiao, X.C., Li, K.B., Chen, Z.Q., *et al.* (2014). Transmission of Avian *Influenza* A (H7N9) Virus from Father to Child: A Report of Limited Person-To-Person Transmission, Guangzhou, China, January 2014, *European Surveillance* **19**: 25.

Xie, R.Q., Cheng, J.Q. and Lu, Z.X. (2005). Population Territorial Moving and Malaria Control, *Chinese Journal of Parasitic Disease Control* **18**(3): 227–229.

Yan, Y. (2012). Measures for Control and Prevention of Influenza A (H1N1) Spread in Public Places, *Chinese Medicine Guides* **9**(23): 161–162.

Yu, H., Wu, J.T., Cowling, B.J, *et al.* (2014). Effect of Closure of Live Poultry Markets on Poultry-to-Person Transmission of Avian *Influenza* A H7N9 Virus: An Ecological Study, *The Lancet* **383**(9916): 541–548.

Yuan, J., Di, B., Ma, X.W., *et al.* (2013). Risk Evaluation on H7N9 Avian *Influenza* in Guangzhou, China, *Chinese Journal of Public Health* **34**(5): 488–490.

Yuanji, G. (2002). *Influenza* activity in China: 1998–1999, *Vaccine* **20**: S28–S35.

Zhang, N., Lan, R., Sun, Q., *et al.* (2014). A Genomic Portrait of Evolution and Epidemic Spread of a Recently Emerged Multidrug Resistant

Shigella Flexneri Clone in China, *Journal of Clinical Microbiology* JCM-02669.

Zhang, X.L., Yang, Z.W. and Zhou, J. (2000a). An Analysis on Current Epidemiological Characteristics of Pertussis in China, *Chinese Journal of Vaccines and Immunization* **6**(2): 93–95.

Zhang, X.L., Yang, Z.W. and Zhou, J. (2000b). An Analysis of Current Epidemiological Characteristics of Diphtheria in China, *Chinese Journal of Vaccines and Immunization* **6**(1): 1–4.

Zhang, Y.Z., Xiao, D.L., Wang, Y., *et al.* (2004). The Epidemic Characteristics and Preventive Measures of Hemorrhagic Fever with Syndromes in China, *Chinese Journal of Epidemiology* **25**(6): 466–469.

Chapter Six

Childhood Obesity: The Chinese Perspective

Mu Li and Louise A. Baur

Abstract

Reports of increasing childhood overweight and obesity originally came from developed countries, but in recent years, countries undergoing rapid economic development and urbanization, such as China, have joined the trend. A recent inter-country study shows that younger Chinese children have experienced greater increases in body mass index (BMI), a measure of fatness, than their counterparts in the United Kingdom (UK), the United States of America (USA) and Australia. Larger body size or rapid growth in the first couple of years of life is a predictor of increased obesity later in life. Furthermore, childhood obesity can lead to long term adverse health effects, such as metabolic and cardiovascular risks. This chapter examines the trend of the childhood obesity epidemic in China and outlines the actions required to curb this public health concern.

6.1 Introduction

Childhood obesity has become a significant public health problem in many countries, as a result of a series of changes in health, diet, nutrition, and physical activity known as the 'nutrition transition'. Childhood obesity has increased in recent decades worldwide, from 4.2% in 1990 for children aged under five years, to 6.7% in 2010, representing a relative 60% increase in 20 years (de Onis *et al.*, 2010). High rates of childhood obesity have been evident for some time in many high income countries, such as the USA, the UK, and Australia (Lobstein *et al.*, 2004, Wang and Lobstein, 2006). In the past one to two decades some low and middle income countries, including many Asian countries, such as Vietnam, Indonesia, and China, have joined the trend (Li and Dibley, 2012). Such countries are experiencing a transition from under-nutrition to over-nutrition. As a result, the absolute number of children who are overweight or obese is now much higher in low and middle income countries, than in high income countries, and they carry the larger share of the global burden of childhood overweight and obesity. The distribution of this global burden is unequally distributed. Recent World Health Organization (WHO) statistics show that, in 2013, 42 million preschool-aged children were overweight or obese globally, among them 31 million living in low and middle income countries (WHO, 2014). Of even greater concern, the number of overweight or obese infants and young children is predicted to rise to 70 million by 2025 if the current trend continues (WHO, 2014). Childhood obesity prevention is now an international public health priority.

The prevalence of overweight and obesity in Chinese children has increased markedly in the past three decades (Zong and Li, 2014). In 2010, about one in ten Chinese school-aged children and adolescents was overweight and a further one in twenty was obese. This translates to 30.4 million Chinese 7–18 year olds being overweight or obese (Ji *et al.*, 2013). Additionally, younger Chinese children have experienced larger increases in BMI in recent decades compared with those in the USA, the UK, and Australia (Popkin, 2010).

Obesity is the result of an imbalance between energy intake and energy expenditure. Being overweight, and particularly being obese in childhood are not simply 'shrugged off' in adulthood; they have been linked to a range of immediate and long-term adverse effects on health and well-being (Gardner *et al.*, 2009, Friedemann *et al.*, 2012). The immediate effects, particularly for older children and adolescents, include cardiovascular disease risk factors, such as high cholesterol levels or high blood pressure, fatty liver disease, musculoskeletal problems, pre-diabetes, and psychosocial problems (Daniels, 2009). Overweight and obese children and adolescents are also more at risk for the development of a range of non-communicable diseases in adulthood, such as cardiovascular disease, type 2 diabetes, stroke and several types of cancer, and they have a higher all-cause mortality (World Health Organization, 2014b, Must and Struss, 1999).

6.2 Measurement of Childhood Overweight and Obesity

BMI is the most commonly used method to measure overweight and obesity at the population level for both adults and children. Unlike the situation for the adult population, BMI differs by age, sex, and developmental stage in children and adolescents. No consensus definition of childhood obesity exists; several internationally recognized references have been used in assessing childhood obesity. In addition, some countries, such as China and Thailand, have developed their own references.

6.2.1 *The international obesity task force (IOTF) cut-off*

The IOTF age- and sex-specific BMI thresholds are based on pooled data of children and adolescents aged 2–18 years from six countries – Brazil, Great Britain, Hong Kong, the Netherlands, Singapore, and the USA. The cut-offs used to designate overweight and obesity were based on statistical methods that drew centile lines corresponding to a BMI of 25 and a BMI of 30 at age 18 years. They thus provide continuity in definition from childhood into adulthood (Cole *et al.*, 2000).

6.2.2 *The World Health Organization (WHO) child growth standard and the WHO growth reference for school-aged children and adolescents*

The WHO Growth Standard for children aged 0–59 months (WHO, 2006) is based on the WHO Multi-Centre Growth Reference Study with participants from Brazil, Ghana, India, Norway, Oman, and the USA. In children <5 years, being overweight and obesity are defined as having a BMI-for-age >2 SDs and >3 SDs, respectively, from the WHO Growth Standard median. In addition, there is another category for being 'at risk' of overweight or obese, defined as having a BMI-for-age >1 SD and <2SDs (WHO, 2008). The advantage of this WHO Child Growth Standard, based on the observed growth of healthy breastfed children, is that it shows how infants and children should grow, rather than how they grow in a certain time or geographic location.

The WHO Growth Reference for School-aged Children and Adolescents is a reconstruction of the 1977 US National Center for Health Statistics (NCHS)/WHO reference (de Onis *et al.*, 2007). In children and adolescents between five and 19 years, overweight, obese and severely obese are defined as having a BMI-for-age >1 SD, >2 SDs and >3SDs, respectively, from the WHO Growth Reference median (WHO, 2008). However, there is no continuity between this WHO Growth Reference and the WHO Growth Standard for children 0–59 months, particularly at the age of five. Further, this growth reference does not link with the adult definitions, that is, where BMI >25 and <30 is defined as overweight, and >30 as obese. The lack of continuity with both the younger age and adult definitions makes it difficult for long-term follow up of adverse health outcomes from childhood and adolescence to adulthood.

6.2.3 *BMI reference norm for screening of overweight and obesity in Chinese children and adolescents*

This reference is based on survey samples conducted with children aged 7–18 years in the year 2000, in the coastal developed cities of

China. The cut-off points for overweight and obesity are defined as the 85th and 95th centiles, respectively (Group of China Obesity Task Force, 2004). At age 18, these correspond to a BMI of 24 and 28, respectively, for both males and females (WHO Expert Consultation, 2004). These cut-offs are consistent with the BMI definition for screening for overweight and obesity in Chinese adults. This means there is a continuity of measurement into adulthood (Group of China Obesity Task Force, 2004).

The rapid secular growth trend in Chinese children in recent decades and the divergence from the WHO growth references of Chinese children's weights and heights at various ages for both sexes are well recognized. Questions have been raised about the application of the WHO Children Growth Standard in China, as there are no participants from eastern Asian countries in the original study upon which the standard is based (Zhang *et al.*, 2013). It has been suggested that a new growth reference for China should be considered (Zong and Li, 2013). Caution is warranted, however, when attempting to redefine a growth reference as it may run the risk of 'normalizing' obesity.

6.3 Secular Trends in, and Prevalence of, Childhood Obesity in China

6.3.1 *School-aged children and adolescents*

The China National Survey on Students' Constitution and Health commenced in 1985 and is conducted every five years in randomly selected school-aged children and adolescents (7–18 years of age) nationwide (except Tibet), with samples exceeding 200,000 in each survey. The prevalence of overweight and obesity in children and adolescents, using the Chinese BMI Reference Norm for Screening Overweight and Obesity in Chinese School-aged Children, (Group of China Obesity Task Force, 2004) has steadily increased. The prevalence of overweight and obesity was 25.5% and 14.3 % in 2010, up from 1.8% and 0.3% respectively in 1985, when the survey first started. It is estimated that in 2010, 30.43 million Chinese school-aged children and adolescents were overweight or obese (Yang *et al.*, 2013). Furthermore, the prevalence of overweight and obesity is linked to the level of urbanization and associated socio–economic development (Table 6.1). In 2010, the prevalence of combined overweight and obesity was greatest in large coastal cities — 32.6% and 19.1% for males and females, respectively. Increased overweight and obesity prevalence was found in all other cities and rural areas, including the western rural areas — 19.0% and 10.4% for males and females, respectively. The rates in most of the rural areas started to rise around the year 2000, and have progressed at a faster pace in comparison with the cities, over the last decade.

6.3.2 *Preschool-aged children (under seven years)*

There are no nationally representative data for assessing childhood obesity in younger children. Nor has a Chinese growth reference been developed for this age group. Two large sample-sized epidemiological survey series have been in place since the mid-1980s for children living in major cities. The Nine Cities Physical Growth and Development Survey for children under seven years of age has been carried out three times at approximately 10 year intervals since 1986 (Coordinating Group of Nine Cities Study on the Physical Growth and Development of Children, 2008). The nine cities, namely Beijing, Harbin, Xi'an, Shanghai, Nanjing, Wuhan, Guangzhou, Fuzhou, and Kunming, are, except Beijing, capital cities of their respective provinces, with the average annual per capita income ranging from RMB 10,766 to 19,978 (approximately US$1800 to 3300). Six of these cities had an average income per capita above the national average of RMB 11,757 in 2006 (National Bureau of Statistics of China, 2006). Using the US NCHS/WHO reference, and yet another definition of obesity (>20% of the standard weight-for-height), the overall prevalence of obesity was 0.9%, 1.77%, and 3.4% in 1986, 1996, and 2006, respectively, indicating that obesity prevalence had nearly tripled over the 20 year period (Zong and Li, 2012). There was also a clear sex difference in prevalence, with boys carrying a larger burden than girls. In the most recent 2006 survey, 4.1% of boys were obese, compared with 2.7% of girls.

Table 6.1. Prevalence of overweight and obesity in 7–18-year-old children and adolescents by regions, 2010

Regions	Male			Female		
	Overweight	Obese	Overweight + obese	Overweight	Obese	Overweight + obese
Group I (Large coastal city)	18.9	13.7	32.6	11.2	7.9	19.1
Group II (Other upper class/large city)	15.8	10.2	26.1	9.1	5.0	14.1
Group III (Middle class/city)	15.1	8.3	23.4	9.0	3.8	12.8
Group IV (Lower class/city)	11.6	6.0	17.6	6.6	2.8	9.4
Group V (Upper class/rural)	15.5	8.9	24.4	9.5	5.2	14.7
Group VI (Middle class/rural)	9.8	5.3	15.1	6.1	2.6	8.8
Group VII (Lower class/rural)	9.4	4.0	13.4	6.3	2.3	8.6
Group VIII (Western/lower class/rural)	12.3	6.7	19.0	7.5	3.9	10.4

Source: Ji *et al.*, 2013.

A parallel epidemiological survey of childhood obesity in children aged 0–6 years was carried out over the same time period in 11 cities (Shenyang, Jinan, Qingdao, Zhengzhou, Changsha, Chongqing, Xi'an, Chengdu, Shenzhen, Haikou, and Wenchang), eight being capital cities, representing three regions, northern, central, and southern China (National Task Force on Childhood Obesity and National Center for Women's and Children's Health, 2008). The prevalence of overweight and obesity (2006 WHO reference, BMI >1SDS and BMI >2SDS) was 19.8% (22.2% for boys and 17% for girls) and 7.2% (9.9% for boys and 5.3% for girls), respectively. These two surveys cover more than 50% of Chinese capital cities on the mainland. However, because of the different reference standards and definitions being used, there is a marked discrepancy in prevalence in the two series, making it impossible either to combine or compare the data accurately. Child overweight and obesity in China should also be viewed within the greater context of world trends in child growth, reflecting changes in economic development. Mean body weight increased in both sexes and all age groups (0–18 years) from 1985 to 2010, and the average height of children and adolescents increased steadily between 1975 and 2010, with no sign as yet of a plateau (Zong and Li, 2014).

6.4 Identified Risk Factors of Childhood Obesity in the Chinese Context

Childhood obesity is a result of a complex web of biological, behavioral, contextual and socio–economic risk factors that affect children's weight (WHO, 2014b).

6.4.1 *Biological and behavioral factors*

In the Chinese context, factors associated with overweight or obesity in young children include maternal overweight (Jiang *et al.*, 2006) and high parental BMI or parental overweight (Jiang *et al.*, 2006, Coordinating Group of Nine Cities Study on the Physical Growth and Development of Children and Capital Institute of Pediatrics,

2008, Zhang *et al.*, 2013). They also include higher total dietary energy intake, mixed or formula feeding in the first four months, and an introduction to semi-solids before four months of age (Jiang *et al.*, 2008, Zhang *et al.*, 2013), caesarean section delivery (Coordinating Group of Nine Cities Study on the Physical Growth and Development of Children, 2008), birth weight >3,000 grams (Zhang *et al.*, 2009), and sleeping <11 hours per night in three-to-four year olds (Jiang *et al.*, 2009). It is worth noting that all of the studies of younger children were in urban settings. While many factors are likely to hold true in both urban and rural populations, issues such as low breast-feeding rates and high caesarean delivery rates are more prominent in urban areas. Frequent snacks (≥3 times per week), frequent consumption of Western fast foods and short sleep time (<10 hours for 6–12 year olds and <8.5 hours for 13–18 year olds) were significantly associated with obesity in a study of school-aged children in Beijing (Shan *et al.*, 2010). For boys, the consumption of sweetened soft drinks ≥4 times per week or >1,100 ml per day and having a medium to high energy intake, and for girls, eating breakfast outside the family home were strong dietary risk factors in Xi'an, a major metropolitan center in north-western China (Li *et al.*, 2008, Li *et al.*, 2010).

Many of these overlap with biological factors, such as inadequate physical activity and overconsumption of foods that are high in calories. In a study of Beijing school-aged children, those who were physically inactive (<1 hour per day physical activity, including physical education class, physical activity after school, walking or bike riding to and from school) and had a high level of sedentary behavior (≥2 hours per day screen time, including watching television, using a computer or playing video games) were more likely to be obese (Shan *et al.*, 2010).

6.4.2 *Contextual, socioeconomic factors*

The prevalence of childhood obesity is higher in urban than in rural settings, and in higher income families in China (Cui *et al.*, 2010). A study of socio–economic influences and dietary habits of adolescents (11–17 years) in Xi'an Metropolitan Area and surrounding areas found that adolescents from families of high socio–economic status and those having permission to purchase snacks with pocket money were 1.7 and 1.5 times more likely, respectively, to be overweight or obese than their respective counterparts. Interestingly, maternal tertiary education was also associated with increased overweight or obesity in boys (Li *et al.*, 2008).

6.5 Major Drivers of China's Childhood Obesity Epidemic

6.5.1 *Modernization and urbanization*

China's national strategy of achieving the 'Four Modernizations'[1] has led to rapid urbanization and uneven development. This has been associated with a temporal trend of increasing prevalence of childhood obesity in recent decades, but also a strong geographic gradient of childhood obesity, with a higher prevalence in the most developed large coastal cities such as Shanghai and a lower prevalence in the western rural areas (Yang *et al.*, 2013, Zong and Li, 2014). Such a spatial distribution suggests that the childhood obesity epidemic in China is largely driven by economic development. Relative to their rural counterparts, urban living exposes children to an unhealthy food environment. Parents may be too busy to prepare food at home and, coupled with a higher family income, children eat pre-prepared food or eat out more often, and have pocket money to buy their own snacks (Li *et al.*, 2008). They live in much more confined spaces and, as parents and grandparents are concerned about their safety, they have limited opportunities to walk to and from school or play outside (James, 2008). Such factors might have influenced both their energy intake and output.

6.5.2 *Dietary changes and nutrition transition*

It was as recently as the eve of the Chinese economic reforms and 'open door' policy at the beginning of the 1980s that most food items

[1] Modernization of agriculture, industry, national defence and science and technology.

such as sugar, oil, and meat were rationed in urban areas (Chan, 1992). The relaxation of food restrictions, the rise in family disposable income and the availability and abundant supply of a range of foods in many regions of China are likely contributors to the obesity epidemic. Further, the increased consumption of pre-prepared foods, including snacks, and more opportunities to eat out may also have led to an increased intake of unhealthy foods (Kim *et al.*, 2004).

6.5.3 *Change in food composition*

A traditional Chinese diet is characterized by plant-based protein, low cholesterol, and some dietary fat. The food composition of the diet of many Chinese families has changed into one that has high fat and animal protein content (Zhai *et al.*, 2009). The China Health and Nutrition Survey in children aged 7–17 years demonstrated a steady decline between 1991 and 2009 in daily carbohydrate intake (from 382.5 to 254.1 grams) and in the proportion of energy from carbohydrates (10% reduction, from 667% to 56.8%). In contrast, daily fat intake steadily increased (from 54.8 to 66.0 grams) and the proportion of energy from fat increased (from 21.5% to 30.0%) (Cui and Dibley, 2012). Children from urban areas tend to consume more fat than their rural counterparts (Chen, 2000). Our study of 550 9–11 year old children in Harbin, in north-eastern China, found that all children bought snacks, often high in sugar, fat or salt, and over 80% bought sweetened beverages in or outside school with their pocket money in the four weeks prior to the survey (manuscript in preparation). With large multinational companies such as Pepsi Co and Coca-Cola eyeing China for expansion, it is expected this will further fuel the epidemic (Lobstein, 2010).

6.5.4 *Change in the food environment*

Since the first Kentucky Fried Chicken (KFC) franchise opened its doors in China in November 1982, Western fast food chains have rapidly penetrated China in the past 30 years. In addition, Chinese-style fast food and small local restaurants are booming, including in less developed rural areas. Data for individual fast food consumption and community level food retail environment, extracted from the 2006 China Health and Nutrition Survey, has revealed that the food retail environment is one of the key factors associated with higher BMI in adults in China (Zhang *et al.*, 2012). Children, particularly from higher income urban families, tend to eat meals in restaurants, including Western style fast food (Cheng, 2003, Lobstein, 2010). Our Harbin study has further revealed that, in the month prior to the survey, 71% and 90% of children consumed Western and Chinese fast foods, respectively (manuscript in preparation).

6.5.4.1 *Food marketing*

Food marketing is a recognized driver of child food preferences and food consumption, and hence, of childhood obesity (Cairns *et al.*, 2013). We recorded three popular television channels in July 2012 between 06.00 and 22.00 hours for four days (two weekdays plus two weekend days), in order to track food and beverage advertisements. Information on the time of day the advertisement was shown, the program it was broadcast in, and the type of food advertised was coded and analyzed. Food and beverage advertisements accounted for 19% of all television advertisements. Noncore foods, such as sweetened drinks, typical fast food, and high fat and salt products, were featured in 84% of all food and beverage advertisements that appeared on television. Among them, 31% were for sweetened drinks (Kelly *et al.*, 2014). More than 70% of children in the survey in Harbin reported that they noticed food advertisements on television, and 63% responded that they would at least occasionally try the advertised food or beverage. Forty six percent of children claimed that they learnt about food from television advertisements and 20% of children said that they were influenced by the television advertisements regarding their preference for snacks and beverages.

6.5.4.2 *Inappropriate infant and young child feeding*

In younger children, exclusive breastfeeding in the first six months of a child's life, prolonged breastfeeding, and appropriate infant feeding not only protect against under-nutrition but may also prevent the development of later childhood obesity (Black *et al.*, 2013). Breastfeeding rates in China, however, have been declining, particularly in major cities (Centre for Health Statistics and Information and Ministry of Health, 2009). The causes of the decline in breastfeeding are multi-factorial and complex. Traditionally, Chinese grandparents take great pride in a well-fed baby, based on the cultural and historical belief that a fat child symbolizes the prosperity of the family (Wang *et al.*, 2002, Cui *et al.*, 2010). Therefore, there may be family pressure to push new mothers to switch to infant formula, a product which many grandparents themselves could not afford to use with their own children when they were young. New mothers have many misconceptions about breast milk: many believe their breast milk is insufficient to meet the child's growth and development needs, both in quantity and quality (Jiang *et al.*, 2012). These beliefs have been influenced by the aggressive marketing of breast milk substitutes, and inferences that formula is superior to breast milk (United Nations Children's Fund, 2014; Harney, 2013). This not only undermines new mothers' determination and confidence in breastfeeding their babies, it also raises anxiety that they may deprive their babies of the 'best' start in a very competitive society. Although China observes the WHO International Code for Marketing for Breast Milk Substitutes, there is a serious lack of enforcement and penalties for violating the Code. Many mothers are targeted during pregnancy or while breastfeeding by salespersons, media, and sometimes health professionals. Breastfeeding is a very private act in Chinese society, and it is difficult for a new mother to breastfeed her baby in public places, most of which do not have private breastfeeding rooms. Many workplaces have not made it easy for women wanting to continue breastfeeding when they return to work (Hu *et al.*, 2013).

6.5.5 *Physical inactivity and sedentary behavior*

Physical inactivity and sedentary behaviors also contribute to the increased prevalence of overweight and obesity. In China over the past three decades, both physical education in the school and physical activity opportunities out of school have decreased (Cui *et al.*, 2011a;

Cui *et al.*, 2011b). The primary aim of schools, often pressured by children's families as well, is for the child to excel academically. The lack of physical activity and sedentary behavior may also be imposed on the children by schools and parents, for example by entering children in extracurricular study programs. The National Health and Nutrition Survey data showed that more than 70% of students engaged in extracurricular study or coaching outside of school. The median value was 420 minutes per week, or 84 minutes a day. At the same time, about 70% of school-aged children engaged in 90–110 minutes per week of moderate to vigorous physical activity in school (around 20 minutes a day), less than 10% participated in any form of moderate to vigorous physical activity outside of school, and less than 20% performed any household chores. (Tudor-Locke *et al.*, 2003) Our study in Harbin discovered that, on average outside of school time, a 9–11 year old child spent 2.2 hours doing homework and 1.2 hours watching television on school days. On weekends and holidays, however, they did not become more physically active. They spent an average 3.2 hours per day attending extracurricular classes, 2.9 hours doing homework and 2.2 hours watching television. Essentially, children could spend up to 11 hours a day during school days and more than eight hours on weekend days indoors, either studying or watching television (manuscript in preparation).

Although private ownership of passenger cars was never forbidden in China, the cost was prohibitive (Riley, 2002). The ownership of private cars has grown from almost none in the early 1980s to in excess of 70 million by mid-2011 (Ministry of Transport of the People's Republic of China, 2011). The distribution of the vehicles, however, is far from uniform. Population growth and urbanization, along with economic development, have been identified as factors influencing car ownership (Riley, 2002). Indeed, car ownership is concentrated in cities, the areas of high economic growth. The country that was once famous for the use of the bicycle as the main means of transport and active travel, and for walking or cycling to school and work, has seen a dramatic decline in these forms of transport. More children, particularly in major cities, are driven to and from school: from 3.6% in 1997 to 14.1% in 2006 (Cui *et al.*, 2011a; Lobstein, 2010).

Travel in motorized vehicles is associated with increased adiposity in the Chinese population (Qin *et al.*, 2012).

Further, one of the consequences of the introduction and enforcement of the family planning policy, commonly known as the 'one-child policy' — which commenced in 1979 (around the same time as the economic reform) — is that the new generation of children is over-protected, discouraged or prevented from engaging in outdoor activities (Cameron *et al.*, 2013) and pampered with food (Lobstein, 2010; Wang *et al.*, 2002).

6.6 Economic and Social Implications if the Trend Continues

China is going through a nutritional as well as an epidemiological transition, with the disease burden shifting from communicable to non-communicable diseases. Amongst the adult population in China, obesity is now a major risk factor for morbidity and mortality. The relative risk of developing hypertension and diabetes is between 2.3 times and 5.2 times higher in overweight and obese adults than in those with a healthy body weight (Chen, 2008). It is estimated that 92 million Chinese adults have type 2 diabetes, with a further 148 million being pre-diabetic (Yang *et al.*, 2010).

Obesity is of great significance from a health policy perspective because of its prevalence in the population and the costs of treating the associated medical conditions in both the short and long terms. However, the emergence of overweight and obesity is as much an economic issue as a public health issue. Under the current Chinese health insurance schemes, most of the direct medical costs of obesity and related health problems are borne by the individuals and their families, many of whom cannot afford them. People suffering from obesity and related health problems also consume more health services, which exerts extra demand on the health system. Based on adult BMI data, it is estimated that 3.6% of the 2000 Chinese Gross National Product (GNP) and 8.7% of the 2025 Chinese GNP was or will be spent on obesity and its associated problems (Popkin *et al.*,

2006). The rapidly growing childhood obesity epidemic in China means that there will be a much higher cost in the future to individuals, and to society as a whole, due to loss of productivity and human capacity, if the trend is not curbed urgently. This urgency should underscore a future research focus of effective interventions to prevent childhood obesity and future health policy that creates an enabling environment.

6.7 Measures to Halt the Trend — Interventions to Prevent or Reduce Childhood Obesity

6.7.1 *Focus on modifiable risk factors at different periods of life course*

The determinants of obesity are complex and vary by countries and regions within a country, socio–economic backgrounds and urban and rural settings. It is important, therefore, to recognize that no single solution is likely to prevent childhood obesity (WHO, 2014b; WHO, 2012). Understanding the major drivers of childhood obesity in China, nevertheless, is the first step to explaining the changes in prevalence and informing the development of effective interventions, targeting modifiable risk factors for childhood obesity.

Numerous intervention studies have been carried out, mostly in developed countries, for preventing childhood obesity in school-aged children, but the results of many remain inconclusive due to lack of long-term follow-up (Summerbell *et al.*, 2005; Waters *et al.*, 2011). In 2009 WHO published a systematic review, *Interventions on Diet and Physical Activity: What Works?* (WHO, 2009), which examined close to 400 publications between 1995 and 2005. It showed multi-component interventions involving the family, school, community and government and adapted to the local context to be the most successful (Bautista-Castano and Doreste, 2004; WHO, 2009; de Silva-Sanigorski *et al.*, 2010). Sadly, the representation of studies from low-middle income countries in the WHO review was extremely low (<13%). The most recently updated Cochrane review of childhood obesity prevention includes studies primarily from high income countries, although a few studies from Thailand, and a number of Latin American countries, for example Brazil, Chile, and Mexico were included (Waters *et al.*, 2011). This indicates that well designed intervention programs urgently need to be implemented in low-middle income countries to gather evidence and to gain experience in order to stop the trend of childhood obesity. Li *et al.*, conducted a systematic review of school-based intervention studies for prevention or reduction of excess weight gain in Chinese literature, and found that most of the published studies (duration varying between 10 weeks to three years) were one-dimensional and mainly focused on improving knowledge, physical activity levels and/or diet (Li *et al.*, 2008). None of the trials demonstrated convincing efficacy.

There is little information from China addressing risk factors occurring during pregnancy or in early life, although it is apparent that interventions implemented from the earliest ages of a child's life will have the greatest potential for cumulative benefits at later stages. For example, improving maternal diet and nutrition status and increasing physical activity are likely to influence child health outcomes. In a cohort study in eastern China we found that pregnant women staying physically active by walking more than 10,000 steps a day in the second and third trimesters could significantly reduce excessive maternal gestational weight gain, a known risk factor for childhood obesity (Jiang *et al.*, 2012).

Exclusive breastfeeding from birth to six months of age is not only beneficial in preventing child under-nutrition and other co-morbidities, but is also recommended by WHO as an important way to help prevent infants from becoming overweight or obese (WHO, 2014). The level of exclusive breastfeeding in the first six months is low in China, particularly in major cities such as Shanghai. We piloted a health promotion program using mobile phone short message services targeting new mothers. The results are encouraging, as they demonstrate prolonged median duration of exclusive breastfeeding and improved exclusive breastfeeding rate at six months in the intervention group compared with controls. We further observed an infant feeding behavior change in mothers in the intervention group, namely a delay in introducing complementary foods to infants.

That means fewer mothers gave complementary foods to their babies in the intervention group compared with the control group (Jiang *et al.*, 2014).

6.7.2 *Responses to the childhood obesity epidemic*

Obesity prevention requires actions to create policies and environments across multiple levels and sectors that influence eating, physical activity, and other behaviors. There should be a holistic response to the obesity epidemic, including childhood obesity, at higher levels, that is global and national. This includes, for example, developing international trade agreements that protect the health of consumers globally while ensuring fair trading, and regulating unhealthy food advertisements targeted at children. At the national level, governments need to provide leadership in setting the agenda and advocating for a multi-sector response. Governments also need to establish the mechanisms for all sectors to engage and coordinate their actions. Further, governments need to develop and implement policies, including laws and regulations, to create healthier environments for food consumption and physical activity (Swinburn, 2008).

The Chinese government is increasingly aware of the obesity epidemic, and has been playing a leading role in obesity prevention in recent years, through a series of policies and regulations. In 2009, the State Council of China issued the National Fitness Regulations, and the 12th Five-Year Plan of National Economic and Social Development (2011–2015) has set preventing chronic diseases, promoting good health and implementing the national health action plan among other key objectives (Wang and Zhai, 2013). There have been several specific guidelines regarding good nutrition and childhood obesity prevention. For example, in 2007 the Ministry of Health published the School-age Children and Adolescents Overweight and Obesity Prevention and Control Guidelines (Wang and Zhai, 2013). The Chinese Nutrition Society revised the Chinese Residents Dietary Guidelines in 2007, which includes dietary guidelines for infants and pre-schoolers 0–6 years old and children and adolescents 7–18 years old (Chinese Nutrition Society, 2007). A policy on reinforcement of physical activity to improve the fitness of children and adolescents has been implemented since 2007; it requires each student to engage in one hour of physical activity at school every day (Central Committee of the Communist Party and the State Council of China, 2007). In reality, the policy has not been enforced effectively and one study showed that very few students fulfilled the requirement (Ying-Xiu *et al.*, 2013). More recently, the Ministry of Education has released the revised the National Students Constitution and Health Standards, stipulating the level of physical fitness all students must achieve (Ministry of Education, 2014).

As the prevalence of childhood obesity is high in major cities, local governments are supportive of school-based childhood obesity interventions. Two more recent comprehensive school-based nutrition and lifestyle intervention trials in Beijing, the national capital, and Nanjing, the capital city of Jiangsu Province, one of the most developed provinces in China, are yet to be fully evaluated (Xu *et al.*, 2012; Li *et al.*, 2010). The effectiveness of many of these types of studies needs to be evaluated rigorously. This will provide strong evidence, and allow the design and implementation of interventions on a larger scale, in order to make a big impact on halting the childhood obesity epidemic. In the meantime, there is a need for strong government support for creating a healthy food environment in schools and in the community at large, restricting unhealthy food advertisements targeting children, and legislating the mandatory nutrition labeling of food.

Benefits from prevention and control of childhood obesity are multi-dimensional, ranging from improvements in maternal and child health, greater human capital gain through academic achievements in young people today and in the next generation, to improvements in productivity, longevity, and the health and wealth capital of a nation. Like many other countries that are going through rapid economic as well as health and nutrition transitions, China is at a very critical time in the fight to end childhood obesity. Having a better understanding of the major drivers of childhood obesity, and being able to measure the magnitude and severity accurately and consistently are important for successfully addressing the problem of childhood obesity. However, actions are required from all stakeholders, such as government policy makers, the food industry, employers, school teachers, parents, children, and adolescents. There is also a need for strong scientific evidence to inform and guide the interventions that are likely to be the most effective.

References

Bautista-Castano, I. and Doreste, J. (2004). Effectiveness of Interventions in the Prevention of Childhood Obesity, *European Journal of Epidemiology* **19**: 617–622.

Black, R., Victora, C., Walker, S., *et al.* (2013). Maternal and Child Undernutrition and Overweight in Low-Income and Middle-Income countries, *The Lancet* **382**(9890): 427–451.

Cairns, G., Angus, K., Hastings, G., *et al.* (2013). Systematic Reviews of the Evidence on the Nature, Extent and Effects of Food Marketing to Children, a Retrospective Summary *Appetite* **62**: 209–215.

Cameron, L., Erkal, N., Gangadharan, L., *et al.* (2013). Little Emperors: Behavioral Impacts of China's One-Child Policy, *Science* **339**: 953–957.

Central Committee of the Communist Party and the State Council of China (2007). *Strengthen Physical Activity to Improve the Fitness of Children and Adolescents.* Available at http://www.gov.cn/jrzg/2007-05/24/content_625090.htm [Accessed 15 January 2015].

Centre for Health Statistics and Information and Ministry of Health (2009). *An Analysis Report of National Health Services Survey in China, 2008*: 409.

Chan, K. (1992). Economic Growth Strategy and Urbanisation Policies in China, 1949–1982, *International Journal Urban and Regional Research* **16:** 275–305.

Chen, C. (2000). Fat Intake and Nutritional Status of Children in China, *American Journal of Clinical Nutrition* **72**(5 Suppl): 1368S–1372S.

Chen, C. (2008). Overview of Obesity in Mainland China, *Obesity Reviews*, **9**(Suppl 1): 14–21.

Cheng, T. (2003). Fast Food and Obesity in China, *Journal of the American College of Cardiology* **42**(4): 773.

Chinese Nutrition Society (2007). *Chinese Residents Dietary Guidelines*, Tibetan People's Publishing House, Lhasa.

Cole, T., Bellizzi, M., Flegal, K., *et al.* (2000). Establishing a Standard Definition for Child Overweight and Obesity Worldwide: International Survey, *British Medical Journal* **320**(7244): 1240–1243.

Coordinating Group of Nine Cities Study on the Physical Growth and Development of Children (2008). A National Epidemiological Survey on Obesity of Children Under 7 Years of Age in Nine Cities of China, 2006, *Zhonghua Er Ke Za Zhi* **46**(3): 174–178.

Cui, Z., Bauman, A. and Dibley M. (2011a). Temporal Trends and Correlates of Passive Commuting to and From School in Children from 9 Provinces in China, *Preventive Medicine* **52**(6): 423–427.

Cui, Z. and Dibley, M. (2012). Trends in Dietary Energy, Fat, Carbohydrate and Protein Intake in Chinese children and Adolescents from 1991 to 2009, *British Journal of Nutrition* **108**(7): 192–199.

Cui, Z., Dibley, M. J. Huxley, R., *et al.* (2010). Temporal Trends in Overweight and Obesity of Children and Adolescents from Nine Provinces in China from 1991–2006, *International Journal of Pediatric Obesity* **5**(5): 365–374.

Cui, Z., Hardy, L., Dibley, M., *et al.* (2011b). Temporal Trends and Recent Correlates in Sedentary Behaviours in Chinese Children, *International Journal of Behavioral Nutrition and Physical Activity* **8**: 93.

Daniels, S. (2009). Complications of Obesity in Children and Adolescents, *International Journal of Obesity* **33**(Suppl 1): S60–S65.

de Onis, M., Blossner, M. and Borghi, E. (2010). Global Prevalence and Trends of Overweight and Obesity Among Preschool Children, *American Journal of Clinical Nutrition* **92**(5): 1257–1264.

de Onis, M., Onyango, A., Borghi, E., *et al.* (2007). Development of a WHO Growth Reference for School-Aged Children and Adolescents, *Bulletin of World Health Organization* **85**: 649–732.

de Silva-Sanigorski, A., Bell, A., Kremer, P., *et al.* (2010). Reducing Obesity in Early Childhood: Results from Romp & Chomp, An Australian Community-Wide Intervention Program, *American Journal of Clinical Nutrition* **91**(4): 831–840.

Friedemann, C., Heneghan, C., Mahtani, K., *et al.* (2012). Cardiovascular Disease Risk in Healthy Children and its Association with Body Mass

Index: Systematic Review and Meta-Analysis, *British Medical Journal* **345**: e4759.

Gardner, D., Hosking, J., Metcalf, B., *et al.* (2009). Contribution of Early Weight Gain to Childhood Overweight and Metabolic Health: A Longitudinal Study (EarlyBird 36), *Journal of Pediatrics* **123**(1): 67–73.

Group of China Obesity Task Force (2004). Body Mass Index Reference Norm for Screening Overweight and Obesity in Chinese Children and Adolescents, *Zhonghua Liu Xing Bing Xue Za Zhi* **25**(2): 97–102.

Harney, A. (2013). Special Report: How Big Formula Bought China. Available at http://www.reuters.com/article/2013/11/08/us-china-milkpowder-specialreport-idUSBRE9A700820131108 [Accessed 2 March 2015].

Hu, Q., Jiang, H., Li, M., *et al.* (2013). Study on Mothers Return to Work and Supportive Status of Breastfeeding in Workplace in Shanghai, *Maternal and Child Health Care of China* **28**: 1778–1781.

James, W. (2008). The Fundamental Drivers of the Obesity Epidemic, *Obesity Reviews* **9**(Suppl1): 6–13.

Ji, C., Chen, T. and Working Group on Obesity in China (WGOC) (2013). Empirical Changes in the Prevalence of Overweight and Obesity Among Chinese Students from 1985 to 2010 and Corresponding Preventive Strategies, *Biomedical and Environmental Sciences* **26**(1): 1–12.

Jiang, F., Zhu, S., Yan, C., *et al.* (2009). Sleep and Obesity in Preschool Children, *Journal of Pediatrics* **154**(6): 814–818.

Jiang, H., Li, M., Qian, D., *et al.* (2012). Awareness, Intention and Needs Regarding Breastfeeding: Findings from First-time Mothers in Shanghai, China, *Breastfeeding Medicine* 7(6): 526–534.

Jiang, H., Li, M., Wen, L., *et al.* (2014). Effect of Short Message Service on Infant Feeding Practice: Findings From a Community-Based Study in Shanghai, China, *JAMA Pediatrics* **168**(5): 471–478.

Jiang, H., Qian, X., Li, M., *et al.* (2012). Can Physical Activity Reduce Excessive Gestational Weight Gain? Findings From a Chinese Urban Pregnant Women Cohort Study, *International Journal of Behavioral Nutrition and Physical Activity* **9**(12): DOI:10.1186/1479-5868-9-12.

Jiang, J., Rosenqvist, U. and Wang, H. (2008). Relationship of Parental Characteristics and Feeding Practices to Overweight in Infants and Young Children in Beijing, China, *Public Health Nutrition* **12**(7): 973–978.

Jiang, J., Rosenqvist, U., Wang, H., *et al.* (2006). Risk Factors for Overweight in 2- to 6-year-old Children in Beijing, China, *International Journal of Pediatric Obesity* **1**(2): 103–108.

Kelly, B., Hebden, L., King, L., *et al.* (2014). Children's Exposure to Food Advertising on Free-to-air Television: An Asia-Pacific Perspective, *Health Promotion International* pii: dau055 [Epub ahead of print].

Kim, S., Symons, M. and Popkins, B. (2004). Contrasting Socioeconomic Profiles Related to Healthier Lifestyles in China and the United States, *American Journal of Epidemiology* **159**(30): 1129–1136.

Li, M. and Dibley, M. (2012). Child and Adolescent Obesity in Asia, in Baur, Louise Twigg, Stephen and Magnusson, Roger, *Modern Epidemic — Expert Perspectives on Obesity and Diabetes*: 171–190, Sydney University Press, Sydney.

Li, M., Dibley, M., Sibbritt, D., *et al.* (2008). Factors Associated with Adolescents' Overweight and Obesity at Community, School and Household Levels in Xi'an City, China: Results of Hierarchical Analysis, *European Journal of Clinical Nutrition* **62**(5): 635–643.

Li, M., Dibley, M., Sibbritt, D., *et al.* (2010). Dietary Habits and Overweight/Obesity in Adolescents in Xi'an City, China, *Asia Pacific Journal of Clinical Nutrition* **19**(1): 76–82.

Li, M., Li, S. Baur, L., *et al.* (2008). A Systematic Review of School-Based Intervention Studies for the Prevention or Reduction of Excess Weight Among Chinese Children and Adolescents, *Obesity Reviews* **9**(6): 548–559.

Li, Y., Hu, X., Zhang, Q., *et al.* (2010). The Nutrition-based Comprehensive Intervention Study on Childhood Obesity in China (NISCOC): A Randomised Cluster Controlled Trial, *BMC Public Health* **10**: 229.

Lobstein, T. (2010). China Joins the Fatter Nations, *International Journal of Pediatric Obesity* **5**(5): 362–364.

Lobstein, T., Baur L. and Uauy, R. (2004). Obesity in Children and Young People: A Crisis in Public Health, *Obesity Reviews* **5**(Suppl1): 4–85.

Ministry of Education (2014). The Announcement of the 2014 "National Students' Constitution and Health Standards". Available at http://www.csh.edu.cn/MOETC/home/homeAction!toPublicInfoDetails.action?publicInfoId=2c959595472fa7fa0147866a85850064 [Accessed 2 March 2015].

Ministry of Transport of the People's Republic of China (2011). *China Transport Statistical Yearbook 2011*, China Statistics Press, Beijing.

Must, A. and Struss, R. (1999). Risks and Consequences of Childhood and Adolescent Obesity, *International Journal of Obesity* **23**(Suppl2): S2–S11.

National Bureau of Statistics of China (2006). Statistics Bulletin of the People's Republic of China 'Capital Cities' Economic and Social Development of 2006. Available at http://www.stats.gov.cn/tjsj/tjgb/qttjgb/qgqttjgb/200705/t20070518_30630.html [Accessed 2 March 2015].

National Task Force on Childhood Obesity and National Center for Women's and Children's Health (2008). National Epidemiological Survey on Childhood Obesity, 2006, *Zhonghua Er Ke Za Zhi* **46**(3): 179–184.

Popkin, B. (2010). Recent Dynamics Suggest Selected Countries Catching up to US Obesity, *American Journal of Clinical Nutrition* **91**(1): 284S–288S.

Popkin, B., Kim, S., Rusev, E., *et al.* (2006). Measuring the Full Economic Costs of Diet, Physical Activity, and Obesity-Related Chronic Diseases, *Obesity Reviews* 7(3): 271–293.

Qin, L., Stolk, R. and Corpeleijn, E. (2012). Motorized Transportation, Social Status, and Adiposity: the China Health and Nutrition Survey, *American Journal of Preventive Medicine* **43**(1): 1–10.

Riley, K. (2002). Motor Vehicles in China: The Impact of Demographic and Economic Changes, *Population and Environment* **23**(5): 479–493.

Shan, X., Xi, B., Cheng, H., *et al.* (2010). Prevalence and Behavioral Risk Factors of Overweight and Obesity Among Children Aged 2–18 in Beijing, China, *International Journal of Pediatric Obesity* **5**(5): 383–389.

Summerbell, C., Waters, E., Edmunds, L., *et al.* (2005). Interventions for Preventing Obesity in Children, *Cochrane Database Syst Rev* **3**: CD001871.

Swinburn, B. (2008). Obesity Prevention: The Role of Policies, Laws and Regulations, *Australia and New Zealand Health Polic* **5**(1): 12.

Tudor-Locke, C., Ainsworth, B., Adair, L., *et al.* (2003). Physical Activity and Inactivity in Chinese School-aged Youth: the China Health and Nutrition Survey, *International Journal of Obesity and Related Metabolic Disorders* **27**(9): 1093–1099.

United Nations Children's Fund (2014). *Nutrition*, Available at http://www.unicef.cn/cn/index.php?m=content&c=index&a=show&catid=53&id=20031 [Accessed 2 March 2015].

Wang, Y. and Lobstein, T. (2006). Worldwide Trends in Childhood Overeight and Obesity, *International Journal of Pediatric Obesity* **1**: 11–25.

Wang, Y., Monteiro, C. and Popkins, B. (2002). Trends of Obesity and Underweight in Older Children and Adolescents in the United States, Brazil, China and Russia, *American Journal of Clinical Nutrition* **75**: 971–977.

Waters, E., de Silva-Sanigorski, A., Hall, B., *et al.* (2011). Interventions for Preventing Obesity in Children, *Cochrane Database of Systematic Reviews* **12**: CD001871.

WHO Expert Consultation (2004). Appropriate Body-Mass Index for Asian Populations and its Implications for Policy and Intervention Strategies, *The Lancet* **363**(9403): 157–163.

World Health Organization (2006). *WHO Child Growth Standards: Methods and Development: Length/height-for-age, Weight-for-age, Weight-for-length, Weight-for-height and Body Mass Index-for-age*, WHO, Geneva.

World Health Organization (2008). *WHO Child Growth Standards: Training Course on Child Growth Assessment*, WHO, Geneva.

World Health Organization (2009). *Interventions on Diet and Physical Activity: What Works.* Available at www.who.int/dietphysicalactivity/whatworks/en/ [Accessed 2 March 2015].

World Health Organization (2012). *Prioritizing Areas for Action in the Field of Population-Based Prevention of Childhood Obesity*, WHO, Geneva.

World Health Organization (2014). *Facts and Figures on Childhood Obesity.* Available at www.who.int/end-childhood-obesity/facts/en/ [Accessed 2 March 2015].

World Health Organization (2014b). *Report of the First Meeting of the Ad Hoc Working Group on Science and Evidence for Ending Chilhood Obesity*, WHO, Geneva.

Xu, F., Ware, R., Tse, L., *et al.* (2012). A School-Based Comprehensive Lifestyle Intervention Among Chinese Kids Against Obesity: Rationale, Design and Methodology of a Randomized Controlled Trial In Nanjing City, China, *BMC Public Health* **12**: 316.

Yang, G., Wang, Y., Zeng, Y., *et al.* (2013). Rapid Health Transition in China 1990–2010: Findings From the Global Burden of Disease Study 2010, *The Lancet* **38**(9882): 1987–2015.

Yang, W.Y., Lu, J.M., Weng, J.P., *et al.* (2010). Prevalence of Diabetes among Men and Women in China, *New England Journal of Medicine* **362**(12): 1090–1101.

Ying-Xiu, Z., Jing-Yang, Z., Jin-Shan, Z. *et al.* (2013). The Role of 1-h Physical Activity Every Day in Preventing Obesity in Adolescents in Shandong, China, *European Journal of Pediatrics* **172**(3): 325–330.

Zhai, F., Wang, H., Du, S., *et al.* (2009). Prospective Study on Nutrition Transition in China, *Nutrition Reviews* **67**(Suppl1): S56–S61.

Zhang, J., Himes, J., Guo, Y., *et al.* (2013). Birth Weight, Growth and Feeding Pattern in Early Infancy Predict Overweight/Obesity Status at Two Years Of Age: A Birth Cohort Study of Chinese Infants, *PLoS One* **8**(6): e64542.

Zhang, X., Liu, E., Tian, Z., *et al.* (2009). High Birth Weight and Overweight or Obesity Among Chinese Children 3–6 years old, *Preventive Medicine* **49**(2–3): 172–178.

Zhang, X., van der Lans, I. and Dagevos, H. (2012). Impacts of Fast Food and the Food Retail Environment on Overweight and Obesity in China: A Multilevel Latent Class Cluster Approach, *Public Health Nutrition* **15**(1): 88–96.

Zong, X. and Li, H. (2012). Secular Trends in Prevalence and Risk Factors of Obesity in Infants and Preschool Children in 9 Chinese Cities, 1986–2006, *PLOS One* 7(10): e46942.

Zong, X. and Li, H. (2013). Construction of a New Growth References for China Based on Urban Chinese children: Comparison with the WHO Growth Standards, *PLOS One* **8**(3): e59569.

Zong, X. and Li, H. (2014). Physical Growth of Children and Adolescents in China Over the Past 35 years, *Bulletin of the World Health Organization* **92**(8): 555–564.

Chapter Seven

Urbanization and Health Inequalities: The Social Determinants of Health and Vulnerable Social Groups in China's Cities

Beatriz Carrillo Garcia

Abstract

China's rapid urbanization has triggered a broad range of processes that have had negative consequences on both access to healthcare services and on health outcomes. The ensuing health inequities are related to changes within the public health care system and to social health insurances, but also to the widening socio–economic inequalities prevalent in urban China. After providing an outline of the main health care reforms, this chapter examines the links between the socio–economic status of specific social groups and their access to medical care and social health insurances. The analysis concentrates on two vulnerable social groups, rural-to-urban migrant workers and older urban laid-off workers.

7.1 Introduction

Urbanization as process and urbanicity[1] — the urban condition — have been identified as factors affecting public health since the industrialization process of 19th century Europe. The study of these two analytical variables, however, only became more salient from the second half of the 20th century, as global urban growth peaked. At the start of the 21st century, the United Nations World Population Prospects (United Nations, 2013) established that over half the world's population (52.1%) was already living in an urban area, and the prediction was for the urbanization rate to go up to 67% by 2050.[2] It is now well established that most of the urban growth since the 1950s has taken place in the developing world, and that the urbanization rate in those countries will continue to grow fastest, at least until 2050 (WHO, n.d.).

China's rapid urbanization process has been a large contributor to this global trend. Since the introduction of the Reform and Opening program in 1978, China has shown consistently high rates of urban growth, with the highest growth rate taking place during the first half of the 1990s (Chan, 2010: 71). During the 1990s alone China added 200 new cities and 8228 towns to its urban system, and by the year 2000 China had a total of 663 cities and 20,312 towns. Subsequently, between 2000 and 2005, the number of Chinese cities remained relatively stable and experienced a slight decrease thereafter due to urban mergers (Chan, 2010: 73). China's impressive urbanization rate is partly the result of its low starting point. At the start of the reform period only about 17% of the Chinese population (around 167 million people) lived in urban areas, but by 2011 the size of the urban population had, for the first time in China's history, surpassed that of

---

[1] Vlahov and Galea (2002) define urbanization as 'the dynamics of agglomeration of individuals, effected by factors such as industrialization and population mobility'. Urbanicity is defined as 'the impact of living in urban areas at a given point in time'; it refers to the conditions particular to urban areas, which in turn make it complementary to the process of urbanization (Vlahov and Galea, 2002: S4–S5).

[2] World Population in 2050 is expected to surpass the 9.6 billion mark, while the urban population is expected to surpass the 6.2 billion mark (United Nations, 2013).

the rural population. In 2012 China's urban population constituted 52.3% (711.8 million) of the total population (*China Daily*, 1 August 2013); this entailed an unprecedented addition of over 500 million people to the urban system over three decades.

Around the world, population agglomeration in cities not only made urban health issues more salient, but it also established cities as the main sites of medical facilities, health research and health funding. National health care systems have, to a large extent, been shaped by the institutional, economic and socio–demographic characteristics of the city. For a long time, health-related research tended to concentrate on the role that public health interventions played in the control of urban disease epidemics (Vlahov and Galea, 2002: S2). The expansion of a therapeutic revolution — spread through new medical technologies and drugs — and the epidemiological transition towards a higher prevalence of non-communicable diseases (NCDs) subsequently broadened the research agenda to include the social and economic determinants of health. Empirical studies from around the world had noted that while overall life expectancy experienced a dramatic increase throughout the twentieth century, socio–economic disparities in morbidity and mortality persisted (Williams, 1990; Wilkinson and Marmot, 2006; Wilkinson and Pickett, 2006). It was increasingly recognized that health inequalities amongst the population were as much the result of the quality of care available to individuals through the health care system, as they were the result of the socio–economic structures in which individuals were enmeshed (Couburn, 2010; Phelan *et al.*, 2010). China's health trajectory during the reform era corroborates the strong causal link between socio–economic status and health inequalities.

China's current health care system contrasts with that which prevailed during the Maoist era, which — though poorly funded and also biased towards urban areas — through its emphasis on preventive care and egalitarian access, achieved substantial improvements in health indicators and life expectancy. For example, while by the late 1970s China's per capita gross domestic product (GDP) was one of the lowest in the world, its life expectancy (68 years) ranked alongside that of middle income countries such as South Korea, Mexico, and Brazil

(Cai, 2009: 145). From 1978, however, the principle of egalitarianism and the focus on preventive medicine were dropped in favor of market mechanisms for the provision of health care services, and increased individual responsibility over access to those services. In tandem China also experienced a dramatic rise in socio–economic inequalities that left many unable to afford medical care.

7.2 Migration and Urban Growth in China

Before the start of the reform process, strict controls over urban growth were seen as necessary, in order to guarantee full employment and the provision of a wide range of entitlements for the urban proletariat under the socialist regime. The urban work unit or *danwei* was responsible for providing lifetime employment, housing, education, health care and other in-kind benefits to its workers and their dependents. The priorities of the *danwei* were mainly social and political, with economic considerations being secondary. Such a tight and inclusive system could only be sustained by limiting those who could live and work in cities. Rural-to-urban migration was discouraged; individuals were largely tied to their place of birth, which determined their household registration or *hukou* status. The state's virtual monopoly over urban work (through the *danwei* system and urban collectives) acted as yet another barrier that guaranteed peasants stayed in the countryside. Organized into rural communes, the rural population, unlike its urban counterpart, remained largely self-sufficient and received little or no financial assistance from the central government.

It was, nonetheless in the countryside where economic reforms were first introduced. In the early 1980s communes were dismantled and agricultural land was redistributed to rural households (under the Household Responsibility system), even though the land remained under collective ownership. After complying with state grain quotas farmers were allowed to sell their agricultural surplus in the newly formed rural markets. The most important outcome of this process, however, was that it allowed for surplus labor to seek work outside agriculture.

Meanwhile, the emergence of an incipient urban manufacturing industry, largely around the export-oriented coastal areas, began to attract the surplus rural labor. Chan and Hu (2003) estimate that about half the population growth in China's cities during the 1990s was due to migration from the countryside.[3] During that decade some cities in the Pearl River Delta, such as Dongguang, Shenzhen, Zhongshan, and Zhuhai, developed from small towns into bustling metropolises largely as a result of inbound-migration.[4] Shenzhen's annual urban growth rate, for example, averaged an impressive 23% (Chan, 2010: 74). Overall, however, it was high ranking cities that grew the fastest, again largely due to inbound-migration. According to figures from the 2010 National Population Census between 2000 and 2010 more than 90% of population growth in the cities of Beijing, Shanghai and Tianjin was the result of inbound-migration (Cai, 2013: 390).

Off-farm opportunities sprouted all around the country, making rural to urban migration the main factor behind China's rapid urban growth at all levels of the urban hierarchy. Small cities with populations less than 200,000 also experienced high growth rates (Chan, 2010: 77). According to the National Bureau of Statistics, by the end of 2013 the number of rural migrant workers had reached 268.94 million, accounting for 19.76% of China's total population (*Xinhua*, 17 March 2014). That same year 53.7% of China's population was said to be living in an urban area, even though only 37.5% held an urban *hukou* (*Xinhua*, 17 March 2014).

Despite having become a common fixture of Chinese cities and even though their contribution to the urban economy has been highlighted since the Hu Jintao leadership, rural migrant workers continue to be perceived and treated as temporary dwellers in the cities. Their rural *hukou* precludes them from enjoying the same citizenship rights and entitlements as their urban counterparts, which limits their economic opportunities, makes them the target of discrimination and abuse, and excludes them from existing social safety nets. Kam Wing

[3] Urban growth also took place through the expansion of urban administrative areas and to a lesser extent through the natural growth of cities.

[4] Their large proportion of in-migrants resulted in their being some of the early pioneers in the introduction of social security schemes for rural migrant workers, including health insurance. See for example: Mou *et al.*, 2009 and Zhu *et al.*, 2008.

Chan (2010: 66) asserts that it was precisely by restricting the legality and entitlement to services of rural migrant workers that China was able to afford the costs of rapid urbanization, as urban governments were not obliged to provide services such as health care, education, affordable housing, and social insurances to these workers and their families.

7.3 Economic and Social Inequalities and Their Effect on Health Equity

The more diverse economic, cultural, educational and other opportunities offered by urban areas remain a big pull factor for rural workers, despite the disadvantages and discrimination they face there. Not only have economic reform, urbanization and urban conditions in China put rural migrant workers at a disadvantage, but also the rise in income and socio–economic inequalities at the regional level; between rural and urban areas; between cities of different sizes; between employees and those not employed; and along gender, age and class lines, has created new vulnerabilities in a variety of social groups. These inequalities tend to overlap with health inequalities such as access to health care and medicines and have become increasingly dependent on individual capacity to pay for those services (Duckett, 2007; Gao, 2002; WHO, 2005; Tang *et al.*, 2008). Reduced government funding for the public health sector, and the introduction of market mechanisms to elicit greater efficiency in the use of health resources, has had the unintended consequence of turning public health facilities into profit-seeking entities that rely on user fees and medicine sales to sustain their operations.

During the first two decades of reform, the Chinese government's share of total health expenditure consistently declined, dropping from 36.2% in 1980 to 15.5% in 2000. Meantime, private out-of-pocket expenses for health services rose from 21.2% to 59% over the same period (MOH, 2012). Cost escalation of medical care and medicines has also resulted in a substantial rise in total health expenditure, from 3.15% of GDP in 1980 to 4.62% in the year 2000 (MOH, 2012). The reliance of public hospitals and their medical practitioners on the fee-for-service principle has resulted in over-prescription of drugs and unnecessary or even dangerous procedures (Tang *et al.*, 2008: 1496; Gao *et al.*, 2002). Studies cited by Hsiao (2014: 62) estimate that around half of all antibiotic prescriptions are medically unnecessary, and that those prescriptions and the use of IV injections are at least double the World Health Organization (WHO) standards. By the mid-1990s, drug sales had already become the main source of income for public hospitals, accounting for as much as 60% of the total revenue (Liu and Hsiao, 1995: 1100). By 2011 half of China's health care spending was devoted to medicines, compared to only 10% in the USA (Hsiao, 2014: 57).

Equally problematic is the fact that, despite the continuous expansion of medical resources throughout the reform era, health indicators showed only moderate improvements (WHO, 2005). Some regions had actually started to show a deterioration in endemic disease controls (Cai, 2009: 145), at the same time that China was having to deal with new health epidemics, such as HIV/AIDS, SARS and bird flu (Kaufman, 2010; Kleinman and Watson, 2006). Regional economic disparities in a highly decentralized system also resulted in unequal spending on public services, including health. A 2003 World Bank report on China's poverty and inequality pointed out that the public spending of the richer counties was on average 48 times greater than that of the poorest counties. The report also showed that Shanghai, the provincial-level entity with the highest GDP per capita, spent over eight times more per capita on public services than Guizhou, the poorest province (Dollar, 2007).

Examining data from the China Health Nutrition Survey (CHNS), Baeten *et al.*, (2012) also found region to be a major determinant of health, due to the unequal distribution of health resources across regions. This was reflected in a range of health indicators and life expectancy. In 2000, for example, life expectancy in Shanghai (78 years) was 13 years higher than that of Guizhou (65 years) (Tang *et al.*, 2008: 1494). Similarly, a report on health disparities by the Institute for Health Economics of the Ministry of Health pointed out that while infant and childhood mortality rates in the more developed coastal areas were on par with those of developed countries, mortality rates in China's western provinces were three to five times higher (cited in WHO, 2005: 8–9).

At the household and individual level, utilization of health services became tightly linked to socio–economic status, resulting in a growing number of people foregoing medical care. The third National Health Services Survey of 2003 found that close to 50% of respondents did not seek out-patient treatment when ill, and that 30% of those referred to a hospital had refused in-patient care; the main reason given to forego treatment was cost (WHO, 2005). Throughout the reform era household health expenses grew faster than income in both urban and rural areas;[5] between 1979 and 2004 the average per capita expenditure on health increased nearly eight fold (WHO, 2005: 19). In the countryside catastrophic health expenses became one of the main factors behind household impoverishment (Liu, Rao and Hsiao, 2003; Wagstaff, 2005; Tang *et al.*, 2008).[6] In its 2000 ranking of national health systems, WHO described China's health system as one of the most unequal in the world, ranking it at 188 for its fairness in financial contribution and at 144 for its overall health system performance, among WHO's 199 member states (WHO, 2000: 152). At the same time China was experiencing high levels of inequality, with its Gini coefficient, a measure of income distribution amongst the population of a country, reaching 0.479 in 2003, which contrasted with its 0.22 starting point in 1978 (*Xinhua*, 21 January 2013).

7.4 Health Reform and Access to Health Care Services and Insurances

As stated above, national health care systems around the world have been greatly influenced by the institutional, economic and socio–demographic characteristics of the city; China's health care system is no different. This is reflected in the persistent urban bias in health

[5] According to a nationally representative survey, by 2010 health expenses accounted for 8% and 14.32% of urban and rural households' total expenditure respectively (CHF, 2013). However, on average, urban residents spent three times more on health care than their rural counterparts (Hsiao, 2014: 59).

[6] Liu *et al.* (2008: 1920) also found that between 1998 and 2003, the fraction of rural households in the lowest income quintile that incurred catastrophic medical spending increased from 21.5% to 25.7% respectively.

funding and promotion, but also in the development of social health insurances that provide more generous support to the urban population. Furthermore, fiscal arrangements throughout the administrative hierarchy have guaranteed better funding for medical facilities in the larger cities. Inequalities in availability, medical capabilities and quality of care are thus not only observable between urban and rural health facilities, but are equally present amongst urban areas of different sizes (Liu, 2004a; Eggleston *et al.*, 2008).

Health inequities brought about by these supply-side disparities were further exacerbated by the steep cost escalation in health care services and medicines, which took place alongside a significant decline in health insurance coverage.[7] Many amongst the old working class, as well as younger cohorts such as dependent children, lost their insurance entitlements as state owned enterprises (SOEs), underwent bankruptcy and ownership restructuring; this resulted in massive lay-offs, and in enterprises resigning their responsibility over employees' insurances. At the same time, those employed outside the state sector or in the informal economy, as well as the self-employed remained largely uninsured. As early as 1993 just over half of China's urban residents still had health insurance coverage; by 1998, as the state owned sector underwent a major overhaul, that figure dropped to 42.1% (Liu, 2004: 160). Coverage continued to decrease thereafter to 39% in 2003 (Tang *et al.*, 2008: 1497). Meanwhile, a growing number of rural migrant workers in urban areas remained without entitlement to social insurances or welfare benefits (Carrillo, 2004; Gong, 2012).

Amongst those who lost their health insurance entitlements, women and workers in smaller underfunded work units and urban collectives tended to be over-represented. Women were usually the first to be laid-off, or else they were encouraged to retire early, to allow for younger workers to be hired. Largely unskilled, these middle-aged women found it difficult to find employment, and often had to compete with younger rural migrant women for menial jobs as

[7] Meantime, from the early 1980s the vast majority of the rural population remained uninsured until 2003 when the new rural cooperative medical system was re-established.

cleaners or nannies for middle class families. From the mid-1990s onwards, a growing number of middle-aged male workers also found themselves laid-off from their SOEs without much prospect of re-employment. This older working class section of the urban population thus experienced downward social mobility, and became part of China's new urban poor (Wu, 2004; Solinger, 2006).

Age and gender, alongside socio–economic status became an important predictor of the health outcomes of reform in China. Analyzing data from 1991 to 2006 in the China Health and Nutrition Survey (CHNS) Baeten *et al.*, (2013: 13) found that income related health inequalities were almost entirely explained through the income mobility pathways of individuals according to their age and gender, which, together with regional position accounted for 70% to 90% of the total evolution in income related health inequalities. They observed that the strongest effects were amongst those over 50 years of age who were downwardly mobile, but also that the effect was particularly strong amongst women. Conversely, a study cited by Tang *et al.* (2008: 1497) found that amongst the urban population men and those in high income groups were more likely to have health insurance. Other studies have also found differentiated effects on individuals based on age, gender and socio–economic circumstances, pointing to a cumulative disadvantage over the life course of those of a lower socio–economic status and in particular, amongst older cohorts (Chen *et al.*, 2010).

By the late 1990s, the Chinese government was aware that the health system was in crisis and that the existing insurances, provided and funded through work units (including state owned enterprises, urban collectives, government departments and public service units such as hospitals, schools and universities), were no longer adequate or sustainable.[8] A new socialized system of insurances — funded by employees, employers, and government — was introduced in

[8] Civil servants and other public employees, however, maintained their insurance entitlements, which provided more generous benefits (including free medical care without co-payments) than the insurance schemes that covered workers in state owned enterprises and urban collectives (Huang, 2014: 21).

1998. The new insurance schemes, however, only covered urban *hukou* holders in formal employment, and thus continued to leave a large proportion of the urban population uninsured. Moreover, coverage expansion under the new employee social insurances was very limited. In the case of the newly established Urban Employee Basic Medical Insurance (UEBMI) the number of enrolled employees experienced very limited growth and even retrenchment, with coverage decreasing from 42.1% in 1998 to 39% in 2003 (Tang *et al.*, 2008: 1497). According to Xian Huang's calculations (2014: 12) a further decrease of about 4% was observed between 2004 and 2010, even though in a selected number of places, such as Beijing, Tianjin, and Shanghai, more than half of health insurance beneficiaries were formal employees. Nonetheless, the provincial UEBMI coverage average had reached 95.88% by 2009.

The relatively slow rate of enrollment of employees in some parts of the country was partly due to the fact that enterprises outside the state owned sector — including foreign owned enterprises — were not enrolling their workers into the new insurance schemes (Wu *et al.*, 2005). Though compulsory by law, local labor, and social security bureaus often did not have the incentives or the resources to enforce the law, which also did not establish specific sanctions for non-compliance (Carrillo, 2011: 93–94). Huang's findings, for example, showed that being employed by the state or by a large enterprise increased an employee's chances of being covered by UEBMI, while being employed in the private sector decreased the likelihood of being insured (Huang, 2014: 19). UEBMI enrollees were also more likely to be of a higher socio–economic status (that is, holding higher levels of education and income) and to hold an urban *hukou* (Huang, 2014: 18).

The slow expansion rate of UEBMI was also due to the fact that a growing number of urban residents were being hired on a part-time basis or on temporary contracts, which allowed employers to circumvent the social insurance law that made enrollment of full-time permanent employees compulsory. This policy of flexible employment was first promoted under the leadership of Jiang Zemin as an antidote to the mass lay-offs and unemployment of the late 1990s and early

2000s, but continued to be supported by the more socially oriented Hu Jintao regime (Zhang and Navarro, 2014: 184). Rather than alleviating the problem of affordability and access to health care, the underlying goal of the UEBMI was to protect the entitlements of a section of the working population, while lessening the burden of insurance expenses for many SOEs. However, despite government promises, the even more generous entitlements of civil servants and other public employees were never undermined. In about two thirds of Chinese provinces, government insurance schemes were integrated into local UEBMI, but only as a subcategory or supplementary insurance program for privileged groups (Huang, 2014: 21).

For Zhang and Navarro (2014: 181–183) health reform and social insurance policies were being primarily deployed by the Party-state as a political instrument, to accommodate social instability and the continued popular discontent with the failings of the health care system. In various opinion polls run by government, people identified escalating medical costs and inadequate health care provisions as a key public policy issue. A report by the Centre for Health Statistics and Information of the Ministry of Health pointed out that between 1998 and 2003 dissatisfaction amongst those who had received hospital in-patient treatment in urban areas had increased from 12% to 61% (Liu *et al.*, 2008: 1914).[9] During that same period another survey found that out of pocket expenditure for hospital care had increased for all income groups, with people in the lowest income group paying the highest proportion (over 60%) of their hospital costs out of pocket (Tang *et al.*, 2008: 1499). Tang *et al.* (2008), also point out that low income groups spent less on hospital care than higher income groups, despite the fact that the former were more likely to experience worse health and thus have greater health care needs.

In order to tackle these inequalities and, more broadly, to address the problems within the health care system and the challenges of a rapidly aging population with increased health care needs, pilot programs were deployed in both rural[10] and urban areas to include the

[9] The dissatisfaction rate in rural areas went from 7% to 54% during that same period.

[10] In the countryside pilots have been run since the early 1990s, but the New Rural Cooperative Medical System (NRCMS) was not made into national policy until 2006.

non-insured population with the ultimate goal of achieving universal coverage. First piloted in 2007 and launched nationally in 2010, the Urban Resident Basic Medical Insurance (URBMI) aimed to cover dependents, students, the disabled, the elderly, and other non-working urban residents (Lin *et al.*, 2009; Barber and Yao, 2010). A limited number of cities included the self-employed and rural migrant workers in local URBMI.

Unlike the UEBMI, enrollment into the URBMI is voluntary, and the scheme is funded through Central and local government subsidies, as well as from contributions by participating households.[11] According to the 'Guidelines for deepening health system reform' announced in April 2009 by the State Council, the main aim of the reform was to establish universal coverage that provides 'safe, effective, convenient, and affordable basic health services' to all urban and rural residents (Meng and Tang, 2013: 331). In the government financial commitment for 2009–2011, of the 850 billion RMB (US$124.26 billion), 46% was specifically allocated to subsidize enrollment into both the URBMI and the NRCMS (Barber and Yao, 2010). At the end of 2010, insurance coverage of the three social health insurances (UEBMI, URBMI and NRCMS) had reached 92% of the Chinese population (Yip *et al.*, 2012: 836). Apart from health insurances, other key areas for development identified in the Guidelines included public health care, service delivery and essential pharmaceuticals (Barber and Yao, 2010; Meng and Tang, 2013).

Two thirds of the newly committed funds for health reform had to come from local governments, with the Central government providing the other third[12] (Yip *et al.*, 2012: 836). For the URMI the Central government establishes a minimum local government annual per capita contribution for enrollees; URBMI reimbursement premium ceilings are set lower than those of the UEBMI (Lin, Liu and Chen, 2009: S84). Otherwise, local governments are allowed to exercise their discretion over the design and implementation of local URBMI plans, a situation that has resulted in wide differences in

[11] Like in the NRCMS, enrolment into URBMI is done at the household level.

[12] A higher rate of Central government funding is allocated to low income western provinces and to some central provinces (Meng and Tang, 2013: 333).

insurance plans across provinces and cities. Local URBMI plans tend to have different eligibility criteria, varying financing rates by various levels of government, as well as different reimbursement rates for in-patient services (Lin, Liu and Chen, 2009; Barber and Yao, 2010), as most local plans tend not to cover out-patient services. By 2010 URBMI enrollees still had to pay over 50% of in-patient and 60% to 70% of out-patient expenditure out of their own pocket (Yip *et al.*, 2012: 836). There is, however, evidence that social health insurance coverage amongst the urban population did improve health care utilization rates, especially among low income URBMI enrollees (Meng and Tang, 2013: 334; Yip *et al.*, 2012).

From 2009 government contributions to the URBMI and to the NRCMS increased year on year, while reimbursement rates also gradually increased in order to make those health insurances real safety nets against health expenditure. The commitment to the goals of the 2009 reform were further reinstated by the State Council in 2012, with the setting of new health reform targets for the 12th Five Year Plan (2011–2015), including larger subsidies for both the NRCMS and the URBMI (Liang and Langenbrunner, 2013). Urban residents nonetheless, continue to bear the heavy burden of medical costs, in particular those who are still uninsured, as the fee-for-service principle and over-prescription in public hospitals prevails. Yip *et al.* (2012: 838), points out the unsustainable nature of the various social health insurances as long as health care costs are not contained.

7.5 Socio–economic Inequalities, Vulnerable Social Groups and Health Outcomes

The picture presented thus far points to the importance of mapping and understanding the links between socio–economic inequalities and health outcomes amongst different regions and social groups within contemporary China. China's case also illustrates the fact that through rapid economic growth countries may be able to experience overall improvements in some health outcomes and health insurance coverage, at the same time they may show persistent socio–economic and class inequalities in health that are avoidable or unfair. The difficulty in examining the relationship between socio-economic status and health lies with the multiplicity of variables that affect it. These include the individual's genetic make-up, lifestyle and health behaviors, education, employment and occupation, social capital, access to quality health care services and housing, through to the political, cultural and environmental context, all of which affect health in different ways throughout life (de Maio, Mazzeo and Ritchie, 2013: 17).

7.5.1 *The impoverished aging working class*

Thus far the social determinants of health studies carried out in China have consistently shown a strong relationship between income inequality and health outcomes (Cai, 2009; Chen *et al.*, 2010; Baeten *et al.*, 2012; Liu *et al.*, 2012). For example, using data from the China Health and Nutrition Survey (CHNS) Baeten, van Ourti and van Doorslaer (2012) found that the degree to which health is associated with income (as a rank-based measure of absolute inequality) more than tripled between 1991 and 2006. Furthermore, the hierarchical social structures within which income inequalities are embedded have had the added effect of increasing the incidence of psychological illness among those of lower social status. This has been particularly the case with rural migrant workers in cities, but also amongst the urban poor, each of whom have experienced the double burden of limited access to health care services and insurances, as well as social stigma. In the case of the impoverished older working class, SOE restructuring not only undermined their economic situation, it also diminished the social standing of this urban proletariat, which suddenly became a disposable class (Carrillo and Goodman, 2012). Having experienced downward social mobility and a loss of social status, these workers also tended to report worse health outcomes. For example, the 2010 East Asian Social Survey found that in China, those who had experienced or expected to experience downward social mobility did report worse health outcomes, particularly in regard to mental health (Jin and Tam, 2012).

As has been outlined, numerous studies and surveys have shown that not only are foregone health care and early discharge from hospital related to inability to pay, but also that up until recently, the bottom income deciles of the Chinese population were less likely to be covered by health insurance (Barber and Yao, 2010; Liu *et al.*, 2012). In the case of population cohorts that entered old age in the 1990s and early 2000s, health care access was particularly affected due to declining state support for health care provision during that period (Chen, Yang and Liu, 2010: 145). Among urban residents, between 1998 and 2003, foregone care and early discharge had indeed increased in tandem with the massive SOE overhaul and the resulting mass lay-offs (Liu *et al.*, 2008: 1921). Moreover, urban residents had until recently also shown a higher incidence of chronic non-communicable diseases (NCDs), while the prevalence of diseases such as diabetes and lung cancer have been higher than in rural areas (Meng and Tang, 2013: 335; Yip *et al.*, 2012: 848). This higher incidence of NCDs and the concomitant increased demand for health care and drugs amongst the elderly presents an extra burden to urban households of lower socio–economic status, even after almost universal health insurance coverage has been achieved. Early pilots of the URBMI showed that although overall utilization of medical services between 2007 and 2009 had increased, particularly for the elderly, for low and middle-income families, and for residents in less developed western provinces, out of pocket expenditure for health services had not been reduced for any income sub-group (Zhao, 2012; Li and Zhang, 2013).

7.5.2 *Rural migrant workers*

While rural migrant workers have consistently tended to report better health, and show better health measures than urban residents, due to the fact that they are, on average, younger than the urban population (Chen, 2011; Niu and Qi, 2013), everything from their lower socio–economic status, their working and housing conditions, their *hukou* status and their resulting lack of health insurance, makes them vulnerable to catastrophic health expenses and to long term health problems.

National poverty and human development surveys have shown a high incidence of poverty amongst rural migrant workers — in 2000 around 14% of rural migrant workers were found to be living in poverty (Tang *et al.*, 2008: 1498). A survey investigating the health seeking behavior of rural migrant workers in Beijing found that most of its respondents were of low socio–economic status, and that monthly per capita household income amongst these workers had a significant effect on their health seeking behavior (Peng *et al.*, 2010: 5).

Socio–economic status and income affects the health of rural migrant workers in different ways. These workers are more likely to have lower educational levels and hence be less aware of health risks. In the Peng and colleagues' study of Beijing migrant workers (Peng *et al.*, 2010: 3), 11.3% were found to be illiterate or semi-literate. It was hypothesized that low levels of education led many to underestimate the severity of their illness and to thus underutilize health care services. Their low socio–economic status and income also led them to work longer hours and to carry out unsanitary or unsafe work, posing a direct threat to the health of even young workers. A study cited by Gong and colleagues (Gong, 2012: 848) establishes that rural migrant workers work nearly 50% longer hours, and are also more likely to experience occupational accidents. Over-time work was not only harmful to the physical and mental health of workers, it also meant workers had less time to seek medical services. In Peng *et al.*'s (2012: 4) survey, 26.1% of respondents mentioned lack of free time as their reason for not seeing a doctor when ill.

Lower income levels and precarious work tends also to influence housing decisions amongst rural migrant workers, who often live in crowded rented accommodation or in employer-provided dormitories, which tend either to lack basic sanitation or offer only publicly shared facilities. Gong, (2012: 846) points out, for example, that these crowded living conditions have made migrant workers more susceptible to tuberculosis infection. Moreover, these workers ambiguous status within cities — due to their rural *hukou* registration — also makes them more reluctant to invest in better quality housing, as they prefer to maximize their savings, which are often their only real safety net (Li and Duda, 2011).

Finally, their lack of health insurance is also a strong influencing factor in their health seeking behavior. Using data from the 2008 Internal Migration and Health in China Survey, Niu and Qi (2013: 13) found that rural migrant workers were 1.83 times more likely to be left out of social health insurances compared to their urban counterparts. Since migrant workers are less likely to be engaged in a formal labor contract, they are also less likely to be covered by the social insurances stipulated by law (Cheng and Smyth, 2013). Even migrant workers enrolled into the new rural cooperative medical system (NRCMS) are unlikely to access health care services outside of their rural community, as using providers outside of NRCMS counties involves much higher co-payment rates (Yip *et al.*, 2012: 839). In places like Shenzhen, which in 2006 established a mandated social health insurance for workers without permanent household registration (*hukou*),[13] one study noted that up to 55% of migrant workers were uninsured, and that 62% of those workers who reported illness had not visited a doctor (Gong, 2012: 845).

Urbanization has been linked to higher incidences of neuropsychiatric disorders, which currently affect around 17% of China's adult population (Gong, 2012: 847), and has had a particularly negative effect on rural migrant workers' mental health (Shen *et al.*, 1998; Li *et al.*, 2006). Alongside the economic and institutional barriers faced by rural migrant workers, discrimination and stigmatization has added to the negative health effects and risks experienced by them in urban areas. Migrant workers are viewed by urban residents as illiterate, poor and unruly; their presence in the cities is seen as a burden to existing services, as competition for jobs, and as a threat to safety. A survey carried out amongst rural migrant workers in Beijing found that a higher degree of perceived social inequity and stigmatization amongst migrant workers was strongly associated with mental health problems (Lin *et al.*, 2011). The experience of interpersonal discrimination has been found to have an even more detrimental effect on

[13] This health insurance is funded through employee and employer contributions. However, by 2008 contributions were very low, even compared to the NRCMS. Employees had to contribute 4 *yuan* per month, while employers contributed 8 *yuan* also on a monthly basis (Zhu *et al.*, 2008).

rural migrant workers' wellbeing than formal institutional barriers like the *hukou* system. Chen (2013: 151) found that this type of discrimination had a more negative effect on both migrants' self-rated physical health and depressive distress than institutional discrimination. Stigmatization of rural migrant workers also presents a barrier to their ability to build social networks in urban areas, particularly limiting their capacity to build social capital that can have health protective benefits. Rural migrant workers supposed 'low quality' has rendered them, in the eyes of urban residents, less valuable and thus less deserving of the rights and benefits of urban citizenship (Anagnost, 2008: 513).

7.6 Conclusion

China's rapid urbanization since the early 1980s has been unprecedented. Over three decades, China has added thousands of towns and cities and more than 500 million people to its urban system. At the turn of the 21st century over half of China's population lived in an urban area, and this is expected to continue rising over the coming decades. A large proportion of that urban growth has been the result of an equally unprecedented movement of people from China's countryside into its dispersed network of industrializing cities. However, this rapid and massive movement of people out of agriculture and into the cities has only been enabled by discriminatory practices against rural migrant workers, who even to this day are largely not entitled to the public goods, social insurances, and welfare benefits available to urban citizens. The urban-to-rural dichotomy, however, is not the only one creating inequalities within the urban population; the expansion of regional and income inequalities across the country has fragmented Chinese society and given rise to new and vulnerable social groups. Apart from rural migrant workers, some within China's aging working class have experienced downward social mobility and have lost entitlement to benefits such as health insurance. Urban poverty and unemployment are just two of the social issues that did not exist during the Maoist era, but which the current Chinese government has to deal with.

Throughout the reform era, China's health care system has been influenced and shaped by these broader socio–economic changes affecting its cities. Changing government attitudes towards the funding and provision of public services, the restructuring of the state owned sector, and the resulting dismantling of the old labor insurance system, alongside a marketization drive within the public health system, have together made health care services and medicines unaffordable to a large proportion of the Chinese population. The effect of these changes has overlapped with regional inequalities, and inequalities between cities of different sizes. Larger cities on the more developed eastern coast of China have been in a better financial position to promote the health — and social development, more broadly — of their populations than smaller cities and towns in central and western China. At the household and individual level, up until the early 2000s, the contraction of government funding for health, the prevalence of the fee-for-service principle in public hospitals and health facilities, and the decreasing number of people covered by health insurance have resulted in the underutilization of health services, worse health outcomes and even impoverishment from health expenses among those of lower socio–economic status.

Since 1998, new social health insurance programs have been established with the aim of achieving affordable and quality health care services and medicines for the whole population. Initially only targeted at permanent workers employed in the formal sector, the 2003 SARS epidemic was said to precipitate a more dramatic turn in health reform (Liu, 2004a). Recently, some commentators have contested this, arguing that the reforms implemented after 2003 were not primarily a reaction to SARS or a concern for the health of the population. They assert that the blueprint for health reform had already been established and that the underlying changes for specific health policies were more concerned with maintaining social and political stability. Wei Zhang and Vicente Navarro (2014: 180–181), for example, point out that the implementation of the urban employee basic medical insurance (UEBMI) and the publication of a series of government documents discussing new rural and urban health insurance schemes took place before the onset of the SARS crisis. Moreover, by the late 1990s, it was clear to the government that there was mounting popular dissatisfaction with the public health care system.

Though the SARS epidemic did highlight the shortcomings of the public health care system, Zhang and Navarro (2014) as well as Huang (2014) argue that the subsequent deployment of new social health insurance programs and even the 2009 and ensuing increases in government funding for health were driven by specific economic and political goals. For them the real winners in those reforms were employers, who would be charged with insuring a smaller proportion of the population — the more privileged formal sector workers — while the majority (rural and urban) would need to be covered by voluntary insurance schemes dependent on individual contributions and government subsidies, and which also offered lower benefits than the UEBMI. Huang (2014: 2) contends that the fragmented and uneven social health insurance benefits introduced since 1998 have actually served to reinforce prevailing inequalities in Chinese society. A clear example of this has been the continued exclusion of rural migrant workers from urban social health insurances.

Universal health insurance coverage alone has been insufficient to close the gap in health inequalities within the Chinese population. Instead of 'leveling the playing field', social health insurances continue to link social benefits to household and individual socio–economic status, including the *hukou* status. Continued cost escalation of health care services and medicines has only exacerbated those inequalities. Moreover, while there have been continued increases in government contribution levels to voluntary health insurances (URBMI and NRCMS) and to their reimbursement rates and payment ceilings, these social health insurances are far from constituting, together with the UEBMI, an integrated and equitable national health care system. To date, the unequal access, quality and entitlements provided by the health care system continue to entrench the socio–economic inequalities prevalent in Chinese society. Income-based inequalities within China's socio–economic hierarchy continue to show a strong link with people's health outcomes. Hence, an understanding of those causal links continues to be crucial to build a health care system that can fulfill the goal of the health reform guidelines of 2009 to provide 'safe, effective, convenient, and affordable basic health services' for all Chinese citizens.

References

Anagnost, A. (2008). From 'Class' to 'Social Strata': Grasping the Social Totality in Reform-era China, *Third World Quarterly* **29**(3): 497–519.

Baeten, S., van Ourti, T. and van Doorslaer, E. (2012). Rising Inequalities in Income and Health in China: Who is Left Behind?, *Tinbergen Institute Discussion Paper No. 12-091/V* (13 June): 1–35.

Barber, S.L. and Yao, L. (2010). Health Insurance Systems in China: A Briefing Note, *World Health Report Background Paper No .37.*

Cai, Y. (2013). China's New Demographic reality: Learning From the 2010 Census, *Population and Development Review* **39**(3): 371–396.

Cai, Y. (2009). 'Regional inequality in China: Mortality and health', in Davis, D.S. and Wang, F. (eds.) *Creating Wealth and Poverty in Postsocialist China*, Stanford University Press, California, pp. 143–155.

Carrillo, B. and Goodman, D.S.G. (2012). 'The sociopolitical challenge of economic change: Peasants and workers in transformation', in Carrillo, B. and Goodman, D.S.G. (eds.) *China's Peasants and Workers: Changing Class Identities*, Edward Elgar, London, pp. 1–14.

Carrillo, B. (2011). *Small Town China: Rural Labour and Social Inclusion*, Routledge, New York.

Carrillo, B. (2004). Rural–Urban Migration in China: Temporary Migrants in Search of Permanent Settlement, *Journal of Multidisciplinary International Studies* **1**(2): 1–26.

Chan, K.W. (2010). Fundamentals of China's Urbanization and Policy, *The China Review* **10**(1): 63–94.

Chan, K.W. and Hu, Y. (2003). Urbanization in China in the 1990s: New Definition, Different Series, and Revised Trends, *The China Review* **3**(2): 49–71.

Chen, F., Yang, Y. and Liu, G. (2010). Social Change and Socioeconomic Disparities in Health Over the Life-course in China: A Cohort Analysis, *American Sociological Review* **75**(1): 126–150.

Chen, J. (2013). Perceived Discrimination and Subjective Well-being among Rural-to-Urban Migrants in China, *Journal of Sociology and Social Welfare* **40**(1): 131–156.

Chen, J. (2011). Internal Migration and Health: Re-examining the Healthy Migrant Phenomenon in China, *Social Science and Medicine* **72**: 1294–1301.

Cheng, Z. and Smyth, R. (2013). Happiness and Job Satisfaction in Urban China: A Comparative Study of Two Generations of Migrants and Urban Locals, Discussion Paper 08/13, Department of Economics, Monash University, Melbourne.

China Daily (1 August 2013). *Urban Push*, Available at http://usa.chinadaily.com.cn/business/2013-08/01/content_16865467.htm [Accessed 20 January 2015].

China Household Financial Survey [CHFS] (2013). Expenditure and Income. Available at http://www.chfsdata.org/detail-19,21-30.html [Accessed 20 January 2015].

Couburn, D. (2010). Inequality and Health, *Socialist Register* **46**: 39–58.

de Maio, F., Mazzeo, J. and Ritchie, D. (2013). Social Determinants of Health: A View on Theory and Measurement, *Rhode Island Medical Journal* **July**: 15–19.

Dollar, D. (2007). Poverty, Inequality and Social Disparities During China's Economic Reform, *World Bank Policy Research Working Paper* **4253**: 1–28.

Duckett, J. (2007). 'Local Governance, Health Financing, and Changing Patterns of Inequality in Access to Health Care', in Shue, V. and Wong, C. (eds.) *Paying for Progress in China*, Routledge, New York, pp. 46–68.

Eggleston, K., Ling, L., Quingyue, M., *et al.* (2008). Health Service Delivery in China: A Literature Review, *Health Economics* **17**(2): 149–165.

Gao, J. (2002). Health Equity in Transition from a Planned to Market Economy in China, *Health Policy and Planning* **17**(S1): 20–29.

Gong, P. (2012). Urbanization and Health in China, *The Lancet* **379**: 84–85.

Hsiao, W.C. (2014). Correcting Past Health Policy Mistakes, *Daedalus: Journal of the American Academy of Arts and Sciences* **143**(2): 53–68.

Huang, X. (2014). Expansion of Chinese Social Health Insurance: Who Gets What, When and How?, *Journal of Contemporary China* **23**(89): 1–29.

Jin, L. and Tam, T. (2012). Subjective Social Status, Perceived Social Mobility and Health in China, Paper Presented at the Population Association of America 2012 Annual Meeting, San Francisco, 3–5 May, 2012: 1–14.

Kaufman, J. (2010). Turning points in China's AIDS response, *China: An International Journal* **8**(1): 63–84.

Kleinman, A. and Watson, J.L. (eds.) (2006). *SARS in China: Prelude to a Pandemic?*, Stanford University Press, California.

Li, B. and Duda, M. (2011). 'Life considerations and the housing of rural to urban migrants', in Carrillo, B. and Duckett, J. (eds.) *China's Changing Welfare Mix: Local Perspectives*: 151–170, Routledge, New York.

Li, X. and Zhang, W. (2013). The Impacts of Health Insurance on Health Care Utilization Among the Older People in China, *Social Science and Medicine* **85**: 59–65.

Li, X., Stanton, B., Fang, X., *et al.* (2006). Social Stigma and Mental Health among Rural-to-Urban Migrants in China: A Conceptual Framework and Future Research Needs, *World Health and Population* **8**(3): 14–31.

Liang, L. and Langenbrunner, J.C. (2013). The Long March to Universal Coverage: Lessons from China, *The World Bank's UNICO Studies Series No. 9.*

Lin, D., Li, X., Wang, B., *et al.* (2011). Discrimination, Perceived Social Inequity, and Mental Health Among Rural-to-Urban Migrants in China, *Community Mental Health Journal* **47**(2): 171–180.

Lin, W., Liu, G.G. and Chen, G. (2009). The Urban Resident Medical Insurance: A Landmark Reform Towards Universal Coverage in China, *Health Economics* **18**: S83–S96.

Liu, Y. (2004). Development of the Rural Health Insurance System in China, *Health Policy and Planning* **19**(3): 15–165.

Liu, Y. (2004a). China's Public Health-Care System: Facing the Challenges, *Bulletin of the World Health Organization* **82**(7): 532–538.

Liu, Y., Rao, K., Wu, J., *et al.* (2008). China's Health System Performance, *The Lancet* **372**: 1914–1923.

Liu, Y., Rao, K. and Hsiao, W.C. (2003). Medical Expenditure and Rural Impoverishment in China, *Journal of Health Population and Nutrition* **21**(3): 216–222.

Liu, X. and Hsiao, W.C.L. (1995). The Cost Escalation of Social Health Insurance Plan in China: Its Implications for Public Policy, *Social Science and Medicine* **41**(8): 1095–1101.

Liu, J., Shi, L., Meng, Q., *et al.* (2012). Income-related Inequality in Health Insurance Coverage: Analysis of China Health and Nutrition Survey of 2006 and 2009, *International Journal of equity in Health* **11**(42): 1–11.

Meng, Q. and Tang, S. (2013). Universal Health Care Coverage in China: Challenges and Opportunities, *Procedia: Social and Behavioral Sciences* 77: 330–340.

Ministry of Health (MOH) (2012). *China Health Statistical Yearbook 2012*, China Union Medical University Press, China.

Mou, J., Cheng, J., Zhang, D., *et al.* (2009). Health Care Utilization Amongst Shenzhen Migrant Workers: Does Being Insured Make a Difference?, *BMC Health Services Research* **9**: 214.

Niu, J. and Qi, Y. (2013). 'Population Migration and Health Stratification in Urban China', Paper presented at the XXVII IUSSP International Population Conference, Busan, August 2013: 1–26.

Peng, Y., Chang, W., Zhou, H., *et al.* (2010). Factors Associated with Health-seeking Behavior Among Migrant Workers in Beijing, China, *BMC Health Services Research* 10: 69.

Phelan, J.C., Link, B.G. and Tehranifar, P. (2010). Social Conditions as Fundamental Causes of Health Inequalities: Theory, Evidence, and Policy Implications, *Journal of Health and Social Behavior* **51**(S): S28–S40.

Shen, Q., Lu, Y., Hu, W., *et al.* (1998). A Preliminary Study of the Mental Health of Young Migrant Workers in Shenzhen, *European Archives of Psychiatry and Clinical Neuroscience* **52**: S370–S373.

Solinger, D.J. (2006). The Creation of a New Underclass in China and its Implications, *Environment and Urbanization* **18**(1): 177–193.

Tang, S., Meng, Q., Chen, L., *et al.* (2008). Tackling the Challenges to Health Equity in China, *The Lancet* **372**: 1493–1501.

United Nations (2013). *World Urbanization Prospects: The 2012 Revision*, United Nations, New York.

Vlahov, D. and Galea, S. (2002). Urbanization, Urbanicity, and Health, *Journal of Urban Health* **79**(4): S1–S12.

Wagstaff, A. (2005). Inequality Decomposition and Geographic Targeting with Applications to China and Vietnam, *Health Economics* **14**(6): 649–653.

Wilkinson, R.G. and Marmot, M. (eds.) (2006). *Social Determinants of Health*, Oxford University Press, Oxford.

Wilkinson, R.G. and Pickett, K.E. (2006). Income Inequality and Population Health: A Review and Explanation of the Evidence, *Social Science and Medicine* **62**(7): 1768–1784.

Williams, D.R. (1990). Socioeconomic Differentials in Health: A Review and Redirection, *Social Psychology Quarterly* **53**(2): 81–99.

WHO (n.d.). Urban population growth: Trends, WHO Global Health Observatory. Available at http://www.who.int/gho/urban_health/situation_trends/urban_population_growth_text/en/ [Accessed 20 January 2015].

WHO (2005). *China: Health, Poverty and Economic Development*, Office of the World Health Organization Representative in China and Social Development Department of China State Council Development Research Center, Beijing.

WHO (2000). *The World Health Report 2000. Health Systems: Improving performance*, WHO, Geneva.

Wu, F. (2004). Urban Poverty and Marginalization Under Market Transition: The Case of Chinese Cities, *International Journal of Urban and Regional Research* **28**(2): 401–423.

Wu, M., Vin, Y., Wang, H. *et al.* (2005). Private and Public Cross-subsidization: Financing Beijing's Health-insurance Reform, *Health Policy* **72**(1): 41–52.

Xinhua (21 January, 2013). Gini coefficient release highlights China's resolve to bridge wealth gap. Available at http://news.xinhuanet.com/english/china/2013-01/21/c_132116852.htm [Accessed 20 January 2015].

Xinhua (17 March 2014). China unveils national urbanization plan. Available at http://english.peopledaily.com.cn/90785/8567957.html [Accessed 20 January 2015].

Yip, W, Hsaio, W.C., Chen, W., *et al.* (2012). Early Appraisal of China's Huge and Complex Health-care Reforms, *The Lancet* **379**: 833–842.

Zhang, W. and Navarro, V. (2014). Why Hasn't China's High-Profile Health Reform (2003–2012) Delivered? An Analysis of its Neoliberal Roots, *Critical Social Policy* **34**: 175–198.

Zhao, Z. (2012). Impact of China's Urban Resident Basic Medical Insurance on Health Care Utilization and Expenditure, IZA Discussion Paper (July): **6768**: 1–33.

Zhu, M., Zhang, X., Hassan, H., *et al.* (2008). The Influence of Health Insurance Towards Accessing Essential Medicines: The Experience from Shenzhen Labour Health Insurance, *Health Policy* **88**: 371–380.

Chapter Eight

Major Challenges the Rural China Healthcare System is Facing in the Epidemic of Chronic Diseases

Yang Feng Wu

Abstract

Historically, the urban–rural dual structure in China has led to an under-resourced rural health care system, and many other significant disadvantages affecting access to health services. An effective healthcare system has a critical role in the prevention and control of the chronic disease epidemic that is currently raging out of control. This chapter will review the major challenges that the rural Chinese health care system is currently facing and that it will face in the future, and discuss how urbanization in China has affected the rural health care system and will hence influence the future epidemic of chronic disease in China.

8.1 Healthcare System in Rural China

Chinese healthcare systems provide health services for both urban and rural residents. The systems are multidimensional and complex, with five tiers of operation (Information Office of the State Council, 2012). The first is the public health service system, which in fact consists of many separate and independent sub-systems, covering a wide range of services, such as disease prevention and control, health education, maternity and child care, mental health, emergency response, blood collection and supply, health supervision, family planning, and primary healthcare that provides public health services. The second is the medical care system, which is responsible for delivering various medical services to everyone in China. In the rural areas, the medical care system is a three-level medical service network, comprising the county hospital, the township hospitals and village clinics, and in the cities and towns it provides various types of hospitals at all levels, as well as community healthcare centers. The third is the medical security system. The basic medical security system covers basic medical insurance for working urban residents, basic medical insurance for non-working urban residents, plus a new type of rural cooperative medical care and urban–rural medical aid. These cover, respectively, the employed urban population, the unemployed urban population, the rural population and people suffering from economic difficulties. The fourth tier is the pharmaceutical and medical devices supply system, which covers the research and development, manufacturing, circulation, price control, procurement, dispatching and use of drugs and devices. The fifth and final tier is the healthcare human resources education and training system, which provides qualified professionals to all of the above.

After the establishment of the People's Republic of China in 1949, China followed the former Soviet Union and chose a planned economic and social system to develop its economy. This so-called urban–rural dual system basically divided the whole country into urban and rural classifications and all policies governing society were developed differently according to classification (Zhou, 2009). Because of this dual system, the Chinese rural healthcare system differs from the urban healthcare system in many aspects. Although both are managed centrally by the government, urban and rural healthcare systems, in effect, are different systems altogether, with the advantages almost exclusively aggregating on the urban side. This chapter looks at the rural healthcare system in detail to reveal problems of access for the rural poor.

8.1.1 *Structure*

The Chinese rural healthcare system is a three-level network comprising county hospitals, township (Xiang/Zhen)[1] hospitals and village clinics, and is administrated by county bureaus of health. It provides healthcare for about 700 million rural residents of China — about half of the country's population — living in over 33,000 townships in 2003 county-level rural administrative areas. A township usually consists of 10 to 20 villages, each having a village clinic, commonly serving between 1000 and 2500 residents. On average, the number of medical practitioners in rural China was 1.4 per 1000 residents in 2013, compared with 3.2 per 1000 residents in urban China (China Bureau of Statistics, 2013).

8.1.2 *Functions*

According to the Planning Outlines for the National Healthcare Services System 2015–2020 (Ministry of Health of the PRC, 2014), village clinics are the first level health care providers in rural China, and are responsible for the basic public health services, and ordinary/primary diagnosis and treatment of common or frequently occurring diseases, rehabilitation services, and so on. The township hospitals or health stations are the second level health care providers and are responsible for the basic public health services and comprehensive medical services on diagnosis, treatment, nursing, rehabilitation, and so on of common or frequently occurring diseases for patients in all villages within the same townships. In addition, township hospitals should also be able to perform ordinary surgeries and provide technical support and training to village clinics. The village clinics are often

[1] Townships are called Xiang or Zhen in Chinese. Xiang and Zhen are slightly different in size of economy and population and Zhen are usually bigger. Administratively both are the same level and directly under the leadership of County.

managed through the township hospitals by the county bureaus of health. Both village clinics and township hospitals are classified as primary care providers, and are the service base for both basic public health services and basic medical services. According to the National Basic Public Health Service Specification (Ministry of Health of the PRC, 2009), basic public health services include urban and rural residents' health records management, health education, health management for children 0–36 months old, maternal health management, elderly health management, vaccination, infectious disease reporting and processing, hypertension patient management, type 2 diabetes patient management, and severe mental illness patient management.

The county hospitals are the key basic medical services providers within the county and are responsible for the diagnosis and treatment of common or frequently occurring diseases, emergency care, critical care and medical care of patients referred by township hospitals and village clinics. Traditionally, county hospitals were usually the highest level of healthcare providers in the rural health care system. With the current health care reforms, since the implementation of the New Cooperative Medical Scheme (NCMS) in particular, farmers can be referred to the higher level hospitals at municipal, provincial, and national levels in cases of a complicated disease.

8.1.3 *Human resources*

Primary care health services are provided jointly by village clinics and township hospitals. Many of the health care practitioners working in the primary health care services are not qualified physicians by western standards; they are healthcare workers with limited medical training, basic equipment and a restricted list of medicines.

In 1998, our study showed a huge disparity in medical training of healthcare professionals existed between urban and rural services. For example, the proportion of professionals with a medical bachelor degree or above was 96% and 89% in national and provincial hospitals but only 55% in county hospitals and only 6% in township hospitals and village clinics (Table 8.1). Recent data from a China Rural Health Initiative (CRHI) study generally confirmed the previous reports, and

Table 8.1 Distribution of education attained by doctors, 1988

	National	Provincial	County	Town and village
N	71	487	466	549
Education:				
Bachelor degree and above	95.8	88.9	54.5	5.5
Junior college	4.2	10.1	29.6	21.7
Secondary and technical school	0	1.0	15.9	72.8
Trained in higher medical institutions	52.1	34.5	21.9	10.4

Source: Wu, 2014.

showed that only 27% of village doctors had more than 12 years of education. This means that the likelihood of a patient in rural China receiving medical care from a qualified medical provider is very low.

However, the size of this primary health care workforce is substantial, with an estimated 1.13 million across China, and over 90% of them are living in the same villages of the patients (CRHI unpublished data).

8.1.4 *Equipment and devices*

Village clinics are usually equipped with an interview room, a treatment room and a pharmacy room, with a total of 50 to 100 m^2. Some advanced clinics may have an observation room with one to three beds and a room with video facilities for health education. The typical equipment includes stethoscope, sphygmomanometer, thermometer, stadiometer and weight scale, and high pressure sterilization pot, debridement and suturing package, medical bag (for house-calls), treatment plate, disposable syringes, a portable oxygen device, tourniquet, tongue depressor, IV pole, and so on.

The township hospitals usually have a space ranging from several hundred to several thousand square meters, with from zero to fewer than 100 beds and with no, or one, surgical operation room. They usually have outpatient rooms, inpatient rooms, delivery rooms, medical examination, and test rooms that are equipped with a biochemistry analyzer, electrocardiograph (ECG), X-ray, and ultrasound, in addition to the rooms for vaccination, health education and healthcare records.

The county hospitals are usually fully equipped, with 300 to 800 beds. Some advanced county hospitals even have facilities for angiography and percutaneous coronary intervention (PCI), but generally primary PCI is not possible at county hospitals.

8.1.5 *Healthcare financing*

The healthcare financing of rural China has been constantly improved through the NCMS since its establishment in 2003. By 2011, over 96% of rural residents were covered by the NCMS. Medical care financing and the reimbursable ratio of medical costs have been raised, and the government subsidy standards for the new rural cooperative medical care system were increased from 20 RMB per person per year in 2003 to 200 RMB in 2011 (China News Network, 2011).

In 2011, the total national spending on hospitals and outpatient establishments was 1808.94 billion RMB. Of the total spending on hospitals, that on urban hospitals, county hospitals, community health service centers and township health service centers stood at 64.13%, 21.28%, 5.17%, and 9.3%, respectively (Ministry of Health of the PRC, 2014a), indicating that there is a significant disparity in healthcare expenditure on the rural Chinese; only about 30% of the national total expenditure is allocated to cover half of the total population of China.

8.2 Recent Trends in Chronic Diseases in Rural China

The 'opening up' policy and socio–economic reforms initiated in 1978 have led to marked changes in socio–economic, environmental, lifestyle, nutrition, and health care conditions and have also resulted in rising risks of non-communicable diseases (NCDs). Over the past decades chronic diseases have increased rapidly, at a pace greater than in western countries. Currently, chronic diseases account for more than four out of five of all deaths in China each year, amounting to approximately seven million deaths annually. Approximately 20% of these are estimated to have been premature deaths (that is, before the age of 70). Figure 8.1 shows data on morbidity hospitalization rates (per 1000 individuals) by major disease categories from the series of National Health Services Surveys between 1993 and 2008. While morbidity and hospitalization rates due to infectious diseases have dropped, rates for all major NCDs have risen significantly, with the exception of morbidity due to chronic obstructive pulmonary disease (COPD), which is possibly the result of declining smoking rates and great improvement in living conditions.

With the overall trend of chronic disease in China increasing, marked inequalities exist across urban/rural areas. In the 1980s, rural

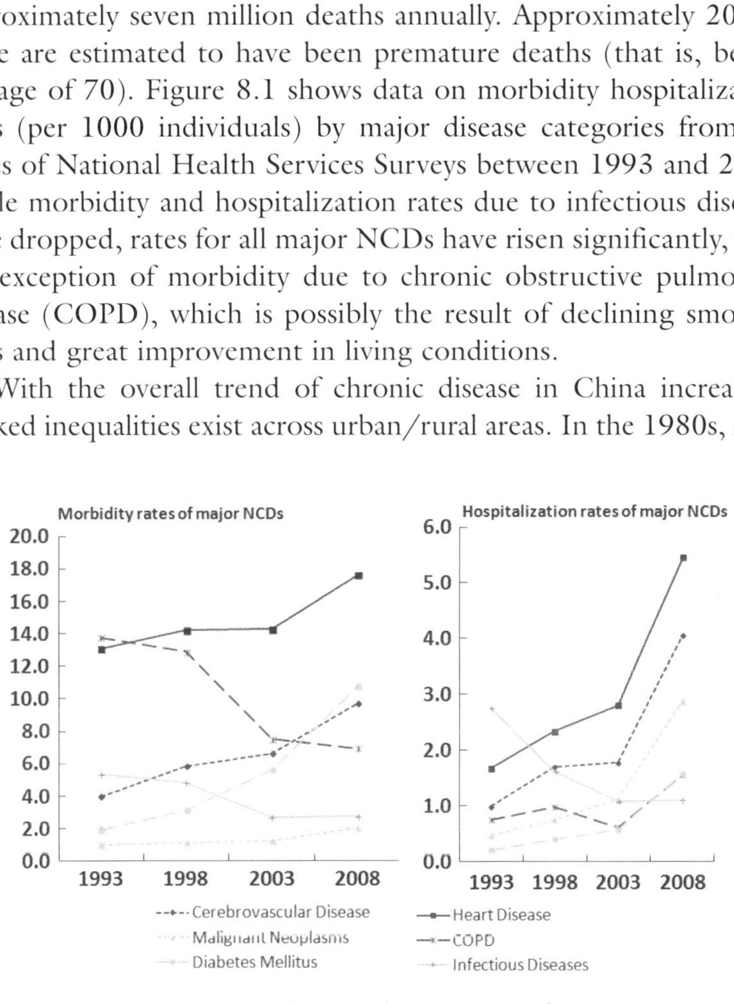

Figure 8.1 Morbidity rates and hospitalization rates of major NCDs.

Note: Morbidity rates of NCDs are defined as the ratio of the total number of being any NCDs half of year before investigation to the total number of the investigated population. Hospitalization rates are defined as the ratio of total number of hospitalization per year to the total number of the investigated population.

***Source*: China National Health Service Survey, 1993, 1998, 2003, 2008.**

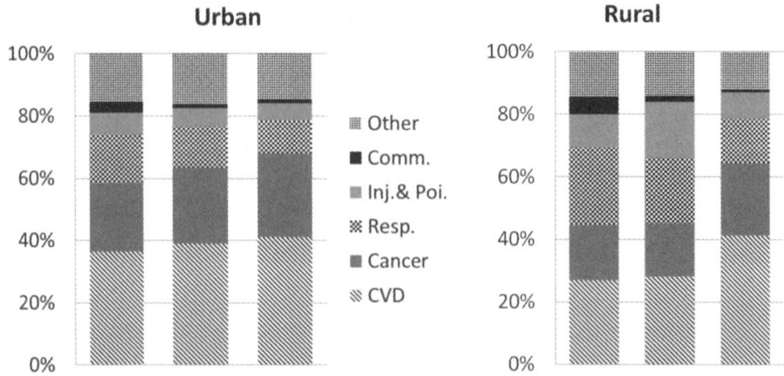

Figure 8.2 Major causes of death in 2000 and 2009 in urban and rural China.
***Source*: Ministry of Health Statistics Yearbook 2000, 2009.**

areas had lower rates of major chronic diseases, except respiratory disease, compared with urban areas. Data on major causes of death in 1990, 2000, and 2010 clearly reveals that a dramatic shift has occurred in the 10 years between 2000 and 2010 (Figure 8.2). Before the year 2000, the profile of the major causes of death in rural China was significantly different from that of urban China. Cardiovascular deaths plus cancer deaths in rural China stood for only about 40% of total deaths, but in urban China the figure was 60% and steadily increasing. In 2010, deaths in rural China from cardiovascular disease and cancer jumped to 64%, very similar to the profile for urban China in 2000, indicating that the lifestyle in rural China had quickly changed direction and followed the path of urban China. Coincidentally, China's urbanization was also in its most rapid stage from 2000 to 2010, increasing by 14% from 36% to 50%. In contrast, the urbanization process increased by only 5% between 1980 and 1990. (Figure 8.3).

In 2008, the age-standardized mortality rates per 100,000 individuals of all four major categories of chronic diseases in rural areas surpassed those of urban areas for both men and women (Table 8.2). This likely reflects the lower capacity and resources of the rural healthcare system in preventing chronic disease. In comparison with their urban counterparts, rural residents are less educated, have less health knowledge and receive much fewer curbs to the unhealthy lifestyle change driven by the improvement in the economy. This is

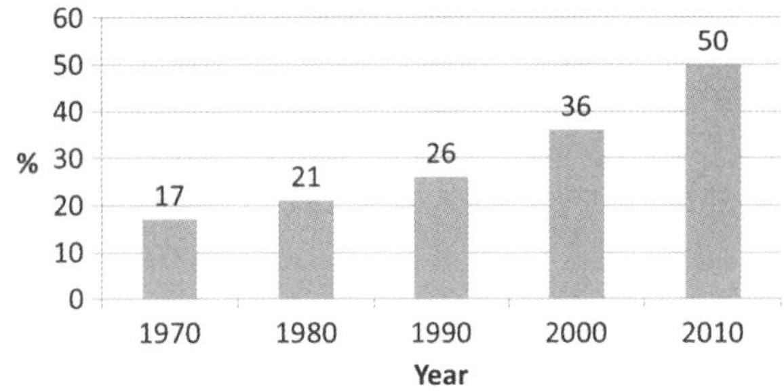

Figure 8.3 Proportion of residents living in the cities.
Source: National Bureau of Statistics of China.

Table 8.2 Age-standardized mortality rate per 100,000 population of major chronic diseases by gender and residence, China, 1990 and 2008

	1990		2008	
	Male	Female	Male	Female
Urban areas				
Cerebrovascular disease	102.07	76.66	131.81	94.78
Heart disease	73.66	60.39	130.13	99.90
Malignant neoplasms	122.12	73.64	201.48	111.37
Diseases of the respiratory system	81.78	57.76	91.87	52.85
Endocrine, nutritional & metabolic diseases	7.16	8.90	1.99	1.50
Infectious diseases	22.09	10.78	8.15	3.53
Injury & poisoning	41.04	28.55	38.09	21.75
Rural areas				
Cerebrovascular disease	91.31	64.35	217.07	143.61
Heart disease	58.46	46.49	140.35	98.41
Malignant neoplasms	123.92	64.05	267.83	121.22
Diseases of the respiratory system	145.97	105.73	182.95	111.10
Endocrine, nutritional & metabolic diseases	4.41	5.45	1.43	1.05
Infectious diseases	39.21	22.13	11.29	4.69
Injury & poisoning	73.68	53.18	78.37	41.79

Source: ***China Health Statistics Yearbook*, 2009.**

probably the reason that rural China now has a greater disease burden from cardiovascular disease and cancer.

National surveys (Li *et al.*, 2011) show that the smoking rate has always been higher in rural than in urban areas and the prevalence of hypertension in rural areas is almost the same as in urban areas except for those extremely under-developed rural areas (Wu *et al.*, 2008). The prevalence of pre-diabetes is also much higher in rural than in urban areas, indicating a higher prevalence of diabetes in the near future (Yang *et al.*, 2010). The surveillance of NCDs is further discussed in Chapter Three of this volume.

8.3 Major Challenges the Rural Chinese Healthcare System Faces in the Epidemic of Chronic Diseases

In a relatively short period, rural China has started to face a very different healthcare challenge: huge demand for the prevention and control of chronic diseases. This type of healthcare is very different from the prevention and control of communicable and infectious diseases that the rural system most commonly dealt with in the past. The government, society, and the rural healthcare system are not yet fully aware of the challenges brought by chronic disease or the ways to contain the problem.

8.3.1 *Challenges to the healthcare system*

Firstly, chronic diseases pose new demands on the poorly resourced rural healthcare system. The system is used to deal with communicable and infectious diseases with vaccination and antibiotics, the two most widely used and easy-to-apply medical interventions. Unlike communicable and infectious disease, chronic disease prevention and control are much more complex. Chronic disease cannot be cured, only controlled. To control chronic disease requires continuous management and lifetime care rather than just acute care and hospitalization. Management requires multiple and comprehensive treatments, covering almost all types of medical techniques, due to the multiple causes of disease, multiple complications, and multiple consequences. Management also relies on the patient's compliance and proactivity, because the roots of NCDs are in the patient's lifestyle and living environment. The rural healthcare system is currently, however, far from ready to meet the challenges in terms of healthcare policies, facilities and equipment, and human resources with new knowledge and technology required to tackle NCDs.

As noted above, the CRHI study revealed that only 20% of village doctors are certified and only 40% received more than 12 years education. With such low technical capacity, rural patients with chronic disease are significantly disadvantaged, as they often do not receive appropriate treatments and quality care. For example, 70% of the patients at high risk of cardiovascular disease have never received aspirin, 36% of them have never received anti-hypertension medication, and very few of them have received healthy lifestyle advice (Table 8.3). Thus, the burden that chronic disease puts on the rural healthcare system is huge.

Table 8.3 Clinical management received by 1701 patients at high risk of cardiovascular disease in 120 villages in northern China, CRHI study baseline data

See doctor for the disease in past 12 months	
>= once	40
Every month	14
Aware of own hypertension (having blood pressure measured)	66
Never taken anti-HTN drugs	36
Prescribed anti-HTN by village doctors	22
Never taken Aspirin	71
Prescribed Aspirin by village doctors	8
Received lifestyle advices at the most recent visit	
Less salt intake	20
Smoking cessation	6
Reduced alcohol	10
Physical exercise	20
Weight loss	8

***Data source*: CRHI study unpublished data.**

Secondly, the rapid increase in the number of patients with chronic disease requires a huge number of healthcare services that are far beyond the capacity of the current rural healthcare system. For example, the CRHI study found that there is one village doctor for every 1000 residents, and 10% of people living in the rural villages were identified as at high risk of developing cardiovascular disease. These patients typically require a monthly clinic visit for their disease risk management. This means that there would be 1200 clinic visits to the village doctor annually. Considering the many other responsibilities of the village doctor, this is clearly more than the doctor could handle. Without increasing the healthcare resources at village clinics, the effective prevention and control of chronic disease will not be realistic or possible.

8.3.2 *Challenges to the society*

Thirdly, the high cost of treatment of chronic diseases has caused catastrophic spending for rural families of patients suffering from serious chronic diseases. One hospitalization with a major chronic disease often costs one to several years of the disposable income of a rural resident (Table 8.4). Although the NCMS is helpful in relieving the economic burden to these families (Figure 8.4), recent statistics show that 34% of healthcare expenses still need to be covered out of pocket (Ministry of Health of the PRC, 2014b).

Fourthly, chronic diseases do not only impose a direct cost to patients and their families due to medical expenses, they also have significant indirect costs due to economic losses from the consequent reduction in productivity. Because chronic disease is much more prevalent in older people, this may particularly impact more on rural families where the younger generation has migrated to a city for a better life, and the older generation is left behind. In Chinese culture, people rely on the younger generation for support in old age. Families where the younger generation has migrated to the cities are often the poorer ones. When the older generation is affected by major chronic disease and loses the ability to work the only choice is often not to seek treatment. The NCMS and urban–rural medical aid are somewhat helpful, but clearly not enough in this situation.

Table 8.4 Average disposable income per capita and average medical expenses of selected Chronic Diseases for one time inpatient care, China, 2011

Income and medical expenses	RMB (yuan)
Average disposable income per capita	
Urban	21,809.8
Rural	6,977.3
Average medical expense per hospitalization	
AMI (Acute Myocardial Infarction)	16,793.1
Congestive Heart Failure	6,732.1
Cerebral Hemorrhage	11,802.1
Cerebral Infarction	7,325.3
Stomach cancer	15,459.2
Lung Cancer	11,536.4
Oesophageal cancer	14,631.2
CABG (Coronary Artery Bypass Grafting)	38,802.2

Source: China Health Statistics Yearbook, 2012 and National Bureau of Statistics of China.

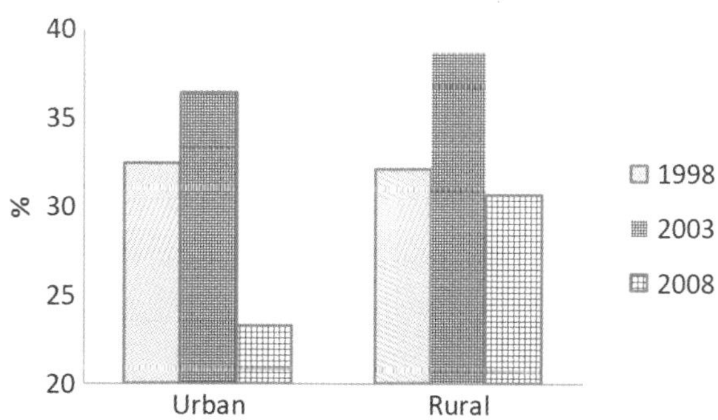

Figure 8.4 Patients who did not seek care in the past two weeks due to financial difficulty.

Source: National Health Services Surveys.

Lastly, urbanization, encouraged by the central government as a means to stimulate economic growth, has accelerated in the past 20 years and more. From 1978 to 2013, the percentage of people living in urban areas in China increased from 17.9% to 53.7% (National Bureau of Statistics of China, n.d.). Compared with the lifestyle in rural areas, life in cities is generally much more sedentary and requires much less physical activity, people tend to eat more fast food and food with high energy density, and have a more rapidly paced life with more pressure and competition. In addition, they also endure a much worse living environment with air pollution, water pollution, and unsafe food. Although health care facilities are better in urban areas, access to health services is often hard for those rural-to-urban migrants due to the barriers in health insurance policies. Current healthcare reform is trying to remove those policy barriers, but it will take a long time before a real equality in accessing healthcare can be achieved since the insurances are designed differently for rural and urban residents. What is even more concerning is that the rural-to-urban migrants or temporary city dwellers, often known as the 'floating population', contribute to the economic development of the cities in their young lives, but then are likely to take chronic diseases with them back to rural areas in their old age, adding a further burden to the struggling rural healthcare system. A universal health insurance for all Chinese would finally eliminate the barriers and secure the rural residents' rights in accessing healthcare to battling chronic disease, wherever they reside.

Urbanization does not only mean farmers migrating into cities, it also involves many other transformations; for example, moving industries to countryside, transforming single-floors housing into multistorey buildings, building more highways and roads for motor cars, gathering small villages to form big townships, and so on. In these cases, although people stay in the countryside, the risk of chronic disease has moved to them; for instance air, soil, and water pollution appears, physical activity reduces, sedentary lifestyles increase. Building a new healthy lifestyle and better planning are crucial if the Chinese government's two development strategies for the 'construction of a new countryside' and 'urbanization' are to succeed in realizing the sustainable development of rural China.

8.4 Summary and Conclusion

The urban–rural dual structure in China has led to an under-resourced healthcare system in rural China, along with many other significant disadvantages, such as the distance to travel that affects access to health services. An effective healthcare system has a critical role in the prevention and control of the chronic disease epidemics, currently raging out of control in rural China. The major challenges that the rural Chinese healthcare system is currently facing and will face in the future are very low technical capacity, and low health financing resources. Urbanization might be helpful in the development of the national economy, but it also has a negative impact on the risks of chronic disease in rural China. Due to the huge economic cost of chronic diseases, a charging urbanization process that does not incorporate effective chronic disease prevention and control strategies will in turn damage economic development and make it unsustainable. Instead of accelerating urbanization, it is better to remove the urban–rural dual structure and develop a universal society with better health equity and to protect long term economic gains by making the rural healthcare system much stronger and the rural labor force much healthier.

References

China Bureau of Statistics (2013). *China Health Statistics Yearbook.* Available at www.nhfpc.gov.cn/htmlfiles/zwgkzt/ptjnj/year2013/index2013.html [Accessed 2 March 2015].

China News Network (2011). Farmers in China to Share 832 million, New Standard Subsidy Raised to 200 Yuan. *ifeng.com* 10 June. Available at http://news.ifeng.com/mainland/detail_2011_06/10/6932480_0.shtml? [Accessed 2 March 2015].

Information Office of the State Council (2012). White Paper: Medical and Health Services in China. Available at http://english.cntv.cn/20121226/105945.shtml [Accessed 2 March 2015].

Li, Q., Hsia, J. and Yang, G. (2011). Prevalence of Smoking in China in 2010. *New England Journal of Medicine* **364**: 2469–2470.

Ministry of Health of the PRC (2009). *National Basic Public Health Service Specification.* Beijing.

Ministry of Health of the PRC (2014a). *Planning Outlines for the National Healthcare Services System (2015–2020)* (Draft for Comment). Available at www.gov.cn/xinwen/2014-10/29/content_2772400.htm [Accessed 2 March 2015].

Ministry of Health of the PRC (2014b) *China Health Statistics Yearbook* 2013. Beijing. China News Network (2011). Farmers participating in the New Rural Cooperate Medical Scheme in China increased to 832 million, new standard subsidy raised to 200 yuan. Available at: http://news.ifeng.com/mainland/detail_2011_06/10/6932480_0.shtml?_from_ralated [Accessed 2 March 2015].

National Bureau of Statistics of China (n.d). *Official website.* Available at http://data.stats.gov.cn/workspace/index?m=hgnd [Accessed 2 March 2015].

Wu, Y. (2014). A Survey on Perception and Knowledge of Chinese Health Care Professionals in Prevention and Control of Hypertension, *Chinese Journal of Cardiology* **32**(3): 264–269.

Wu, Y., Huxley, R., Li, L., *et al.* (2008). Prevalence, Awareness, Treatment, and Control of Hypertension in China: Data from the China National Nutrition and Health Survey 2002, *Circulation* **118**: 2679–2686.

Yang, W., Lu, J., Tian, H., *et al.* (2010). Prevalence of Diabetes Among Men and Women in China. *New England Journal of Medicine* **362**(12): 1090–1101.

Zhou, Z. (2009). The Establishment of Urban–Rural Dual System: The Dividing Line of the System between Peasants and Citizens. *Journal of Social Science of Hunan Normal University* **2**: 5–8.

Chapter Nine

New Villages on the Urban Fringe: Spatial Planning, Lifestyle Changes, and Health Implications

Duan Fang Lu and An Rong Dang

Abstract

This chapter provides an analysis of how peasants' daily lives (space, time, and lifestyle) have been radically restructured in the process of China's rural relocation program. By looking into the planning and design of the new villages, their effects on villagers' everyday lives, and residents' perceptions of the effects of these changes, the chapter offers a unique angle from which to view the changing rural lifestyle in the context of rapid Chinese urbanization. The chapter provides a discussion on the health implications of the new village life.

9.1 Introduction

Under China's extraordinary economic boom, rapid urbanization is set to continue. While the agriculture sector played a significant role in feeding a large population and funding industrialization until the 1990s, its impact on the economy has declined. Yet it would be a mistake to conclude from these phenomena that rural communities are no longer critical to China's future. Given the fact that agriculture still provides about half of the employment, and rural areas still accommodate about half of the total population, rural China will continue to have an important economic, political, and social impact on the nation's future.

The past three decades have witnessed both the positive and negative impact of marketization upon rural development. On the one hand, with continuous growth in non-farm employment, the development of rural industry, and enhanced agricultural productivity, rural incomes in many areas have risen significantly. On the other hand, the urban–rural income gaps have widened, most villages are still struggling with poor infrastructure, and large segments of the population in western and central China still suffer from a dearth of consumer goods. With the rural health care system built during the Mao era collapsing, rural families have to be self-supporting. Many of those who need medical treatment cannot afford it. There is limited capacity to deal with a variety of environment-related health issues.

To address a wide range of challenges in rural China, 'building a new socialist countryside with Chinese characteristic' was introduced at the third Plenary Session of the 15th Central Committee of China's Communist Party (CCP) in 1998. Various policies, programs and strategies were developed in the years that followed (Ahlers and Schubert, 2009). For example, the 1998 revision of the Organic Law of Village Committees led to enhanced transparency in village committee election and administration. The Rural Cooperative Medical Care and Insurance coverage for major illnesses was first introduced in 2002 and extended to 40% of counties at a cost of 4.7 billion RMB in 2006 (Su, 2009:135). One of the most significant policy changes was the reduction of agriculture taxes in 2004, which reduced peasants' annual tax burden by ¥120 billion RMB Yuan, and poverty alleviation subsidies went directly into peasants' accounts. The State also took responsibility for local salaries, compulsory rural education and the direction of major infrastructure development, including road construction, electrification, and water conservation.

'Building a new socialist countryside' as a concept and a program has been studied by scholars in disciplines ranging from sociology to political science (Schubert and Ahlers, 2012). Most existing literature focuses on its socio–political aspects; disciplinary limitations have made many social researchers reluctant to include the spatial dimension in their interpretations. To plug the gap, this chapter will focus on spatial changes and their impact on rural lifestyle and health. Specifically, it will examine the changes brought by rural relocation in new villages on the urban fringe in recent years. With industrial and residential developments continually spreading into rural hinterlands, the city fringe has become the 'restless urban frontier' — a most dynamic sphere in terms of social and spatial changes (Ma and Fulong, 2005). Notably, the policy of 'linking the increase with decrease in land used for urban and rural construction' (*chengxiang jianshe yongdi zengjian guagou*) was introduced in 2004 (Ren and Zhou, 2013), which further sped up the transition of the city fringe. In essence, the new policy allowed local governments to convert the land currently occupied by peasants for housing into arable land. In turn, based on the increased size of arable land, they received the same quota of land for urban construction. The policy gave rise to intensive local initiatives to carry out large scale projects of rural relocation and combination (*qiancun bingju*) (Fang, 2012). As a result, many villages with age-old histories have been razed to the ground and redeveloped into cultivable land. Villagers are moved from vernacular dwellings to modern apartment flats in newly constructed residential districts. What are the social, cultural, political, and economic impacts of these radical spatial changes? How have peasants' lifestyles changed along with them? What are the implications of new village life for rural health?

To answer these questions, this chapter provides an analysis of how peasants' daily lives (space, time, and lifestyle) have been radically restructured in the process of rural relocation based on findings from 120 semi-structured interviews and surveys conducted in 2013 in urban fringe areas of Hubei Province (Jiangxia District, Wuhan), Hebei Province (Yongqing County, Langfang) and Jiangsu Province (Nanjing, Nantong, Xuzhou, Jiangyin, Yancheng, Wuxi, Xuzhou, Changzhou, Taizhou, Yangzhou, Suzhou), as well as pilot field research in Shandong Province in 2012. By looking into the planning and design of the new villages, their effects on villagers' everyday lives, and residents' perceptions of the effects of these changes, the chapter provides a unique angle from which to view the changing rural lifestyle in the context of rapid Chinese urbanization. The chapter will close with a discussion on the health implications of the new village life.

9.2 Background: Building a New Socialist Countryside

In the early years after the socialist revolution in 1949, the agriculture sector was regarded as the foundation of the nation's overall revitalization (Hsu, 2000). The 1950 Land Reform Law allowed the seizure of land from landlords and rich peasants for massive land redistribution. As a result, agricultural output grew as much as 41% during the period 1949–1952 (Su, 2009). Yet as most agricultural produce was used to feed the urban population and the development of heavy industry grew, peasants remained economically marginalized despite the fact that they were categorized politically by CCP as the most loyal and dependable of China's citizens (*ibid.*). In the years that followed, the Unified Purchase and Sales System kept the prices of agricultural products low, and the establishment of the household registration system (HRS) and the associated ration coupon systems in urban areas, limited peasants' mobility (Chan, 1994). After three decades of structural bias against the rural sector, the late 1970s saw most rural families on the brink of desperate poverty.

In January 1981, the Chinese government, led by Deng Xiaoping, endorsed the policy of contracting agricultural production to the household (*baogan daohu*), thus replacing the collective as the basic unit of farming production and management with the individual household. Agricultural productivity increased dramatically shortly after the onset of this reform, but the aggressive taxation practices adopted by local governments as a result of coping with the 1994 national fiscal reforms adversely affected the rural population's capacity to further improve their quality of life. The rural–urban inequality reached an alarming level by the turn of the millennium. Issues related to agriculture and peasants once again became the top items on the national agenda. Following the release of the document 'Decisions

About Several Major Issues on Agriculture and Rural Work' at the CCP third Plenary Session of the 15th Central Committee in 1998, measures for poverty relief were trialed in Anhui and other provinces (Su, 2009). In addition, the State Council introduced the Rural Cooperative Medical Care and Insurance coverage for major illnesses in 2002. Under the new guideline of 'Give more, take less, and don't interfere' (*duoyu, shaoqu, fanghuo*), the central leadership abolished the agriculture tax and all other associated fees in 2004, rekindling rural enthusiasm for farming.

First introduced in 1998, the concept of 'building a new socialist countryside' was further developed in China's 11th Five-Year Plan (2006–2010), which called for a multifaceted set of solutions, including advancing production, improving livelihood, building a civilized social atmosphere, and achieving efficient management (Pan, 2007). In 2006 alone, 339.7 billion RMB was spent in rural China, accounting for 21.4% of the total state fiscal spending of the year, from which 53 billion RMB was spent on rural construction (Su, 2009:134). The central government also invested 20 million RMB each year to send five million books to libraries and culture centers in villages and towns from 2006 to 2008 (*ibid.*).

The village relocation and combination movement, as part of the 'building socialist new countryside' program, was driven by a number of factors against this background. First, land has increasingly become the new scarcity after three decades of rapid urbanization, including spatial expansion of urban areas (Hsing, 2010). China is facing a double crisis. On the one hand, there is deep concern about the loss of arable land to urbanization, industrialization, and commercial land development, believed to be affecting national food security (Cartier, 2001). On the other hand, while most local governments heavily depend on land revenue to balance their finances, they have exhausted their existing land stock and thus face a deadlock in economic growth (Zhang and Gai, 2009). Through village relocation, local governments receive much-needed land quotas for urban development.

Second, village relocation is considered an important way to enhance the living standards of the rural population. A large proportion of peasants still live in villages with conditions similar to ancient times: open-pit toilets, muddy roads with unsanitary run-off, and solid waste scattered everywhere. As of the mid-2000s, more than half the villages did not have running water, about 40,000 villages did not have any roads, while another 300,000 had roads and streets but remained unpaved (Su, 2009:125).

Third, with many villagers moving to cities for job opportunities or better education, some rural settlements have become empty villages (*kongxin cun*), resulting in the deterioration of local schools, health clinics and other facilities (Fang, 2012). It is considered, therefore, more cost effective to provide social services and facilities by combining several villages with few residents into one.

9.3 Planning and Design of New Villages

The spatial planning of new rural settlements follows the same micro-district (*xiaoqu*) principles as those adopted in the development of urban residential districts, although the scale is often much smaller. Main planning principles include scattered villages being relocated and designed into concentrated residential districts; housing and facilities (shops, parks, etc.) being integrated in each district; through traffic being discouraged; and the provision of community facilities being determined by the number of residents they serve (Lu, 2011 [2006]). The master plan for Yijiayuan Village (Tongzhou, Jiansu Province), for example, integrates dwellings, public facilities, and greenery for 182 households in one residential district. The circular layout of the dwellings discourages through traffic, and groups dwellings into several clusters. Each cluster has a small park for entertainment and exercise. Facilities such as the community center and the convenience store are located near the intersection of main roads, and within walking distance from each dwelling.

Ironically, the spatial planning and design strategies adopted in new rural settlements are quite similar to those adopted in the people's commune movement in 1958–1960. During the commune movement, concurrent with sweeping institutional changes, architects and planners boldly experimented with modernist design in rural

China (Lu, 2011 [2006]). However, as little state funding was available for rural construction at the time, those proposals rarely progressed from the drawing board to reality. In contrast, today, driven by high land revenue, local governments take active initiatives to ensure fast resettlement. The design of new settlements often features modernist apartment buildings with rationalist façades and layouts, without resorting to vernacular architectural styles and construction techniques (Figure 9.1). Most dwellings are walk-up apartment buildings with up to six floors, but townhouses and detached single-family houses are not uncommon. In new villages near the city, high-rise apartment buildings are adopted. The design is similar to that of urban residential districts. Facilities such as children's playgrounds and sports fields can be found in most new villages (Figure 9.2). In other words, people in the newly urbanized rural communities are now enjoying similar living environments and facilities to their city counterparts without moving away from their origin.

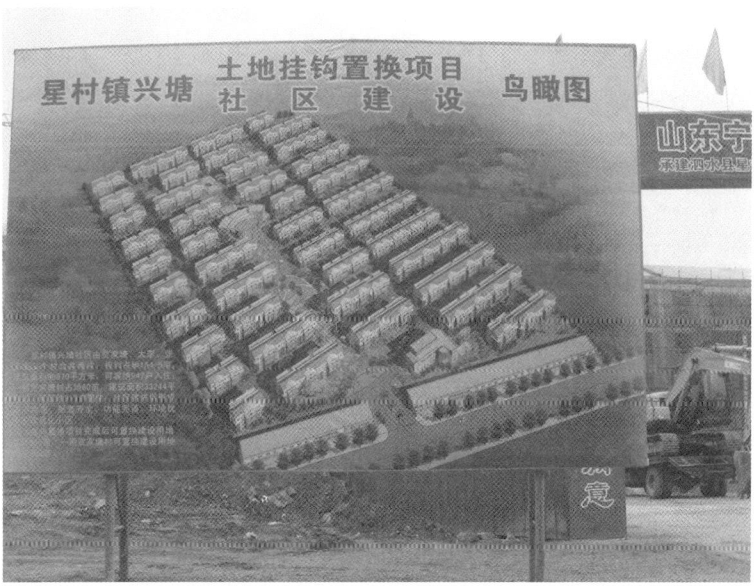

Figure 9.1

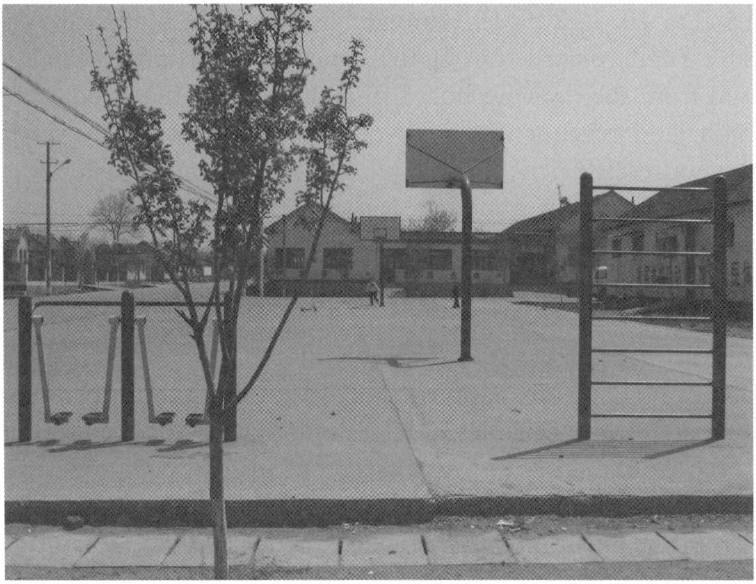

Figure 9.2

9.4 People's Perceptions of the New Village

In order to understand the effects of the new settlement on the everyday life of the residents, and to elicit their perceptions about these effects, we interviewed 120 residents of the new settlements in three of the provinces that pioneered the program in 2013.

Eighty-two percent of the interviewees reported that their new villages were planned and constructed integrally, while 17% indicated that the villages were planned as a whole, but dwellings were constructed by individual families. Many interviewees indicated that their new village had improved facilities: an open area for exercise (63%), a health clinic (55%), public greenery (48%), a bank (29%), and a post office (29%). In comparison, far fewer interviewees indicated that their old village had these facilities: such as an open area for exercise (10%), a health clinic (24%), public greenery (6%), a bank (5%), and a post office (8%). In terms of community services, 57% of interviewees indicated that their village has an owners' committee, while only

26% indicated its existence before the resettlement. In addition, garbage collection services and security services have reportedly increased from 33% and 31% before resettlement to 79% and 58% after resettlement, respectively. The improvements in social provisions are clearly evident. Most participants agreed that the new village and related services are much better managed. Of course, some aspects of the new village remain unsatisfactory to the people interviewed, notably transport connections to the nearby town or city (52%), residence layout (40%), the provision of greenery (31%), fitness facilities (28%) and library (24%) being the most perceptible aspects.

Seventy-four percent of the interviewees were satisfied with the resettlement program. Among those who were unsatisfied, 39% disliked the fact that they were forced to live in multi-storey apartment buildings (*bei shanglou*), 32% disliked the fact that they had to leave their homestead, 16% could not adapt to living in the new residence, and 35% were unsatisfied for a variety of other reasons. The reasons for dissatisfaction with the new residences or the new village life differ. The least satisfying aspects of the new residences are the lack of courtyards and storage space. Traditionally, rural residences perform a variety of production-related functions apart from residential shelter. Modeled after urban housing, the new apartment buildings in most new villages do not provide adequate space for production and storage. While apartment residents enjoy better lighting and hygienic conditions, they lose space to continue courtyard economy, as most peasants use space around the house to generate extra income in creative ways whenever possible. For example, in Dongjiawu Village (Langfang, Hebei Province) the front yard often fulfils a variety of functions in residents' everyday lives, such as growing fruits and vegetables for their own consumption or for sale at the local market, raising livestock (chicken, pigeons, and sheep), drying agricultural products, and constructing storage spaces for tools or crops, all of which are important to rural households. Further, the lack of sufficient insulation in the roofs and walls in some of the housing designs lead not only to severe thermal discomfort but also to a higher level of energy consumption and higher operational costs.

9.5 Changing Lifestyles

The study shows that radical changes have taken place in various aspects of village life after relocation in terms of the way people live and work, and the local culture. 79% of the interviewees considered their way of life had changed since resettlement. For example, 82% of the interviewees experienced reduced time in agricultural production, which might be due to the fact that many lost their farmland. Thirty-three percent of interviewees had used the internet, among whom 80% considered their online time had increased after the resettlement. 88% of interviewees reported that they knew their neighbors, but 66% indicated that they visited their neighbors less frequently than before.

The survey reveals that the resettlement program has greatly increased the distance from the new residence to farmland (Table 9.1). Before resettlement, 67% of interviewees' main mode of traveling to the farmland was walking, but this has reduced to 22% after resettlement. While the distance to farmland has increased, the transport connections with nearby towns and cities have been improved after resettlement. Seventy percent of interviewees considered that it is more convenient to go to the city after moving to the new village, and 50% reported that their children have better access to education now.

Notably, 48% of the interviewees lost their farmland after resettlement. These now had to seek alternative ways of making a living, most engaging in non-agricultural work, such as running a small business, working in nearby factories, establishing small workshops and so on. As mentioned before resettlement, most households grew vegetables

Table 9.1. Distance from residence to farmland

Distance to farmland (Km)	Percentage of interviewees before relocation (%)	Percentage of interviewees after relocation (%)
≤1	74.2	24.2
1–2	12.5	8.3
2–3	4.2	8.3
≥3	3.3	10.8
NA	5.8	48.3

near their residence or on farmland, partly for the consumption of the family and partly for market exchange. They also raised chickens and other livestock in their courtyards. After the resettlement, most villagers had much smaller or no space to grow vegetables or raise livestock. Only very few new villages would provide adequate areas for raising livestock. Nevertheless, the younger generation have adapted to new village life relatively well, as many of them now work in non-agriculture sectors with higher salaries. This has contributed to the overall household income. Before the resettlement, the average monthly household income was 3860.19 RMB (approximately US$640), which has increased to 4347.96 RMB (approximately US$720) after the resettlement.

There has been reduced participation in traditional cultural activities such as ancestor worship, seeking advice from Master Fengshui and traditional handicraft production, while participation in folk and other local cultural activities has increased slightly. The chances of using traditional techniques to build houses have been greatly reduced, given the fact that most new developments adopt modern construction methods and materials. 46% of interviewees believed that resettlement would affect the development of local culture, and among those 72% were concerned that traditional culture would gradually disappear.

The great majority of interviewees (91%) considered that their living costs had increased since the resettlement. Expenses such as bigger bills for electricity, water, cable TV, gas and broadband services were most notable (Table 9.2). For example, before the resettlement, most villages had wells, so water supply was free. In contrast, residents now had to pay for tap water. Gas was also identified as expensive, so they still used traditional stoves instead of using gas for heating in the winter. Items such as cable TV and broadband Internet connection are the new additions to living costs. The rise in basic household expenses such as for food, education, and health are relatively modest. Interestingly, the study shows that 69% of interviewees considered their spending desires have been enhanced after the resettlement. While most families already owned a variety of household appliances, many added new items when they moved to new the residence.

Table 9.2. Increased living costs

Increased living costs	Percentage of interviewees (%)
Running water	80.7
Electricity	83.5
Gas	42.2
Heating	13.8
Transport	16.5
Education	8.3
Health	5.5
Cable TV	44.0
Broadband	32.1
Strata management	11.0
Phone	3.7
Food	4.6
Other	7.3

9.6 Urbanized Village Life and Implications for Health

Our data show that most residents have adapted to the new village life fairly well, and their quality of life has been greatly improved. There are significant improvements in terms of housing quality and the provision of greenery, social services, and public facilities. Notably, as the new villages are modeled after urban residential districts, the conventional spatial needs of the relocated peasants are ignored. Design improvements may be made in key aspects of village planning and design including transport connections, dwelling layout, and the provision of storage space. On the one hand, the new residences are designed to support the urbanized lifestyle, but lacking the space to develop their traditional courtyard economies, the agricultural income of peasants has suffered. On the other hand, radical changes have taken place in patterns of consumption and leisure activities, which require a higher level of financial capacity. As a result, many younger-generation residents now work in non-agricultural sectors in nearby towns and cities earning better incomes to support their new lifestyle. The sense of local community is diluted, while connections with cities have become stronger. The empirical evidence on changes in production, travel and consumption patterns, lifestyle and cultural attitudes indicates that peasants have become increasingly urbanized through the relocation program.

The findings have important implications for rural health. First, the improved settlement quality will have positive effects on health. The infrastructure provision, services, and housing design have been brought up to modern standards. For example, new villages have running water and proper sanitation. In most cases, people and farm animals no longer live side by side. These lead to better food hygiene and environmental hygiene. The improved housing, water, and sanitation conditions help reduce infectious disease transmission. Second, with better transport connecting villages to nearby towns or cities, people have better access to urban hospitals and other medical facilities. Despite increased state investment, rural clinics remain with limited capacity. Most health resources are concentrated on hospitals in large and medium-sized cities. Although the government encourages doctors to practice in the countryside, few are willing to do so. There is a major inequality in health services between rural and urban areas. Therefore, access to urban hospitals remains crucial for rural residents. Third, with wider use of computers and the internet, residents have better access to health-related knowledge. The expanding rural perception of environmental health issues may help reduce related risks (Fang and Bloom, 2010).

There are, however, new challenges for health resulting from newly urbanized village life. Similar to residents in urban China, villagers have generally reduced their physical activity due to changes to their everyday lives. For example, in the past, peasants usually walked to their fields. Increased distance between the new settlements and the fields today means that it is no longer feasible to walk, but instead, some peasants now ride motorcycles. As shown in our research, household appliances have been widely adopted. Reduced physical activities and social isolation especially for the elderly are of particular concern. Before relocation, older people often actively participated in activities such as raising livestock and growing household vegetables. Due to the lack of space for the courtyard economy in the urbanized new settlements, the elderly now spend more time indoors. In addition, many of them have now moved to multi-story buildings and become increasingly isolated. Peasants used to grow and consume fresh vegetables from their own yards regularly. However, many have lost land for growing vegetables after relocation. This means that they have to buy vegetables from the local market, which is likely to lead to a change in diet patterns.

During the first three decades after the establishment of the People's Republic in 1949, infectious diseases, which have been gradually eliminated or brought under control, were the main health threat in rural China. Today, more and more Chinese are facing a set of different epidemics: diabetes, high blood pressure, and heart disease. For example, a recent national survey on diabetes shows that 11.6% or 114 million Chinese adults are suffering from diabetes, which means nearly one quarter of diabetes sufferers worldwide live in China (Xu *et al.*, 2013). Considering it was estimated at 1% in 1980, the increase in the prevalence of diabetes in China is as phenomenal as the nation's rapid pace of urbanization. There is evidence of the new epidemics being closely associated with rapid changes in urban lifestyle: over-nutrition, lack of physical exercise, and sedentary behavior such as extended periods of time sitting in front of a computer. From this perspective, if no effective preventative measures are adopted, in the near future the increasingly urbanized village lifestyle is likely to have such a negative impact on rural health that the current health system will be unable to cope.

References

Ahlers, A.L. and Schubert, G. (2009). "Building a New Socialist Countryside" — Only a Political Slogan? *Journal of Current Chinese Affairs* **38**(4): 35–62.

Cartier, C. (2001). Zone Fever, the Arable Land Debate, and Real Estate Speculation: China's Evolving Land Use Regime and Its Geographical Contradictions, *Journal of Contemporary China* **10**(28): 445–469.

Chan, K.W. (1994). *Cities with Invisible Walls: Reinterpreting Urbanization in Post-1949 China,* Oxford University Press, Hong Kong.

Fang, J. and Bloom, G. (2010). China's Rural Health System and Environment-Related Health Risks, *Journal of Contemporary China* **19**(23): 23–35.

Fang, X. (2012). The Main Problems and Strategies of Rural Relocation and Combination in Our Country, *Journal of Shenyang Agricultural University (Social Science Edition)* **14**(6): 652–654 (in Chinese).

Hsing, Y. (2010). *The Great Urban Transformation: Politics of Land and Property in China*, Oxford University Press, New York.

Hsu, I.C.Y. (2000). *The Rise of Modern China*, Oxford University Press, New York.

Lu, D. (2011 [2006]). *Remaking Chinese Urban Form: Modernity, Scarcity and Space, 1949–2005*, Routledge, London.

Ma, L.J.C. and Fulong W. (eds) (2005). *Restructuring the Chinese City: Changing Society, Economy and Space*, Routledge, London.

Pan, J. (2007). New Countryside Construction, Urbanisation and the Problem of Floating Population, *Journal of Zhejiang Normal University* **32**(1): 20–29 (in Chinese).

Ren, P. and Zhou J. (2013). The Policy of Linking the Increase with Decrease in Land Used for Urban and Rural Construction: Policy Review and Research Perspectives, *Chinese Agricultural Science Bulletin* **29**(5): 97–102 (in Chinese).

Schubert, G. and Ahlers, A.L. (2012). County and Township Cadres as a Strategic Group: "Building a New Socialist Countryside" in Three Provinces, *The China Journal* **67** (January): 67–86.

Su, M. (2009). *China's Rural Development Policy: Exploring the "New Socialist Countryside"*, First Forum Press, Boulder, CO.

Xu, Y., Wang, L., He, J., *et al.* (2013). Prevalence and Control of Diabetes in Chinese Adults, *Journal of the American Medical Association* **310**(9): 948–958.

Zhang, Q. and Gai, H. (2009). The Origin and Reform of China's Land Finance, *Financial and Trade Economy* **9**: 77–81 (in Chinese).

Chapter Ten

Migrant Health: Reproductive Health Awareness and Access

Chao Guo, Li Hua Pang, Gang Zhang and Xiao Ying Zheng

Abstract

As urbanization progresses more and more of the rural population is migrating to urban areas. This chapter focuses on the reproductive health of Chinese rural-to-urban migrants, especially youth and married women of childbearing age. It offers a comprehensive and detailed analysis of their reproductive health knowledge attitudes and behaviors and their access to reproductive healthcare services from two nationally representative data sets.

10.1 Introduction

Reproductive health is a basic human right. As stated at the International Conference on Population and Development 1994 this "implies that people are able to have a responsible, satisfying and safe sex life and that they have the capability to reproduce and the freedom to decide if, when and how often to do so" (UN, 1994). The Millennium Development Goals (MDGs) further emphasize the target of universal reproductive health by 2015 (UN, 2000). However, migrants in many parts of the world have limited access to reproductive health care and may face specific and serious threats to their reproductive health and rights (UN, 1994). Since China's economic reforms and opening up in the late 1970s, the level of urbanization in China has increased sharply. Especially between 1996 and 2011, the urbanization rate, that is the proportion of people living in urban areas, jumped from 30.48% to 51.27%, with an annual growth of 1.39% (National Bureau of Statistics of the people's Republic of China, 2012.)

The growth of the urban population is the most basic characteristic of urbanization. With its unprecedented rate of urbanization, China is facing a significant challenge from extensive internal migration (Zhou *et al.*, 2009). This has resulted in a large 'floating population'. These are the people not permanently registered in their current place of residence, and form the main component of the urbanization-related population. By 2012, the floating population had reached 236 million, according to The Department of Services and Management of Migrant Population of National Population and Family Planning Commission of China (2012). Most of these people are villagers who have moved from rural areas to urban areas in search of improved employment opportunities (Wang *et al.*, 2013). These rural-to-urban migrants face especially acute risks to their well-being and dignity, including their reproductive health, due to aspects of their status and their reduced social power (High-Level Task Force for ICPD, 2013). In addition, the 'village in the city'[1] population may retain the fertility behaviors and fertility culture of the rural areas they have left behind, such as high fertility aspirations (Smith and Qian, 2010). The reproductive health characteristics of migrants do not only affect the health of the current generation, but also the new cycle of demographic transition. Special attention should therefore be given to the study of all aspects of reproductive health including knowledge, attitudes, and behaviors of migrants.

[1] The 'village in the city' (chengzhongcun) is a term used to describe a form of urban development which first emerged in the Pearl River Delta region of China and refers to many villages that are not fully fledged urban areas, but are nevertheless swallowed up by urban sprawl (Lin *et al.*, 2011).

In this chapter, important studies on the reproductive health of Chinese migrants are reviewed. Two nationally representative sets of data are used to discuss two types of migrants in particular, youth and married women of childbearing age.

10.2 Review of Existing Studies on the Reproductive Health of Chinese Migrants

With increasing interest in reproductive health in China, reports on the reproductive health-related knowledge, attitudes, and behaviors of Chinese rural-to-urban migrants have, in recent years, become more widely available in international and Chinese journals. Married women and unmarried youth are usually the key target population for researchers. The literature shows that migrants are lacking in reproductive health-related knowledge, have a more tolerant attitude towards unsafe sex, and are more at risk from abortion and sexually transmitted diseases (STDs) or HIV/AIDs.

10.2.1 *Inadequate reproductive health-related knowledge*

In a population-based sample of internal migrant workers in China, Zhou *et al.* (2009) found that there was limited sexual and reproductive health knowledge, and extensive unmet reproductive health services needs among migrant workers. Wang *et al.* (2005) profiled the changing characteristics of female migrants based on data collected from multiple sources in Shanghai from 1998 to 1999. The study reported a relatively high level of ignorance in relation to STDs, and found ample evidence that female migrants' access to urban health care was limited due to a number of institutional barriers, such as inadequate insurance and ineffective treatment. Similarly, Lu *et al.* (2012) and Qu *et al.* (2010) investigated the sexual and reproductive health status among 1346 female migrant workers in Huangpu district, Guangzhou city and 1056 married female migrants in Dalian city, respectively. Limited knowledge of reproductive health and contraceptive methods was found among the respondents.

He *et al.* (2012) and Wang *et al.* (2013) assessed the knowledge, attitudes and behaviors related to sexual and reproductive health among 1690 young unmarried female migrants in Qingdao in 2012, and 944 unmarried rural-to-urban female migrants 16–27 years old in Shanghai, respectively. Both studies revealed that most respondents had limited knowledge of sexual and reproductive health. Huang *et al.* (2005) investigated 1,981 female migrants 15–35 years old in Guangdong province and found a low level of contraceptive and reproductive health knowledge. The study by Zhao *et al.* (2008) among 137 unmarried female floating adolescents aged from 15–24 years indicated that knowledge about reproductive health was quite low, especially knowledge about contraception.

10.2.2 *Sexual and contraceptive behaviors and consequences*

Zhou *et al.* (2009) conducted a cross-sectional survey of 4900 rural-to-urban migrants in six provinces of China in 2004 and reported about three-quarters of internal migrant workers had not used any contraception at sexual debut. Among migrants who were sexually active one month prior to the survey, only 14.0% reported that they had used condoms. Qu *et al.* (2010) and Xie *et al.* (2006) focused on married female migrants of childbearing age in Dalian and Shenzhen, respectively. The former found that the long-term contraception rate was 61.74% among 1056 respondents. The latter found that the proportion of high-risk behaviors was significant among 2936 participants, that is 50.47% had sexual experience before marriage, 42.78% of females under 20 years of age had already had their first sexual experience, and 11.33% had had several sexual partners. Huang *et al.* (2005) investigated 1981 female migrants 15–35 years old in Guangdong province and found that sexual activity before marriage among young female migrants was widespread, and the rate of unsafe sex was very high.

Inadequate knowledge and unsafe behaviors render migrants more at risk of some reproductive diseases. Lu *et al.* (2012) reported a high prevalence of self-reported symptoms of reproductive tract infection (RTI) (27.2% of 831 unmarried respondents and 40.2% of

515 married respondents) among young female migrant workers 18–29 years old in Guangzhou, and further, that unmarried migrant workers are more vulnerable to sexual and reproductive health problems. Qu *et al.* (2010) revealed that the gynecological morbidity rate was 51.52% among 1056 married female migrants in Dalian. Furthermore, Xie *et al.* (2006) reported that among 2936 married female migrants of childbearing age in Shenzhen, 17.77% underwent induced abortion. The repeat abortion rate was 28.29%, and 26.33% suffered RTI. The status of young migrants may be even more concerning. Unsafe reproductive health behaviors among youth, such as sexual debut at an early age and low rates of contraceptive use, result in high rates of unwanted pregnancies and induced abortion. For example, the research of He *et al.* (2012) revealed that unmarried female migrants 16–27 years old were among the most vulnerable groups, with 10.4% participants reporting an unwanted pregnancy, with 95% of them reporting an abortion.

10.2.3 *Factors that impact reproductive health behaviors*

Researchers have concluded that there are some factors that can impact the reproductive health behaviors of female migrants. Huang and Wang (2010) investigated the effect that certain factors had on the reproductive health knowledge and behaviors of 1189 female migrants 18–49 years old in Fujian province in 2010, and concluded that education level and economic status were the most important factors, followed by age, time of migration, marriage status and lifestyle. Zhang *et al.* (2013) researched the influential factors in preventing genital tract diseases and related behaviors of 493 female migrants in Chengdu, based on the theory of the health belief model (HBM), and indicated that age, marriage, monthly income, perceived barriers and self-efficacy have a direct influence on reproductive health-related behaviors. Pei *et al.* (2013) studied the association between contraceptive choice and the risk of induced abortion among 1796 floating married females of childbearing age in five cities of China, and found that age, short-acting contraceptive methods, having to pay for access to contraceptive devices and ignorance of emergency contraception might largely contribute to the increased risk of induced abortion among these women, a finding that calls for future attention. The study by Zhao *et al.* (2008) indicated that the factors associated with the reproductive health knowledge of 137 female adolescent floating population 15–24 years old in Qingdao were age, monthly income and education level.

Throughout, the literature reveals that while there has been a great deal of research on the reproductive health of migrants, it has been limited to regional or small populations. That makes the results difficult to compare with other countries. It is necessary to collect more nationally representative data to evaluate the reproductive health-related knowledge, attitudes and behaviors of migrants, especially of women and youth.

10.3 Results of a Nationally Representative Survey on Reproductive Health Among Migrant Youth

As revealed in the literature, in China it is the floating population, made up predominantly of young people, that is exposed to reproductive health risks such as unprotected sex, pregnancy outside marriage and STDs including HIV. The reproductive health of youth not only affects their physical and mental health, but also their stability and security in the near future. The 2009 Survey of Youth Access to Reproductive Health in China was the first nationally representative survey to measure the knowledge, attitudes and practices of reproductive health among youth, and their requirement for and use of reproductive health information and services (Zheng *et al.*, 2010). The survey included 22,288 unmarried youths of both sexes, born in the years between 1985 and 1994, regardless of whether they were part of the floating population or not. The survey employed multistage stratified random cluster sampling, with probability proportional to size, to derive a nationally representative sample. The youth were categorized into floating population and non-floating population groups according to their residence time in cities, that is, more or less than six months. The differences relating to sexual knowledge, attitude, and behaviors between the floating and non-floating youth were examined.

The study made several findings. In terms of knowledge, the floating youth were lacking in sexual knowledge. The correct rate of each question (the percentage of respondents who got a single question right) about reproductive health knowledge was from 15.1% to 69.1% (Table 10.1). However, there was no significant difference between the sexual knowledge of floating and non-floating youth. In terms of attitude, the floating youth may have a more open attitude towards sex, with a higher acceptance level of premarital sex, and most of them were not concerned about contracting HIV/AIDS (Table 10.2). In terms of behavior, the prevalence of high risk sexual behaviors (30.1%) and the abortion rate (9.0%) among floating youth were higher than that of youth who were non-floating. The odds ratios of high-risk sexual behaviors and abortion among floating youth were 36% and 66% higher than that among non-floating youth, respectively (Table 10.3).

10.4 Results of the Recent National Monitor Survey of Migrants

Married women of childbearing age account for a large proportion of migrants. The reproductive health of the women migrants is important for them, their children, and their families. To identify the reproductive health of women of childbearing age, data was extracted from the 2012 Monitor Survey of Migrants, a comprehensive survey on the demographic information, employment, residence, family planning, availability of reproductive health services and other public services, and the social participation and social integration of the urban floating population (The Department of Services and Management of Migrant Population of National Population and Family Planning Commission of China, 2012). The survey sampled all provinces, autonomous regions and municipalities of mainland China using a stratified, multiphase and cluster probability sampling design. The final total sample size of the survey was 158,556. Among the surveyed population, 56,542 married females of childbearing age were targeted for analysis.

Table 10.1 The rate of accurate sexual knowledge of floating and not floating youth

Questions		Floating youth N (%)	Not floating youth N (%)	P-value
Reproductive knowledge	A woman may get pregnant once she has sexual intercourse	1607 (53.0)	9388 (50.0)	0.002
	Masturbation causes serious damage to health	574 (18.9)	2828 (15.1)	0.000
	Abortion can't impact women's subsequent pregnancies	1607 (53.0)	9315 (49.6)	0.000
HIV/AIDS knowledge	Only having a sexual relationship with one healthy person who has no other sexual partners can reduce the risk of having HIV/AIDS	2094 (69.1)	12064 (64.2)	0.000
	Using condom every time you have sexual intercourse can reduce the risk of having HIV/AIDS	2067 (68.2)	11765 (62.6)	0.000
	Can a healthy looking person possibly be HIV/AIDS infected?	1482 (48.9)	9417 (50.1)	0.206
	Can mosquito bites transmit HIV/AIDS?	1004 (33.1)	7348 (39.1)	0.000
	Can eating with a HIV/AIDS infected person transmit HIV/AIDS?	1645 (54.3)	10992 (58.5)	0.000
Contraceptive knowledge	Do you know which method can effectively prevent pregnancy and also STDs and HIV/AIDs?	2074 (68.4)	11685 (62.2)	0.000
	Do you know what to do if you have unprotected sexual intercourse?	1694 (55.9)	8819 (46.9)	0.000

Table 10.2 The sexual attitudes of floating and not floating youth

Questions		Floating youth N (%)	Not floating youth N (%)	P-value
What do you think of sexual intercourse before marriage by a male youth?	Can never have	561 (18.6)	4687 (25.1)	0.000
	Can have if he loves the girl	1134 (37.7)	5473 (29.3)	
	Can have if he is ready to marry the girl	864 (28.7)	4829 (25.8)	
	Can have with or without love	135 (4.5)	733 (3.9)	
	Others and 'Don't know'	6 (0.2)	35 (0.2)	
	Don't know	311 (10.3)	2952 (15.8)	
What do you think of sexual intercourse before marriage by a female youth?	Can never have	757 (25.1)	6127 (32.7)	0.000
	Can have if she loves the boy	1007 (33.3)	4775 (25.5)	
	Can have if she is ready to marry the boy	924 (30.6)	5112 (27.3)	
	Can have with or without love	90 (3.0)	462 (2.5)	
	Others and 'Don't know'	3 (0.1)	35 (0.2)	
	Don't know	239 (9.7)	2236 (11.9)	
I never want things like abortion happen to myself or my sexual partner	Agree	2280 (75.2)	14644 (77.9)	0.003
	Uncertain	649 (21.4)	3561 (19.0)	
	Disagree	103 (3.4)	585 (3.1)	
Most of my friends don't want things like abortion happen to themselves or their sexual partner	Agree	1725 (56.9)	10677 (56.8)	0.207
	Uncertain	1157 (38.1)	7307 (38.9)	
	Disagree	151 (5.0)	807 (4.3)	
Abortion is simple, not a big deal	Agree	151 (5.0)	935 (5.0)	0.000
	Uncertain	960 (31.7)	4800 (25.5)	
	Disagree	1922 (63.4)	13055 (69.5)	

Table 10.3 High-risk sexual behaviors and abortion of floating and not floating youth

Variables		Not floating youth N (%)	Floating youth N (%)
High-risk sexual behaviors	No	16253 (84.4)	2120 (69.9)
	Yes	3003 (15.6)	913 (30.1)
	Adjust OR (95%CI)	1	1.357 (1.236~1.490)
Abortion	No	9275 (97.1)	1289 (91.0)
	Yes	279 (2.9)	127 (9.0)
	Adjust OR (95%CI)	1	1.662 (1.322~2.090)

Descriptive analysis was used to report the status of contraceptive behaviors (including the contraceptive methods used, the place where contraceptives were accessed and the main source of contraceptive services), abortion behaviors, and use of reproductive health services among married female migrants of childbearing age.

The survey results reveal that 89.3% of the respondents used some form of contraception. Among them, 75.6% of women chose long-term contraceptive methods such as male sterilization, female sterilization, intrauterine devices (IUDs) and subcutaneous implants, while 24.4% used short-term methods. Further, 55.5% reportedly accessed the contraceptives from their permanent registered residence, and 40.3% from their current residence. Family planning institutions (for example county-level and town-level family planning service stations and centers) and medical institutions (for example general hospitals, specialized hospitals, clinics, nursing homes, maternal and child health hospitals and so on), were the main sources of contraceptive services for women, accounting for 51.9% and 34.1%, respectively. Furthermore, 3.3% of the respondents had undergone induced abortion in the previous 12 months, among them 64.3% undergoing abortion once, 33.4% twice and 2.3% three or more times. In addition, during the previous year, 73.5% of the respondents had received a regular check of their IUD (to determine whether the IUD was correctly positioned), 83.9% had received information literature and advisory services, 77.0% had received information about the addresses and telephone numbers of family planning or medical institutions, and 33.7% had received condoms and other contraceptives from the family planning or medical institution in their current residence. The details are shown in Table 10.4.

10.5 Discussion

The results of our research on the reproductive health of youth in China indicated that the floating youth were lacking in sexual knowledge, and may have a more open attitude to sex with a higher acceptance level of premarital sex. Most of the floating youth were not conscious of the risk of HIV/AIDS, and the incidence of high-risk sexual behaviors and abortion in the floating youth were higher than that of youth who were non-floating. These results reinforce the related research mentioned above (Wang *et al.*, 2013; Lu *et al.*, 2012; He *et al.*, 2012; Huang *et al.*, 2005; Zhao *et al.*, 2008) at a national level, and indicate that more effort is warranted to improve reproductive health education among youth, especially among young migrants. However, the recent results for female migrants indicated that although still not very desirable, some of the reproductive and contraceptive behaviors of Chinese married women migrants of childbearing age in 2012 were improved compared with previously reported studies. For example, in our research, 89.3% of the respondents used one or more contraceptive methods at the time of survey, which was higher than Zhou's report that among migrants who were sexually active only 14.0% reported that they had used condoms one month prior to the survey (Zhou *et al.*, 2009). The proportion of our respondents who chose the long-term contraceptive methods (75.6%) was also higher than Qu found (61.74%) (Qu *et al.*, 2010). This contrast may be attributable to the different study population and the time lapse between studies. Our study uses the latest available data from the 2012 nationally representative survey, and the results indicate the latest update of the national situation.

In addition, studies from other countries indicate the same reproductive health status among migrants. A study from Nigeria reported

Table 10.4 The status of contraception and abortion behaviors of women migrants and service

Questions	Contraception and abortion behaviors status
Do you use contraceptive methods at present?	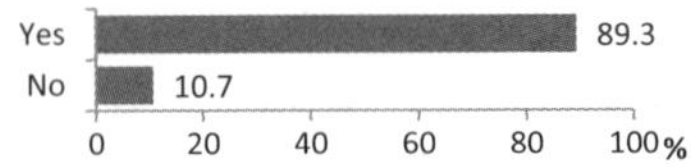
Which contraceptive method do you use mainly at present? (%)	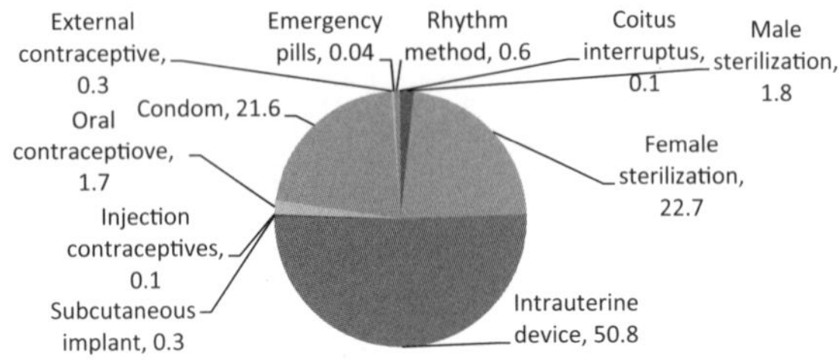
Where do you get your contraceptive method?	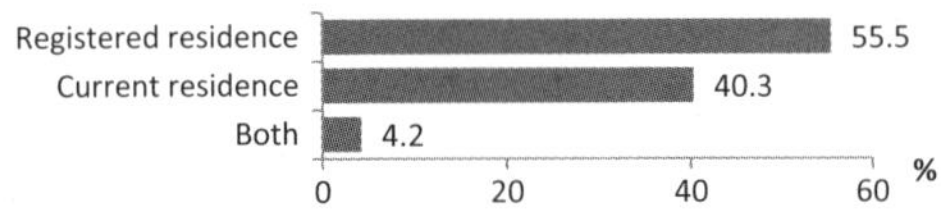
What is the source of your contraceptives?	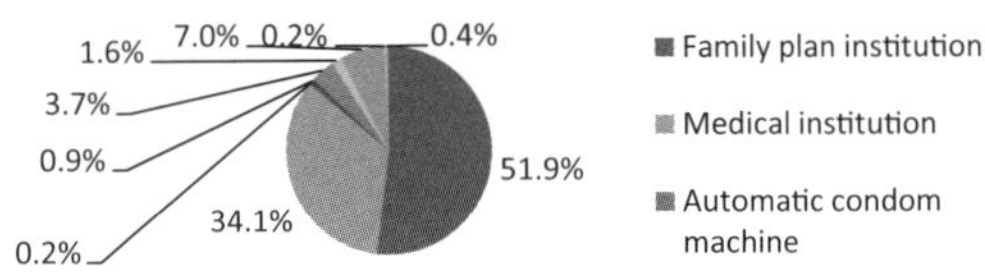
How many times have you undergone induced abortion during the recent one year?	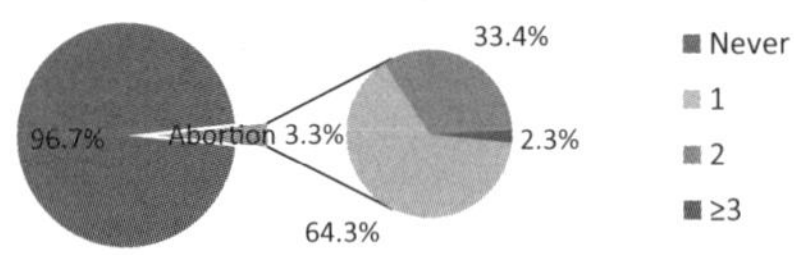
During the last year, did your local family planning clinic or medical institution provide you any reproductive health service?	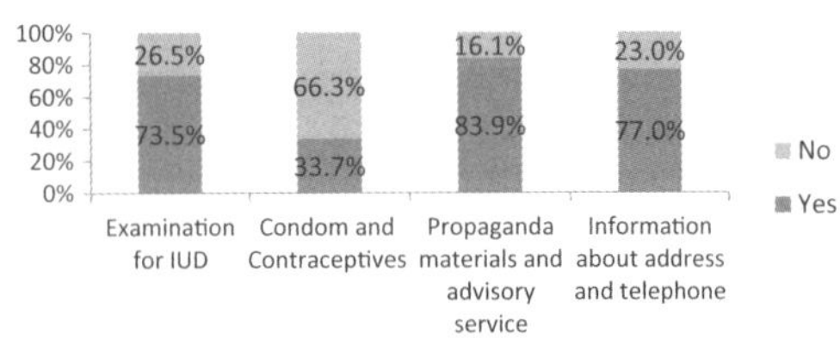

that among female out-of-school adolescents, migrants were less knowledgeable about HIV and AIDS and that migration status is a major basis for social exclusion in this population (Kunnuji *et al.*, 2013). Research from Pakistan found that only 40% of rural migrants were using family planning methods (Akhtar *et al.*, 2009). A cross-sectional study on sexual and reproductive health behaviors in undocumented migrants in Geneva suggested that they engage in frequent and high-risk sexual intercourse with insufficient use of contraceptive methods and suboptimal strategies for the prevention of STIs. Nearly half of the women had had at least one induced abortion and 40% had had an unplanned pregnancy. One in four participants reported a current or past STI or other genital infection (Sebo *et al.*, 2011). These results indicate that the reproductive health of migrants may be a serious concern and a challenge for policy makers and programmers around the world with the development of urbanization and the increase in the number of migrants.

Significantly, the pace of rural-to-urban migration has dramatically increased in China, and some new trends in migration have emerged. Firstly, the new generation of migrants, born after 1980, has gradually become the main component of the working-age population. Secondly, the trend of whole-family migration has significantly increased, and thus population migration has gradually changed from pendular movements of individuals to the movement of whole core families. According to the Report on China's Migrant Population Development by The Department of Services and Management of Migrant Population of National Population and Family Planning Commission of China (2011), the proportion of migrants moving together with their spouses, children, and parents already accounted for 66% of the total migrant population in 2011. As family migration and adult male labor increases, more and more women and adolescents are joining the flow of rural-to-urban migration. Young people now make up a large proportion of these migrant populations. Approximately a quarter of the migrants are 15–24 years old according to the national monitor survey of migrants in 2012. Since the 1994 International Conference on Population and Development (ICPD), the reproductive health of young people has been identified as one of their basic rights, as well as a serious concern and a challenge for policy makers and programmers around the world.

Young migrants have the same developmental needs common to all youth, but they are the group most at risk of reproductive health problems because of inadequate policy support. The primary cause of these barriers is the urban-to-rural dual household registration system, which not only has a negative impact on the basic rights of migrants in such aspects of life as voting, employment, insurance, and education rights, but also weakens the social integration of migrants (Zhang, 2012). Most of the children and adolescents from the floating families cannot enroll in government public schools because of the registration restrictions of the institutions. In addition, their parents are always busy with their work, supporting the family and attempting to realize their dreams in the city, and so their children's physical and mental health tends to be ignored. Exclusion from school and lack of family supervision are strong predictors of unprotected sex among adolescents (Zhang, Temmerman and Li, 2013). Young migrants who leave their homes and communities may suddenly experience a lack of social support from family, friends, and mentors, as well as increased exposure to violence, coercion, and new sources of pressure. These factors can affect the ability of youth to practice safe reproductive health behaviors and create risky situations that may lead to unhealthy and potentially fatal choices (Lane, 2008).

Similarly, there is also an unmet need for reproductive health information and services and a high risk of STDs, RTI, unwanted pregnancy and induced abortion among female migrants according to the findings in our research and previous studies. However, the female migrants are not included in maternity insurance, which prevents them from exercising their social security rights (Wang, 2012). Female migrants do not experience the same rights as urban women during pregnancy and birth, which means that a sizable majority of migrants have to appeal to substandard medical institutes for assistance because they cannot afford the standard medical fee. As a result, maternal and infant mortality rates of migrants remain significantly higher than those of the permanent residents. For example, the maternal mortality rate of migrants in Beijing in 2004 was higher than that of permanent residents (41.9/100,000 and 15.2/100,000 respectively) (Zhang, 2007). The infant mortality rates of migrants and permanent residents in Xiaoshan in 2006 were 13.63% and 4.4%, respectively (Yu *et al.*, 2009). In addition, there are many barriers to maternal and child health care and primary health care after the birth of migrant children. Immunization, for instance, is still a big challenge for children from migrant families (Zeng *et al.*, 2012) and the immunization rate of migrant children is very low (Sun *et al.*, 2010). Although the Chinese government has worked hard to extend the coverage of medical insurance to solve the health problems related to increasing internal migration, the institutional guarantees and financial support for the rural-to-urban migrants are still inadequate (Yip and Hsiao, 2008).

Migrants have been the main contributors to the increase in urban population. The reproductive health of migrants, especially of youth and women, plays a very important role in the lives of those migrants and in the development of the next generation. Moreover, the health of migrants guarantees the accumulation of human capital in the urbanization process. As China changes its focus from urban construction to the quality of life of the people living in cities, the human heart of urbanization is more and more the focus of local and national governments. Here we provide some recommendations to help the government improve reproductive health.

Firstly, the government should equip itself with improved policies to deal with disasters and steady urbanization, and pay more attention to address poverty and disease among migrants in the cities. Therefore, the urban-to-rural dual household registration system is the first challenge that should be faced squarely. Targeted legislation to ensure the rights of migrants should be developed, so that their medical insurance and education problems can be progressively resolved. In addition, special efforts should be made to ensure universal access to sexual and reproductive health information and services for all migrants, and attention given to the elimination of social, legal, and financial barriers to access. Policy makers need to be responsive to the migrant population, with special attention given to youth and women migrants (High-Level Task Force for ICPD, 2013). Young people should be informed and treated through youth-friendly approaches that respect their right to confidentiality, rather than judging them or discriminating against them. In the context of public education barriers, family should play a more active role in educating children, especially floating youth, about reproductive health, and pay more attention to the behavior of their children in the big city. Meanwhile, emphasis should be placed on young migrants as a priority group, including in national plans for sexual and reproductive health, maternal mortality reduction and HIV/AIDS.

Moreover, for female migrants, advice and information about contraceptive methods should be strengthened, to promote the use of long-term contraceptive methods and reduce high-risk sexual behaviors. Migrants should be encouraged to contact the local family planning institution to get safe and affordable contraceptive guidance and help (Wu, 2010). Further, in current residences better services should be provided for migrant women in cooperation with factories and communities.

Finally, the reproductive health of migrants should be meaningfully included in the design of data collection and studies on migrants, so that it can be well evaluated and monitored.

References

Akhtar, S., Rashid, M., Misbah, K.N., *et al.* (2009). Perception, Attitude and Practices of Rural Migrants about their Reproductive Health: A Case Study of Faisalabad city, *Pakistan Journal of Agricultural Sciences* **46**: 3.

He, D., Zhou, Y., Ji, N., *et al.* (2012). Study on Sexual and Reproductive Health Behaviors of Unmarried Female Migrants in China, *Journal of Obstetrics and Gynecology Research* **4**: 632–638.

High-Level Task Force for ICPD (2013). *Policy Recommendations for the ICPD Beyond 2014: Sexual and Reproductive Health & Rights for All.* Available at http://icpdtaskforce.org/beyond-2014/policy-recommendations-for-the-icpd-beyond-2014-sexual-and-reproductive-health-rights-for-all/ [Accessed 15 February 2015].

Huang, J.T., Yu, S.Q. and Yu, X.Y. (2005). Knowledge and Requirement on Reproductive Health of Female Youngsters Floating Population, *Maternal and Child Health Care of China* **6**: 92–93 (in Chinese).

Huang, P. and Wang, D.W. (2010). Investigation on Status of Reproductive Health among Floating Women in Cities of Fujian Province, *Knowledge Economics* **6**: 66 (in Chinese).

Kunnuji, M.O., Adejoh, S., Esiet, U., *et al.* (2013). Migration Status, Reproductive Health Knowledge and Sexual Behaviour Among Female Out-of-School Adolescents in Iwaya Community, Lagos, Nigeria, *African Journal of AIDS Research* **4**: 221–228.

Lane, C. (2008). *Adolescent Refugees and Migrants: A Reproductive Health Emergency*, Pathfinder International. Available at http://www.pathfinder.org/publications-tools/pdfs/Adolescent-Refugees-and-Migrants-A-Reproductive-Health-Emergency.pdf [Accessed 15 January 2015].

Lin, Y., De Meulder, B. and Wang, S. (2011). Understanding the 'Village in the City' in Guangzhou Economic Integration and Development Issue and their Implications for the Urban Migrant, *Urban Studies* **48**: 3583–3598.

Lu, C., Xu, L., Wu, J., *et al.* (2012). Sexual and Reproductive Health Status and Related knowledge among Female Migrant Workers in Guangzhou, China: A Cross-Sectional Survey, *European Journal of Obstetrics, Gynecology, and Reproductive Biology* **160**: 60–65.

National Bureau of Statistics of the People's Republic of China. (2012). *China Statistical Yearbook 2012*, China Statistical Press, Beijing.

Pei, L.J., Zhu, L., Guo, C., *et al.* (2013). Association between Contraceptive Choice and the Risk of Induced Abortion among Floating Married Women of Childbearing age, *Chinese Journal of Epidemiology* **7**: 677–681 (in Chinese).

Qu, A.Z., Li, Z.M., Li, H., *et al.* (2010). Dalian 1056 Mobile Population of Married Women's Reproductive Health Status and Related Factors of Contraceptive Measures, *World Health Digest* **6**: 16–18 (in Chinese).

Sebo, P., Jackson, Y., Haller, D.M., *et al.* (2011). Sexual and Reproductive Health Behaviors of Undocumented Migrants in Geneva: A Cross Sectional Study, *Journal of Immigrant and Minority Health* **3**: 510–517.

Smith, H. and Qian, X. (2010). Migration and Women's Reproductive Health, in Malarcher, S. (ed.), *Social Determinants of Sexual and Reproductive Health: Informing Future Research and Programme Implementation*, WHO, Geneva, pp. 93–113.

Sun, M., Ma, R. and Zeng, Y. (2010). Immunization Status and Risk Factors of Migrant Children in Densely Populated Areas of Beijing, China, *Vaccine* **28**: 1264–1274.

The Department of Services and Management of Migrant Population of National Population and Family Planning Commission of China. (2011). *China's Migrant Population Development 2011*, China Population Publishing House, Beijing.

The Department of Services and Management of Migrant Population of National Population and Family Planning Commission of China. (2012). *Report on China's Migrant Population Development*, China Population Publishing House, Beijing.

UN (1994). *Report of the International Conference on Population and Development (A/CONF.171/13/Rev.1)*. Available at http://www.un.org/popin/icpd/conference/offeng/poa.html [Accessed 15 February 2015].

UN (2000). *United Nations Millennium Development Goals. Goal 6: Combat HIV/AIDS, Malaria and Other Diseases.* Available at http://www.un.org/millenniumgoals/aids.shtml [Accessed 15 January 2015].

Wang, F., Ren, P., Shaokang, Z., *et al.* (2005). Reproductive Health Status, Knowledge, and Access to Health Care among Female Migrants in Shanghai, China, *Journal of Biosocial Science* **5**: 603.

Wang, J.Q. (2012). On the Protection of Maternity Insurance Rights of Newborn Floating Female Population, *Journal of Shandong Women's University* **1**: 20–24 (in Chinese).

Wang, Y., Yao, W., Shang, M., *et al.* (2013). Sexual and Reproductive Health among Unmarried Rural–urban Female Migrants in Shanghai China: A Comparative Analysis. *International Journal of Environmental Research and Public Health* **8**: 3578–3589.

Wu, J.Q. (2010). Current Status of Sexual and Reproductive Health among Migrants in China, *International Journal of Family Planning and Reproductive Health* **6**: 414–417 (in Chinese).

Xie, L.C., Zhong, Y.L., Zeng, X.C., *et al.* (2006). Investigation on Status of Reproductive Health among Floating Married Women Aged Childbearing in Shenzhen, *Chinese Journal of Family Planning* 7: 417–420 (in Chinese).

Yip, W. and Hsiao, W. (2008). The Chinese Health System at a Crossroads, *Health Affairs* **27**: 460–468.

Yu, F.Y., Wang, D.L. and Li, J. (2009). The Infant Deaths of the Registered Population and Floating Population in Xiaoshan, *Chinese Rural Health Service Administration* **1**: 74–76.

Zeng, M., Li, Y. and Wang, X. (2012). Epidemiology of Hand, Foot, and Mouth Disease in Children in Shanghai 2007–2010, *Epidemiology and Infection* **1**: 1–9.

Zhang, D.C. (2012). Analysis on the Social Integration Related System for Floating Population, *Journal of Guangzhou Police College* **4**: 49–51 (in Chinese).

Zhang, R., Liu, Q.L. and Yang, Y. (2013). Research on Influencing Factors of Floating Women's Reproductive Health-related Behaviors, *Modern Preventive Medicine* **1**: 190–193.

Zhang, X., Temmerman, M. and Li, Y. (2013). Vulnerabilities, Health Needs and Predictors of High-Risk Sexual Behaviour among Female Adolescent Sex Workers in Kunming, China, *Sexually Transmitted Infections* **3**: 237–244.

Zhang, Y. (2007). Analysis on Establishing Birth Insurance System for Urban Floating Population, *Soft Science of Health* **4**: 283–285 (in Chinese).

Zhao, Y.X., Wan, J.H., Zhang, C.C., *et al.* (2008). Knowledge and Requirement on Reproductive Health of Unmarried Female Youngsters Floating Population, *Maternal and Child Healthcare of China* **16**: 2248–2250 (in Chinese).

Zheng, X.Y., Chen, G., Han, Y.L., *et al.* (2010). Survey of Youth Access to Reproductive Health in China, *Population and Development* **16**: 2–16 (in Chinese).

Zhou, J.F., Mantell, J.E. and Ru, X.M. (2009). Reproductive and Sexual Health of Chinese Migrants, *Journal of Reproduction and Contraception* **3**: 169–182.

Chapter Eleven

Urbanization in China and Changes to the Environment

Hao Chen Wang, Feng Lu, Jia Min Gao and Xiao Ying Zheng

Abstract

The urbanization level of a country or region is a significant indicator of its level of socio–economic development. Urbanization in China has been gradually gathering pace since the reform and opening up in 1978, and is expected to reach 60% by 2020. Urbanization can promote large-scale industrial and agricultural modernization, along with the development of various services. While China enjoys the dividends of urbanization, it also bears some of its negative impacts. During this process, many environmental issues, such as air, water and soil pollution, the heat island effect and noise pollution in cities have become apparent. This chapter reviews the process of urbanization and the status of several main types of pollution in China with reference to health. It then provides relevant suggestions in order to facilitate a sustainable urbanization process.

11.1 Urbanization in China

In the 65 years since the founding of the People's Republic of China, especially in the last 36 years since reform and opening up in 1978,

China has become the world's second largest economy, behind only to the United States of America in terms of total gross domestic product (GDP). Since the First Census in 1953, the urbanization rate in China grew from 12.8% in 1953, to 17.6% in 1964, 20.4% in 1982, and 25.8% in 1990 (National Bureau of Statistics of China, 1996). It reached 35.4% in 2000 (National Bureau of Statistics of China, 2001). According to the most recent Sixth Census in 2010, the proportion of the urban population reached 49.7%. At the end of 2012, the urbanization rate was 52.6% (National Bureau of Statistics of China, 2013). There is no consensus among researchers or commentators as to how to classify the Chinese urbanization process since 1949. There were suggestions of three stages (Zou, 2004), four stages (Chen, 2009), five stages (Jiang, 2001) or six stages (Bai, 2003), based on different characteristics. Combining statistical data of economic development and historical events, suggests that the five stages classification, which means the period between 1949 and 2012 is divided into 1949–1957, 1958–1965, 1966–1978, 1979–1996, and 1997–2012 is probably the most plausible one. In this chapter, we will use this classification to discuss environmental issues corresponding to the five stages.

11.2 Environmental Issues During Urbanization

The Chinese government promotes urbanization as 'low-cost, high-performance', but in reality there are the drawbacks of 'low quality, high price' (Li and Wang, 2012). Urbanization stimulates social and economic development and industrialization; meanwhile, it inevitably has negative impacts on the environment, including air pollution, water pollution, and soil contamination that in turn have adverse effects on human health. Other issues such as the heat island effect and noise pollution, particularly in cities, also affect people's health. In the fifth stage of Chinese urbanization between 1997 and 2012, the process of urbanization in China accelerated and so did the environmental problems.

11.2.1 *Air pollution*

The composition of atmospheric pollutants is very complex but can be divided into two major categories, particulate matter (PM) and gaseous pollutants. According to diameter, PM can be categorized into the pleural particles (diameter $<10\,\mu m$, PM10), coarse particles (diameter 10-5μm, PM10-2.5), fine particles (diameter $<5\,\mu m$, PM2.5) and ultrafine particles (diameter $<1\,\mu m$, UFPs). Gaseous pollutants include nitrogen oxides (NOx), sulfur dioxide (SO_2), carbon monoxide (CO) ozone (O_3), and volatile organic compounds (VOCs). These pollutants come from different sources and have various effects on human health.

With the rapid development of modern industry and urbanization, as well as the ever-increasing population density and frequency of motor vehicle use, air pollution in China is becoming increasingly serious and is receiving increasing attention from people from all walks of life. In 2010, a nationwide environmental air quality monitoring program carried out in 471 cities revealed that 80 cities out of the 471 (17.2%) failed to meet the Chinese national air quality standard Level 2, which means the air quality index (API) is greater than 50 but less than 100 (Beijing Municipal Environmental Protection Bureau, 2004). This is the second best level of air quality in China. Among the 113 Chinese cities under intensive environmental monitoring, 63 cities (55.8%) failed to meet this standard. From a national perspective, vehicle exhaust emissions have become an important source of air pollution in large (500–1000 thousand people) and medium-sized cities (200–500 thousand people) (National Bureau of Statistics, 2013).

Whereas emissions of sulfur dioxide (SO_2), soot, industrial dust and other major pollutants have declined, nitrogen oxide (NO_2) emissions, one of the main pollutants in car exhaust, have shown an upward trend as the number of private cars continues to grow (Figure 11.1). Results from the monitoring of 31 provincial capital cities on mainland China (excluding Hong Kong and Macau) show that the concentrations of PM10 and SO_2 decreased during 2003–2010, while NO_2 concentrations remained stable (Figure 11.2). However, there were

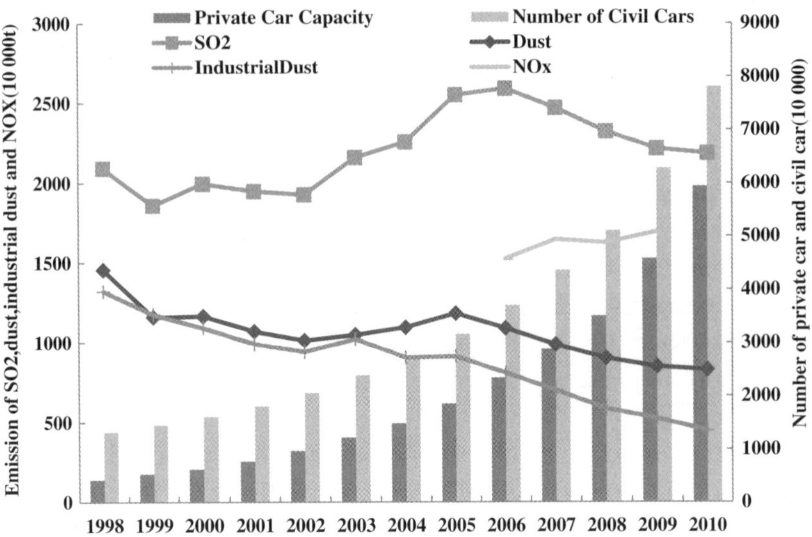

Figure 11.1 Emissions of major pollutants (SO_2, dust, industrial dust and NO_X) in the waste gas and number of private car and civil car during 1998–2010.

Data sources: China Environment Statistical Yearbook (2002–2009), China Environmental State Bulletin (1998) and China Statistical Yearbook (2010).

significant variations among the capital cities. For example, compared with the 2003–2006 period, the average NO_2 concentration in the air in 16 of the 31 capital cities increased during the period 2007–2010 (Figure 11.3). The highest increases were in Guiyang, Guizhou Province in the southwest and Changchun, Jilin Province in the northeast.

The decline in the concentrations of PM10 and SO_2 in the air may be, in part, a result of the decrease in coal consumption. Meanwhile, improved planning of industrial areas and adjustments to industrial design may have also contributed to the reduction in the concentrations of these air pollutants. Take Beijing as an example. In 2013, about 288 high pollutant-generating factories were moved out of Beijing and underwent a technology upgrade. The overall reduction of emissions was estimated to be 4000 tonnes of industrial dust, 7000 tonnes of nitrogen oxide and 8000 tonnes of volatile organic compounds due to the industrial upgrade and transformation that occurred in Beijing in 2013 (Ministry of Environmental Protection of the People's Republic of China, 2013).

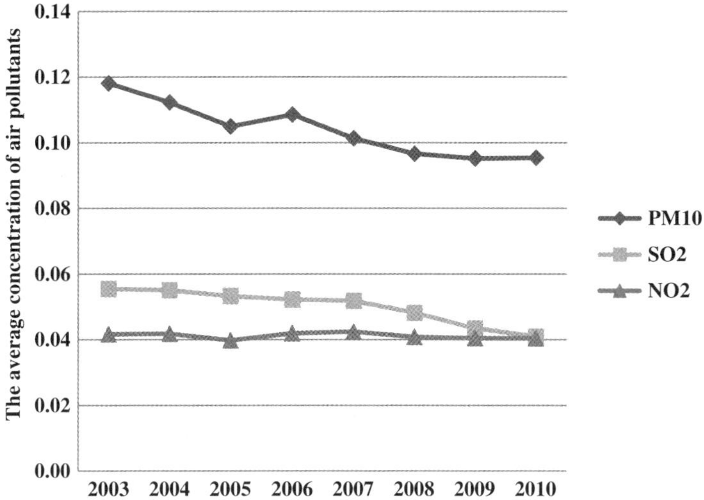

Figure 11.2 Average concentration of air pollutants ($PM_{10}/SO_2/NO_2$) in 31 provincial capital cities during 2003–2010.

Data sources: China Statistical Yearbook (2004–2011). A: The average concentration of PM_{10} during 2003–2006; B: The average concentration of PM_{10} during 2007–2010; C: The percentage of average PM_{10} concentration change; C = (B–A)/A.

However, China is still one of the countries with the highest levels of SO_2 emissions in the world, and is also one of the countries affected by severe acid rain damage. The total amount of damage is of concern. In the national 448 county-level cities' acid rain monitoring, it was found that acid rain occurs in 258 of them. The distribution pattern of the acid rain is mainly in the areas stretching from south of the Yangtze River to the east of the Tibetan Plateau, covering most parts of several provinces, including Zhejiang, Jiangxi, Hunan, and Fujian, and the economically advanced regions of Yangtze River Delta and the Pearl River Delta. Some cities, such as Changde in Hunan province, Dexing in Jiangxi province, and Lishui, Ji'an and Kaihua in Zhejiang province have 100% frequency of acid rain (Zhou and Li, 2010). The areas affected by acid rain are as big as 1.2 million km^2, and the areas severely affected by acid rain cover about 60,000 km^2 (Ministry of Environment Protection, 2010).

Air pollution is becoming one of the major urban environmental problems. The concentrations of nitrogen oxide, carbon monoxide

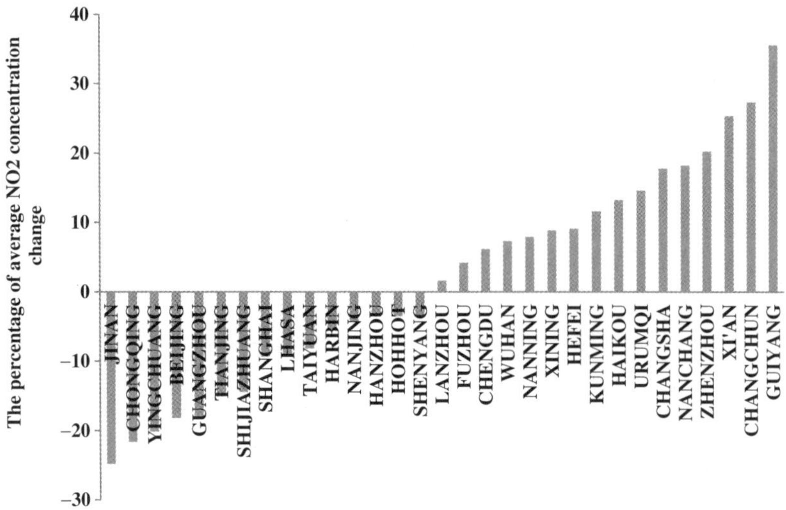

Figure 11.3 Changes of NO_2 concentration in 31 provincial capital cities.
***Data source**: China Statistical Yearbook (2004–2011).* **Calculation of the change values: A: The average concentration of NO_2 during 2003–2006; B: The average concentration of NO_2 during 2007–2010; Change = (B–A)/A.**

and related pollutants in metropolitan air are increasing. As illustrated in Figure 11.1, the rise in concentration of nitrogen oxide is following the rise in the number of motor vehicles in China. The air pollution problem caused by vehicle emissions is particularly prominent in medium and large cities. The concentration of carbon monoxide, hydrocarbons and sulfur dioxide is the highest along major roadways. In 1998, motor vehicle emissions of nitrogen oxide and carbon monoxide were estimated at 120,000 tonnes and 1.3 million tonnes in Beijing, respectively (Hao *et al.*, 2001). According to an official news release, in 2004 carbon monoxide and hydrocarbon derived from the emissions of motor vehicles accounted for 80% of the total urban emissions in Beijing, Shanghai, Guangzhou and other big cities (Ministry of Environmental Protection of the people's Republic of China, 2004). These substances can also cause photochemical smog under certain climatic conditions.

Urban air pollution is also driven by the rapid increase in population and the expansion of cities. Increase in population leads to a high demand for residential housing. The space for and number of houses in city centers is limited, so the urban area is continuously expanding in order to accommodate more people. However, there are limited employment opportunities in the new areas. People who live in the new residential areas need to commute to work. Because of the long distances between work and home, the range of population activities expands. Nationally, the number of private vehicles increased from 816,200 in 1990 to 59,387,100 in 2010, a staggering 72 times growth; civilian vehicles, including privately owned vehicles, official cars, commercial vehicles and farm vehicles, increased from 5,513,600 in 1990 to 78,018,300 in 2010, in just 20 years (Ministry of Transport of the PRC, 2011). It is predicted that in 2020 motor vehicle ownership will reach 13 million and the average annual fuel consumption growth will reach 6%. Take Beijing as an example. The number of private cars was 821,600 in 2000, while in 2010, the number had increased to 4,257,400, a more than four-fold increase in one decade (Beijing Municipal Bureau of Statistics, 2011). However, the area of the city and the roads in Beijing has not increased correspondingly. The rapid increase in the number of private cars has caused tremendous pressure on the city's road traffic system. More roads have to be built which leads to the 'more people–more vehicles–more emissions' path.

It is obvious that the urban area cannot expand infinitely. Coupled with the land shortage, the road network expansion cannot match the fast pace of motor vehicle growth. This of course leads to lower travelling speed, frequent traffic congestion, thus low transportation efficiency. These phenomena perpetuate the environmental pollution problem from car emissions. The highest concentration of nitrogen oxide in air surges when traffic congestion and traffic peak occurs in the city areas. For example, the concentration of nitrogen oxide within the Second Ring Road in Beijing is about four times that outside the Fourth Ring Road. Corresponding to traffic peak times, two daily pollution peaks appear around 8–10 am and 3–5 pm (Hao *et al.*, 2000). As a result, the type of air pollution in urban areas of China has changed from simple smoke pollution into the mixed pollution of coal-burning and vehicle exhaust.

Energy consumption of coal, and industrial and vehicle exhaust are the leading pollutants, and these are consequences of urbanization. Negative impacts of particle matter PM10 and PM 2.5 of total suspended particulate matter (TSP) have attracted many researchers' and government's attention. These pollutants not only contain a large amount of organic and toxic metal components, but can also enter the body more easily than coarse particles and, therefore, present a greater threat to human health. Ironically, human activities are the main source of urban fine particulate matter. A study by the Chinese Academy of Science revealed sources of PM2.5 include vehicle exhaust, burning coal, pollutants from neighboring provinces, restaurants, industry, construction dust and other sources (Wang *et al.*, 2013).

11.2.2 *Water pollution*

Historically, many Chinese cities are located by rivers or lakes for easy access to water. However, due to poor local environmental awareness and inadequate sewage treatment capacities, water pollution in China has reached a critical point. Figure 11.4 shows annual industrial and

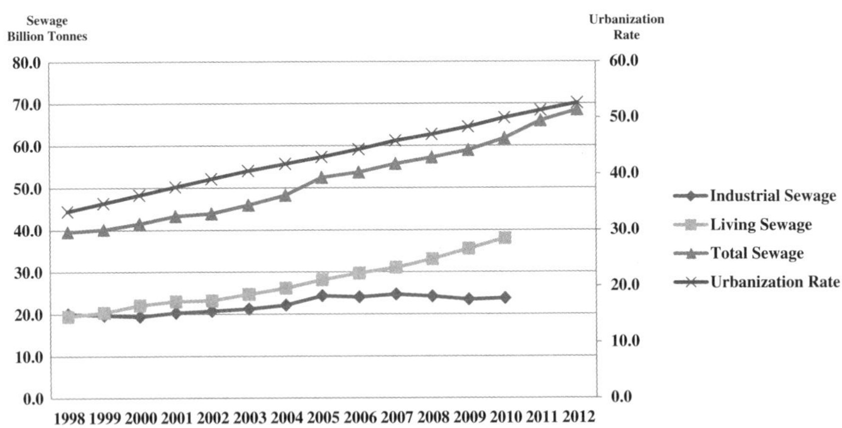

Figure 11.4 The amount of industrial sewage, living sewage and the total sewage with urbanization rate.

Data source: China Statistical Yearbook (1999–2013).

domestic sewage emissions against the trend of urbanization rate from 1998 to 2012.

As demonstrated in Figure 11.4, during the process of urbanization, the amount of human sewage emissions is continuing to increase, and is the dominant source of water pollution. Such a trend parallels the increasing trend of urbanization. Sewage emissions have led to serious contamination in rivers, lakes and underground water bodies, resulting in many health incidents. During the period 1996–2006, there were a total of 271 reported emergent incidents of water pollution, of which 171 were biological and 92 chemical (Wang *et al.*, 2010).

The *2010 Report on the State of the Environment in China* (Ministry of Environmental Protection of people's Republic of China, 2011) revealed the grim truth, that the Songhua River in the northeast, and the Huai River in central China were mildly polluted, the Yellow River in the north and the Liao River in the north-east were moderately polluted, while the Haihe River in the east was severely polluted. Based on Chinese water quality standards, the water quality of major lakes was also very poor, 77% being at level four (the second worst level, only for industrial use) or level five (the worst, for scenic use only) (Ministry of Environmental Protection of people's Republic of China, 2002).

In 2013, the total amount of waste water discharged was 69.54 billion tonnes (National Bureau of Statistics, 2014). Of even greater concern, the quality of nearly a quarter of the drinking water sources monitored was below the national standard. Of the 271 reported water pollution accidents, the overall population affected exceeded seven million; and as many as 31,000 people became ill (Ministry of Environmental Protection of the People's Republic of China, 2011). There are more than 2,000 species of organic pollutants that have been identified in the drinking water, including 114 with suspected carcinogenic, teratogenic, and mutagenic effects; these cannot be eliminated by the traditional chlorination treatment in the water plants. The estimated area of polluted arable land throughout the country has reached more than 10 million hectares. A total of 12 billion kilograms of polluted grains is discarded. Further, up to 45.5 million kilograms of fish die from water pollution (Wang, 2006). The economic losses caused by environmental pollution are estimated at

RMB 187.5 billion; out of which the losses from water pollution account for an estimated RMB 142.9 billion (Lu, 2009).

One of the consequences of urbanization is the amount of sewage discharged from the combined populations in urban areas. In some regions, urbanization is still in its early stage, as people start to use washing machines and flush toilets. However, sewage treatment facilities have not caught up with the large volume of waste water, resulting in most of the sewage being discharged directly into bodies of water or infiltrating the soil. Moreover, urban sewage treatment facilities have reached their capacity in the existing cities. In addition, existing sewage treatment facilities are not effectively utilized. As of September 2005, the operating rate of sewage treatment plants in 40 cities was less than 30%, and in another 30 cities they were not in operation (Qiu, 2006). Meanwhile, heavily polluted industrial discharges beyond the ability of the existing sewage treatment plants to treat, means incompletely treated waste was being released into waterways. This situation has been improved with the building of 2996 sewage treatment plants by the end of March 2011, which means the capability of sewage treatment is up to 133 million m^3/day. The average operating load rate of all plants was 75%, a significant improvement compared with 2005. However, there were still 607 plants with an average operating load rate less than 60% (Beijing Youth Daily, 2011).

The total number of water pollution incidents in urban and suburban areas is rising annually. Biological pollution remains the main cause of drinking water pollution in China. However, in Beijing, studies of 195 water pollution incidents during 1960–1998 showed that chemical pollution incidents rose whereas biological pollution incidents remained stable (Liu *et al.*, 2002). Investigation of the causes of water pollution incidents is consistent with contamination of water supplies, including pipes, and inadequate water treatment as discussed earlier. In Heze city, Shandong Province, the causes of water pollution included infiltration of sewage into the water supply, substandard antiseptic treatment and the contamination of water pipes (Liang and Zhang, 2003). The main reasons for drinking water safety incidents in Anshan city, Liaoning Province were leaking pipes and insufficient protection of water sources (Wang *et al.*, 2005), while the main cause of drinking water pollution in Chengdu city, Hebei Province was from domestic sewage contamination (Li and Yang, 2006).

11.2.3 *Soil pollution*

Soil contamination usually includes inorganic and organic pollution. Inorganic pollution can further be divided into heavy metal pollution and metalloid pollution. Some Chinese cities, for example Hezou, Gansu province (Cheng *et al.*, 2007) and Jinchang, Ningxia province (Jin *et al.*, 2010), were built adjacent to the local metal mining industry. With the urban population increasing, the cities have expanded into the land once used for storing mining products, and substances in metal ores have ended up in urban land via the rain and river, resulting in serious inorganic pollution.

11.2.3.1 *Inorganic pollution*

Heavy metal and metalloid pollution in soils is widely observed in China. Heavy metal–polluted soil means the contents of heavy metals, such as mercury (Hg), cadmium (Cd), lead (Pb), chromium (Cr), and nickel (Ni) in soils are significantly higher than the background contents, resulting in environmentally degraded soil and ecological deterioration. With economic development and urbanization, these heavy metals are in high demand, as mining and processing activities increase. The toxicity of some heavy metals on human health is well recognized (Lin, 2004). Heavy metals in soil may be transferred to plants and affect human health through the food chain. They can also affect drinking water or become atmospheric dust and then enter the human body. Taking nickel (Ni) as an example, it is widely distributed in the environment because its anthropogenic sources include fuel combustion, industrial production and the use and disposal of nickel products (Kasprzak *et al.*, 2003). The main occupational Ni exposure pathways include mining, nickel-alloy products, electroplating and welding. Analyses of soils and wheat in the Jinchang area, 'The Capital of Ni' in Gansu Province, showed elevated nickel concentrations, and the adult daily nickel intake was eight times higher than the current amount recommended by the International Commission on Radiological Protection (ICRP) (Jin *et al.*, 2010). Elevated concentrations of nickel have also been found in the soils of some developed coastal regions and cities. The average soil nickel concentration in some cities in Leizhou Peninsula, Shandong Province is 49.8 mg/kg, higher than Level 2 of the national soil standards (Guan *et al.*, 2007).

Arsenic contamination is another example of inorganic pollution. Arsenic is a metalloid which is considered as poison. China is one of the countries in the world most severely affected by arsenic pollution in the environment. The pollution is particularly prevalent in Guangxi, Yunnan, Guizhou, and Gansu provinces (Cheng *et al.*, 2007; Guo *et al.*, 2001; Li *et al.*, 2005). Arsenic in soil can be transferred to humans via drinking water and food. According to the National Standard of Maximum Levels of Contaminants in Foods, the safe level of total arsenic is less than 0.5 mg/kg in food (Ministry of Environmental Protection, 2012). In vegetables, the main form of arsenic is inorganic arsenic (Díaz *et al.*, 2004). The acceptable daily intake of inorganic arsenic, as set by WHO, is 0.128 mg (for an adult male weighing 60 kg) (Tsuji *et al.*, 2004). In Shanghai, the arsenic level in vegetables has been detected as high as 0.123 mg/kg and the average concentration is 0.019 mg/kg (Sun *et al.*, 2010), while in Dongguan, Guangdong Province, the highest level of arsenic in vegetables is 0.276 mg/kg and the average amount is 0.095 mg/kg (Cai *et al.*, 2010), levels that are certainly hazardous to human health according to the national standards (State Environmental Protection Administration of China, 1995).

11.2.3.2 *Organic pollution*

Persistent Organic Pollutants (POPs) are the main organic pollutants in soil. They are ubiquitous chemicals that can accumulate in the human body because of their resistance to metabolism and lipid solubility. The sources include irrigation by sewage, use of organochlorine pesticides (OCPs), incomplete combustion of coal, petrol or oil (Straif *et al.*, 2005). Organic pollution of soil is mainly the consequence of using organochlorine pesticides (OCPs) since the 1950s in the agricultural sector. Soil is the main reservoir of OCPs and 20–70% of

OCPs in the environment exist in the form of bound residues in soils (Zhang *et al.*, 2006). The Chinese government imposed a ban on the use the pesticides in 1983 due to a range of health concerns. However, the expansion of urban areas into what was previously farmland is still affected by the residual organic pollution in the soil, which is an environmental hazard.

Polycyclic aromatic hydrocarbons (PAHs) are a kind of POPs ubiquitous in the environment. Many PAHs are carcinogenic, teratogenic, and mutagenic (Chen and Liao, 2006). They are widespread in soils in China, and their degradation is very slow in the environment. They can pass through the food chain, and pose a great threat to human health. As PAHs derive from incomplete combustion of coal, oil, chemical fuel and petroleum products (Basheer *et al.*, 2003) research on the health risks of PAHs mainly focuses on the soils where oil or petrochemical products are consumed, such as urban areas, industrial areas and highways. Taking coking plants as an example, incomplete combustion of fossil fuels in the production of the tar, natural gas and other chemical products is likely to cause emissions of PAH substances (Zhi, 2005). PAHs can contaminate soil and atmosphere in the forms of dust, gas, and coke breeze. In coking plants in Beijing and Panzhihua city, Sichuan province in south-western China, the contents of PAHs in the topsoil are spatially variable due to various degrees of contamination made by different processes (Feng *et al.*, 2009; Wang *et al.*, 2011). Due to coal-fired heating, the PAH fallout on topsoil in Handan city, Hebei Province is mainly caused by incomplete combustion of coal (Zhang *et al.*, 2002). Soils near coal gas plants show similar features to soils near coking plants (Xu, 2002). The pollution in deeper soils may also be more seriously affected (Zhang *et al.*, 2012).

Furthermore, in urban areas, the number of petrol stations is increasing because of the rising consumption of petroleum and diesel fuel. Soils near petrol stations may be contaminated by leaked oil (Jia *et al.*, 2012). The soils most polluted by PAHs in Fuzhou city, Fujian Province are found near a gas station and in industrial areas (Ni *et al.*, 2012). Some petroleum storage and processing facilities are located near cities. Soil surrounding these facilities will carry organic pollutants.

In these areas, PAHs contamination poses a high risk to human health. Studies on the bioavailability and ecological risks of this group of pollutants are needed (Tao *et al.*, 2010).

High PAH concentrations in soils are found in areas with high fuel consumption, such as industrialized areas or big cities, densely populated areas and along main roads. The concentration of PAHs in the soils of these areas is greater than that in the agricultural areas or scenic areas (Peng *et al.*, 2010). For example, the soil PAHs pollution level in the agricultural area of Ningbo, Zhejiang Province was lower than the neighboring Hangzhou city, the capital city of Zhejiang Province (Feng *et al.*, 2011; Yu *et al.*, 2009), and Shanghai. However, atmospheric transportation may transfer PAHs pollution from industrial areas or urban areas to agricultural areas and the outskirts of the city and deposit it in the soil. In Zhanjiang, Guandong Province, the rapid development of heavy industry has led to an increase in the PAHs pollution level, and PAHs were detected in soil surrounding the city (Zhao *et al.*, 2012). It is concerning that the concentrations and distribution of PAHs in soils of underdeveloped cities and regions are emerging parallel to rapid development, especially the development of heavy industries. On the positive side, a recent study in Beijing showed that trees and plants can alleviate some of the problem; PAHs content was low in the soils of some schools because more trees were planted (Peng *et al.*, 2012). This offers some evidence for future greener urban planning and as a way of reducing environmental pollution.

Urbanization, population concentration, and economic development lead to the expansion of urban areas. To expand traditional advanced economies, industrialized urban areas need more industrial land or wasteland on the urban fringe. In the meantime, new cities and towns formed by the concentration of the local population in rural areas are also expanding by expropriating nearby agricultural land. According to *2014 National Survey of Soil Pollution Bulletin* (Ministry of Environmental Protection and Ministry of Land and Resources, 2014), among 775 soil pollution monitoring points in industrial wastelands, 35% were classified as polluted points, mainly secondary and mining industry sites. New towns built alongside industrial parks are also polluted by heavy metals and PAHs. Compared with air or water pollution, soil pollution is more concealed and more difficult to remediate (Li, 2009). Therefore, the monitoring of the contents of heavy metals and organic pollutants in soils needs to be enhanced. Moreover, in the process of urbanization, protecting the soil from inorganic and organic pollutions is challenging environmental protection experts and government policy makers alike.

11.2.4 *Other environmental issues*

11.2.4.1 *Heat island effect*

Anthropogenic climate warming is mainly caused by two types of greenhouse gas emissions and land-use changes. Urbanization perpetuates the impact of both these problems. Urban construction which leads to the urban heat island effect has caused widespread concern. Research on regional and urban heat island effect has become the mainstream of research on effects of urbanization on climate change. In relation to the urban heat island effect, there are two schools of thought. Scholars in one school postulate that urban heat island is confined to small regions of big cities and suburbs. This condition will not have a significant impact on changes in the average temperature on a large scale. This viewpoint, the mainstream position, emphasizes the changing trend in the degree of individual urban heat island. The example for this thought is the observed trend of temperature changes in Xi'an, Shannxi Province, northwestern China (Gao *et al.*, 2009). Other scholars point out that in recent decades, urban heat island effect is caused by globalization and urbanization worldwide. It not only affects the trend of climate change in a city itself, but also contributes to a long-term climate trend in the scale of a region, demonstrated by studies in Yangtze River Delta region in southern China (Xie *et al.*, 2007; Cui *et al.*, 2008).

Both schools agree, however, that the impact of urbanization on temperature is seasonal and periodic. The stage of rapid urbanization is accompanied by a stage of temperature warming, which has been confirmed in a study on Beijing urbanization and warming (Zheng *et al.*, 2006). Seasonal warming effects in different regions have varied intensities. For example, in the Yangtze River Delta region, the warming rate is higher in winter and spring, and lowest in summer (Gao *et al.*, 2009), while Xi'an has the largest linear warming trend in the spring, followed by a linear increase in the magnitude of warming in winter, and the trend is minimal in summer (Cui *et al.*, 2008). These conditions suggest the heating system prompts the warming effect by energy consumption and the emission of carbon dioxide and sulfide. In addition, through the analysis of urbanization and climate change some scholars believe the environmental impact of urbanization is complex, and local improvement is only temporary (Ren *et al.*, 2006).

11.2.4.2 *Noise pollution*

In the urban environment, noise pollution has become a major form of pollution, which not only interferes with the residents' work and daily lives, but can also inflict serious harm on human health, such as noise induced hearing loss. Although China has developed noise standards in urban areas and in the development of large-scale industrial production and transportation, urban noise has nevertheless become a serious concern. In 2013, noise monitoring results of the Beijing urban area showed that in 293 major roads in Beijing urban area, the average traffic noise was 69.1 decibels; it was 67.2 decibels in the outer suburbs; and 69.8 decibels in some expressways surrounding residential areas (Table 11.1) (Beijing Municipal Environmental Monitoring Center, 2014).

Noise monitoring of eight major cities' different functional regions reveals that the central business district usually has a long-term high noise level. The peak time for noise in these cities always occurs 8–10am and 4–6pm, times which match the peak traffic hours. The noise level next to roads that met the national standards in these cities is much lower than those in other small cities (Liu *et al.*, 2009). Although the Chinese government is trying very hard to control noise pollution, the result is far from satisfactory (Figure 11.5).

Table 11.1 Average noise levels in Beijing, 2000–2001

	Regional Noise (Decibel (A))			Traffic Noise (Decibel (A))		
Year	Beijing	Urban	Suburb	Beijing	Urban	Suburb
2000	53.9	53.6	55.0	71.0	71.0	69.5
2001	53.9	53.7	54.7	69.6	69.6	70.1
2002	53.5	53.5	54.3	69.5	69.5	69.0
2003	53.6	53.5	54.0	69.7	69.7	69.0
2004	53.8	53.7	54.4	69.6	69.6	69.1
2005	53.2	53.3	53.7	69.5	69.5	68.4
2006	53.9	53.7	53.9	69.7	69.9	69.0
2007	54.0	53.6	53.7	69.9	70.1	68.9
2008	53.6	53.4	53.7	69.6	69.8	68.9
2009	54.1	53.9	53.6	69.7	69.9	68.4
2010	54.1	54.0	53.5	70.0	70.2	68.0
2011	53.7	53.7	53.4	69.6	69.8	67.9
2012	54.0	53.6	53.1	69.2	69.7	67.7
2013	53.9	53.6	53.0	69.1	69.8	67.2

Data source: Beijing Municipal Environmental Monitoring Center-Noise Monitoring (2000–2013).

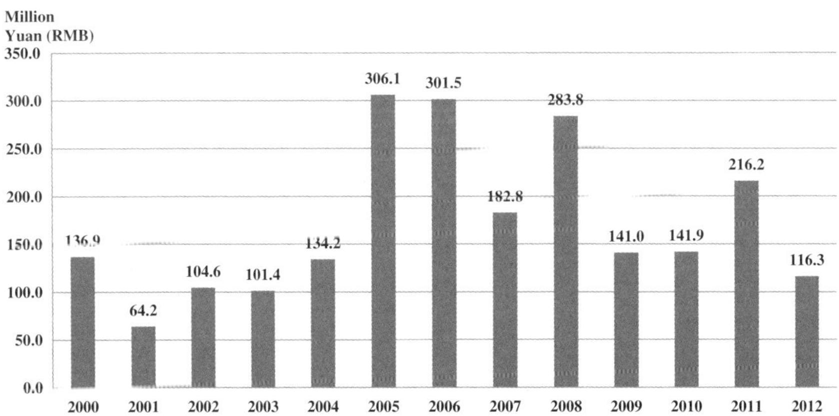

Figure 11.5 Investment on control of noise pollution in Chinese urban areas.
Data source: China Statistical Yearbook (2013).

11.3 Health Effect of Pollution

11.3.1 *Air pollution*

A large number of epidemiological studies have confirmed that air pollution has become one of the major environmental risk factors affecting human health in China (Kan and Chen, 2002). Premature deaths in China due to outdoor air pollution have reached about 30 million annually (Cohen *et al.*, 2005). Based on the "Cost of Environmental Pollution in China" (The World Bank, 2007), an estimated economic burden of 157.3 billion RMB was lost due to air pollution related morbidity and premature deaths, accounting for 1.16% of GDP. According to the Global Burden of Disease Study, ambient particulate matter (PM) pollution was the fourth leading risk factor for disability-adjusted life-years (DALYs) in China, in 2010, leading to 25.2 million DALYs (Yang *et al.*, 2013). The health effects of air pollution include a spectrum of conditions, including death. In China, many studies have been carried out that explore the impacts of these pollutants on population health.

11.3.1.1 *Mortality*

Acute mortality related to air pollution has been the focus of investigations since the 1990s. In the early stages, many studies were concerned with the acute effects of sulfur dioxide (SO_2), nitrogen dioxide (NO_2) and PM10, while many recent studies have focused on PM2.5, carbon monoxide (CO) and ozone.

The acute effects of PM, including PM10 and PM2.5, on mortality have been the subject of several recent reviews (Huang *et al.*, 2012; Yang *et al.*, 2008; Yang *et al.*, 2013). Shang *et al.* (2013) found that PM was significantly associated with increased all-cause and cardiorespiratory mortality risks in the Chinese population. In this study, with 10 $\mu g/m^3$ increase in PM10 and PM2.5 concentrations, the total of all-cause mortality increased by 0.36% (95% confidence interval (CI): 0.26%, 0.46%) and 0.40% (0.22%, 0.59%) respectively. Cardiovascular mortality increased by 0.36% (0.24%, 0.49%) and 0.63%

(0.35%, 0.91%), and respiratory mortality by 0.42% (0.28%, 0.55%) and 0.75% (0.39%, 1.11%).

For gaseous pollutants, including SO_2, NO_2, and ozone, Shang *et al.* (2013) concluded that with per 10 μg/m^3 increases, the total mortality risk increased by 0.81% (0.71%, 0.92%), 1.43% (1.30%, 1.56%), and 0.57% (0.45%, 0.69%), respectively; the cardiovascular mortality risk increased by 0.84% (0.68%, 0.99), 1.54% (1.325, 1.76%), and 0.60% (0.40%, 0.79%), respectively; and the respiratory mortality risk increased by 1.15% (0.75%, 1.56%), 2.05% (1.62%, 2.48%), and 0.89% (0.57%, 1.20%), respectively. Whereas with 1 mg/m^3 increase in carbon monoxide, the estimated mortality risk increases were 3.70% (2.88%, 4.51%) in total mortality, and 4.77% (3.53%, 6.01%) in cardiovascular mortality.

11.3.1.2 *Respiratory system disease*

Inhalation is the main pathway for the PMs and other harmful substances in the air to enter the human body. Therefore, the respiratory system is a target organ directly affected by air pollutants. Epidemiological studies have shown that respiratory morbidity and mortality are closely related to air pollution. For example, SO_2 has a strong stimulating effect on the respiratory mucosa, which is able to invade the respiratory tract, weakening the alveolar, causing or aggravating bronchitis and bronchial asthma. Studies have been carried out on the relationships between air pollution and respiratory diseases, involving different areas, different population groups (for example, children, adults, traffic policemen). Adults in the urban area of Beijing have a higher prevalence of persistent phlegm and asthma than those who live in peri-urban areas (Wang *et al.*, 2011). In Guangzhou city in the south, the higher daily concentration of NO_2 and SO_2 the more daily emergency room visits by residents (Li *et al.*, 2009). In less developed cities, like Nanning, Guangxi Province in the southwest, the morbidity rates of bronchitis, pneumonia, asthma, and rhinitis in pupils living in heavily polluted areas were higher than those living in less polluted areas ($P < 0.05$) (Hu *et al.*, 2004).

11.3.1.3 *Cardiovascular disease*

Epidemiological studies show that the level of air pollutants is positively correlated with the morbidity and mortality of cardiovascular diseases (Adamopoulos *et al.*, 2010; Akinaga *et al.*, 2009; Mills *et al.*, 2007; Mills *et al.*, 2008). Populations with existing cardiovascular diseases, those with diabetes and the elderly are particularly susceptible to cardiovascular diseases caused by air pollution (Simkhovich *et al.*, 2008). However, at present, the mechanism of atmospheric pollutants affecting the cardiovascular system is not well understood. It has been found that air pollution can influence the cardiovascular system by changing the vascular tone, atherosclerosis, autonomic nervous system effects, and systemic inflammatory response (Rom and Samet, 2006). The ambient PM10 concentration is positively associated with daily hospital visits for cardiovascular diseases in Beijing (Wang *et al.*, 2009). PM2.5 concentration in air was significantly positively correlated with the mortalities of cardiovascular diseases, coronary diseases, stroke and chronic obstructive pulmonary disease (COPD) (Zhao *et al.*, 2011).

11.3.1.4 *Carcinogenic effects*

The carcinogenic effects of certain air pollutants have been identified through air toxicology experiments and epidemiological studies. During the past 20 years, a large number of epidemiological studies reported the relationship between air pollution and lung cancer incidence and mortality rate, but the degrees of correlation and statistical significance levels were quite different. This may be related to differences in air pollution levels and composition, the accuracy of the pollution and health data, research methods, and consideration of the incubation period. In general, most studies have found a positive relationship between air pollution and lung cancer (Chen *et al.*, 2011).

In urban areas of Beijing, the strongest correlation was found between SO_2 level and lung cancer mortality rate of seven years later (Zhang *et al.*, 2009). The lung cancer incidence rate in Xiamen City showed a significant correlation with SO_2, which is greater than that with Total Suspended Particulates (TSP) (Huang, 2008). In Jiangsu Province, a positive correlation was found between the lung cancer mortality data and nitrogen oxide concentration in the air (Lu *et al.*, 2003). After adjusting for the level of population exposure, respiratory rate and susceptibility, the general population's attributable score for polycyclic aromatic hydrocarbons (PAHs) for lung cancer is 1.6%, which is equivalent to an approximate increase of 0.65/ 100,000 in the incidence rate of lung cancer among the Chinese population in 2003 (Zhang *et al.*, 2009).

11.3.2 *Other issues*

11.3.2.1 *Water pollution*

Water pollution often causes intestinal diseases, such as typhoid fever, dysentery, or hepatitis. In some areas, incidence rates of intestinal diseases, hepatitis, typhoid and other epidemics keep increasing annually. According to a survey in four municipalities directly under the Central Government, including Beijing, Tianjin, Shanghai, and Chongqing, the incidence of hepatitis, typhoid or other intestinal diseases caused by water pollution in the urban areas was three times higher than that in the peri-urban areas (Cui and Fu, 1998). A typhoid fever outbreak in Guilin city, Guangxi Province was caused by a polluted ground water source from November 9th to 12th, 2004 (Yang *et al.*, 2008). In Guiyang, Guizhou Province, water pollution from the water plant was related to typhoid fever in July and August, 2003, due to incomplete disinfection of the polluted lake water (Zhou *et al.*, 2004).

11.3.2.2 *Heat island effect*

Heat island effect in cities is particularly dangerous for people with existing cardiovascular and respiratory diseases, and the elderly. In Wuhan, Hubei Province, Central China one of the hottest places in China, the average daily death rate of people with circulatory diseases in high temperature periods is 0.92 times more than in normal temperature periods (Cheng *et al.*, 2009). Guo *et al.*, (2009) found that during a heat wave, the greater the increase in temperature on any given day, the greater the number of visits to the emergency room in Haidian District, Beijing. Most of the visitors were elderly people. For those who have respiratory diseases, there is a positive relationship between the increase in daily mean temperature and the rate of upper respiratory disease (Lu, 2003). In Beijing, it was reported that when the temperature was in the range of 15–25°C and above 25°C, every 1°C increase in daily mean temperature may lead to a 7.3% (OR = I.073, 95% Cl:1.002–1.149) and 25.7% (OR = I.257, 95% Cl:1.115–1.416) increase in the mortality rate of people older than 65 with respiratory conditions, respectively (Tao *et al.*, 2011).

11.4 Way Forward

Urbanization is an inevitable trend in the socio–economic development of China. According to "The New Urbanization State Plan (2014–2020)" (The Central People's Government of People's Republic of China, 2014), the urbanization rate will reach about 60% in 2020. This means if existing problems cannot be handled effectively, urbanization will not only exert greater pressure on the environment and natural resources, but will also accumulate and compound into significant environmental problems. Thus, positive responses to environmental pollution issues in both rural and urban areas will achieve sustainable urban development and promote steady urbanization.

The central and local governments have taken a range of measures in recent years to mitigate the current issues brought about by the urbanization process. These include:

- Promoting gas and other clean energy to replace fossil fuel consumption and to reduce dust emissions.
- Building sewage treatment plant capacities to improve urban sewage management and water quality.
- Planning and facilitating industries to relocate to the industrial parks outside major cities, to control urban environmental pollution.

- Increasing investment in public facilities and environmental protection, such as central heating, drainage, landscaping and other infrastructure investment.
- Adopting more stringent environmental protection standards.
- Institutionalizing environmental protection supported by laws and regulation.
- Promoting environmental awareness among residents.

While these are welcome measures and initiatives, the causes of environmental pollution should be addressed when improving the existing cities and constructing new ones.

11.4.1 *Recommendations*

1. Rational planning of urban layout and building the low-carbon city
   Low-carbon city advocates support the development of energy saving transportation and green buildings. These can be achieved by the rational division of functional areas and urban residential areas to reduce unnecessary transportation and the use of low-carbon buildings from both the design and operational management, to reduce energy consumption in buildings. Low-carbon city advocates also support the development of green transportation, which means the implementation of effective public transport systems, to reduce the number of vehicles in cities, and the use of intelligent transport management to reduce traffic congestion.
2. Transformation of economic models
   Models of economic growth need to be transformed to gradually reduce the heavy reliance on resources and high energy consuming industries in cities. Vocational training and technical training should be strengthened, to develop the labor-intensive service industry reducing energy consumption and creating less pollution. The proportion of clean energy in the overall energy structure should be increased.
3. Advancement of technology to reduce energy consumption per unit of GDP Industrial restructure and development of land-intensive

agriculture for mass production will provide opportunities for effective environment protection and pollution control. Further, promoting a technology upgrade and using energy-efficient new technologies in new factories will reduce energy consumption per unit of output.

4. Establishing a long-term mechanism to manage sustainable development. Government, business and the civil society should work together for urban environmental protection and make efforts toward sustainable development. Government should focus on building institutions, establishing management standards and imposing strict implementation of the regulations. Enterprises should use new technologies to reduce resource consumption and low unit production costs. Awareness of environmental protection should be strengthened in the civil society so the public will adopt a low-carbon, green, and healthy lifestyle.

In urbanization, besides measures for promoting environment protection, approaches for reducing the impact on health should also be considered. For example, special health facilities for air pollution related diseases should be set up for people who are vulnerable to air pollution, such as those with respiratory or cardiovascular disease so they can go to such facilities for specialized prevention and treatment.

Urbanization is the result and an important symbol of social and economic development. At the same time, unavoidably, there are also many existing and emerging environmental issues which need to be taken seriously. It is up to the Chinese government, businesses and the civil society to transform the challenges into opportunities, to ensure the sustainable development of Chinese urbanization.

References

Adamopoulos, D., Vyssoulis, G., Karpanou, E., *et al.* (2010). Environmental Determinants of Blood Pressure, Arterial Stiffness, and Central Hemodynamics, *Journal of Hypertension* **28**(5): 903–909.

Akinaga, L.M.Y., Lichtenfels, A.J., Carvalho-Oliveira, R., *et al.* (2009). Effects of Chronic Exposure to Air Pollution from Sao Paulo City on Coronary of Swiss Mice, from Birth to Adulthood, *Toxicologic Pathology* **37**(3): 306–314.

Bai, N. (2003). China's Urbanization, *China Urban Economy* **4**: 7–13.

Basheer, C., Obbard, J.P. and Lee, H.K. (2003). Persistent Organic Pollutants in Singapore's Coastal Marine Environment: Part II, Sediments, *Water, Air and Soil Pollution* **149**: 315–323.

Beijing Municipal Bureau of Statistics, NBS Survey Office in Beijing (2011). *Beijing Statistical Yearbook 2010,* China Statistics Press, Beijing.

Beijing Municipal Environmental Monitoring Center (2000–2013). *Noise Monitoring.* Available at http://www.bjmemc.com.cn/g362.aspx (updated November 2014) [Accessed 20 December 2014].

Beijing Municipal Environmental Protection Bureau (updated April 2004). *Air Quality Index.* Available at http://www.bjepb.gov.cn/news/2004-4/200442894307.htm [Accessed 8 August 2014].

Beijing Youth Daily (updated 10 July 2011). *Operating Load Rates of 607 Sewage Treatment Plants are Less than 60%.* Available at http://finance.ifeng.com/roll/20110719/4285897.shtml [Accessed 19 December 2014].

Cai, L.M., Huang, L.C., Zhou, Y.Z., *et al.* (2010). Arsenic Concentrations in Vegetables and Soils in Dongguan and Potential Risk to Human Health, *Environmental Science & Technology* **33**(1): 197–200.

Chen, F. (2009). Review and Prospect of China's Urbanization and Urban Development since 1978, *Planners* **1**: 10–12 (in Chinese).

Chen, R.J., Zhang, J.L. and Kan, H.D. (2011). Review of Chinese Epidemiological Studies of Air Pollution and Lung Cancer, *Journal of Hygiene Research* **40**(2): 243–245.

Chen, S.C. and Liao, C.M. (2006). Health Risk Assessment on Humans Exposed to Environmental Polycyclic Aromatic Hydrocarbons Pollution Sources, *Science of the Total Environment* **366**: 112–123.

Cheng, J.H., Chen, M.Z., Zhang, G.Z., *et al.* (2007). Epidemiologic Investigation on Endemic Arsenicosis of Hezuo City in Gansu Province, *Chinese Journal of Endemiology* **26**(1): 61–63.

Cheng, Y.B., Jin, Y.L., Li, Y.H., *et al.* (2009). Impacts of High Temperature on Death Caused by Cerebrocardiovascular Diseases in Wuhan, *Journal of Environmental Health* **26**(3): 224–225.

Cohen, A.J., Anderson, H.R., Ostro, B., *et al.* (2005). The Global Burden of Disease Due to Outdoor Air Pollution, *Journal of Toxicology and Environmental Health* **68**(13–14): 1301–1307.

Cui, L.L, Shi, J., Yang, Y.M., *et al.* (2008). Temperature Change Characteristics and its Influence by Urbanization in the Yangtze River Delta, *Geographical Research* **27**(4): 775–786.

Cui, Y.C. and Fu, T. (1998). Water Pollution and the Organic Pollutants in the Source of Drinking Water in China, *Urban Environment and Urban Ecology* **3**: 23–25.

Díaz, O. P., Leyton, I., Muñoz, O., *et al.* (2004). Contribution of Water, Bread, and Vegetables (Raw and Cooked) to Dietary Intake of Inorganic Arsenic in a Rural Village of Northern Chile, *Journal of Agricultural and Food Chemistry* **52**(6): 1773–1779.

Feng, H.Y., Fu, X.Q., Zhao, Q., *et al.* (2011). Health Risk Assessment of Polycyclic Aromatic Hydrocarbons in Soils of Ningbo Area, China, *Journal of Agro-Environment Science* **10**: 1998–2004.

Feng, X., Teng, Y.G., Li, J., *et al.* (2011). Residues Characteristics and Health Risk Assessment of PAHs in Soils on the Shore of Songhua River in Jiamusi City, *South-to-North Water Diversion and Water Science & Technology* **3**: 114–117, 123.

Feng, Y., Lu, Y.L., Jiao, W.T., *et al.* (2009). Distribution and Risk of Polycyclic Aromatic Hydrocarbons in Soils from Different Workshops of an Abandoned Coking Factory in Beijing, *Asian Journal of Ecotoxicology* **3**: 399–407.

Gao, H.Y., Cai, X.L. and He, H. (2009). The Impact of Urbanization on the Surface Temperature in Xi'an, *ACTA Geographica Sinica* **64**(9): 1093–1102.

Guan, H., Wang, J.S., Wan, H.F. *et al.* (2007). Content of Nickel in Agricultural Soils and Crops in Leizhou Peninsula and the Potential Risk to Human Health, *Journal of Agro-Environment Science* **4**: 1411–1416.

Guo, H.R., Yu, H.S., Hu, H., *et al.* (2001). Arsenic in Drinking Water and Skin Cancers: Cell-type Specificity (Taiwan, ROC), *Cancer Causes and Control* **12**: 909–916.

Guo, Y.M., Wang, J.J., Li, G.X., *et al.* (2009). Association between Ambient Temperature and Hospital Emergency Room Visits for Cardiovascular Diseases: A Case-Crossover Study, *Chinese Journal of Epidemiology* **30**(8): 810–817.

Hao, J.M., He, D.Q., Wu, Y., *et al.* (2000). A Study of the Emission and Concentration Distribution of Vehicular Pollutants in the Urban Area of Beijing, *Atmospheric Environment* **34**(3): 453–465.

Hao, J.M., Wu, Y., Fu, L.X., *et al.* (2001). Source Contributions to Ambient Concentration of CO and NOx in the Urban Area of Beijing, *Journal of Environmental Science and Health* **36**(2): 215–228.

Hu, H.S., Huang, L., Zhang, X.Y., *et al.* (2004). Effects of Air Quality on the Respiratory System of Pupils, *Journal of Environment and Health* **21**(6): 386–388.

Huang, W., Cao, J., Tao, Y., *et al.* (2012). Seasonal Variation of Chemical Species Associated with Short-Term Mortality Effects of $PM_{2.5}$ In Xi'an, a Central City In China, *American Journal of Epidemiology* **175**(6): 556–566.

Huang, X.X. (2008). Analysis of Correlation and Generalized Estimating Equation for the Relationship between Atmospheric Pollution and Diseases, *China Preventive Medicine* **9**(2): 96–99.

Jia, H., Wu, X.F., Hu, L.M., *et al.* (2012). *In Situ* Experimental Research on Natural Attenuation of Oil Pollutants in a Gas Station, *Environmental Science* **1**: 163–168.

Jiang, Y.Q. (2001). Century Review and Prospect of China's Urbanization, *Seeker* **2**: 27–30 (in Chinese).

Jin, W.Q., Nan, Z.R., Liu, X.W., *et al.* (2010). Specification and Bioavailability Assessment of Cu, Zn and Ni in Agricultural Soils from Jinchang, Gansu, China, *Environmental Chemistry* **2**: 220–225.

Kan, H.D. and Chen, B.H. (2002). 10-Year Review of Effects of Urban Air Pollution on Health in some Chinese Cities, *Journal of Preventive Medicine* **36**(1): 59–61.

Kasprzak, K.S., Sunderman, J.F.W. and Salnikow, K. (2003). Nickel Carcinogenesis, *Mutation Research Fundamental and Molecular Mechanisms of Mutagenesis* **533**(1–2): 67–97.

Li, H. and Wang, T.L. (2012). Historical Stages of China's Urbanization since 1949, *Urban Planning Forum* **6**: 4–13.

Li, J.F., Li, W., Zhang, Y.C., *et al.* (2010). A Laboratory Investigation of a Dysentery Outbreak Caused by Water Pollution in a Primary School, *Chinese Journal of Health Laboratory Technology* **20**(11): 3038–3039.

Li, L.F., Zeng, X.B., Bai, L., *et al.* (2010). Soil Arsenic Content and its Health Risk Assessment for Agricultural Products in the Region

Surrounding Shimen Arsenic, Sulphide Mine, *Chinese Journal of Applied Ecology* **11**: 2946–2951.

Li, N., Peng, X.W., Zhang, B.Y., *et al.* (2009). Relationship between Air Pollutant and Daily Hospital Visits for Respiratory Diseases in Guangzhou: A Time-Series Study, *Journal of Environment and Health* **26**(12): 1077–1080.

Li, Z.C. and Yang, J. (2006). The Analysis of Drinking Water Pollution Accidents in Chengdu in 2005, *Modern Preventive Medicine* **33**(8): 1468–1469.

Li, Z.H. (2009). Discusses the Soil Pollution Infringement in Human Health, *Journal of Environmental Science and Management* **347**: 192–194.

Liang, B.C. and Zhang, C.X. (2003). A Comprehensive Analysis of Typical Drinking Water Contamination Events over the Years in Heze City, *Chinese Journal of Urban and Rural Industrial Hygiene* **4**: 47–48.

Lin, Q. (2004). The Status and Control Countermeasures of Soil Pollution in China, *Fujian Soil and Water Conservation* **6**(1): 25–28.

Liu, Y.H., Zhang, P. and Gao, X.J. (2009). China's Urban Noise Pollution and the Characteristics of the Status, *Environmental Monitoring in China* **25**(4): 88–90.

Liu, Y.J., Zhang, X.M., Shen, Z., *et al.* (2002). Analysis of 195 Drinking Water Pollution Accidents in Beijing, *China Preventive Medicine* **3**: 136–138.

Lu, C. (2003). Association between Upper Respiratory Infection and Climate Change in Beijing. *Chinese Journal of Epidemiology* **24**(10): 955–956.

Lu, Y.C., Hu, X.S., Zhao, J.K., *et al.* (2003). The Geographic Information System of Air Pollution and the Mortality of Lung Cancer in Jiangsu Province, *Bulletin of Chinese Cancer* **12**(7): 374–377.

Lu, Y.X. (2008). Significance, Challenges and Strategies of Ecological Civilization Construction. Available at http://www.news.zju.edu.cn/lecture.php?id=24386 [Accessed 22 March 2013].

Mills, N.L., Donaldson, K., Hadoke, P.W., *et al.* (2008). Adverse Cardiovascular Effects of Air Pollution, *Nature Clinical Practice Cardiovascular Medicine* **6**(1): 36–44.

Mills, N.L., Tornqvist, H., Gonzalez, M.C., *et al.* (2007). Ischemic and Thrombotic Effects of Dilute Diesel-Exhaust Inhalation in Men with Coronary Heart Disease, *New England Journal of Medicine* **357**(11): 1075–1082.

Ministry of Environmental Protection of the People's Republic of China (2010). *2009 Report on the State of the Environment in China*, MEPC, Beijing.

Ministry of Environmental Protection of the People's Republic of China (2011). *2010 Report on the State of the Environment in China*, MEPC, Beijing.

Ministry of Environmental Protection of the People's Republic of China (2013). *Beijing Excluded 288 High Polluted Enterprises and Complete 3 Goals of Air Cleaning in 2013.* Available at http://www.zhb.gov.cn/zhxx/hjyw/201312/t20131227_265712.htm (updated 27 December 2013) [Accessed 6 June 2014].

Ministry of Environmental Protection of the People's Republic of China (2004). *Light Vehicle Emission Standards of the People's Republic of China, Stage II.* Available at http://www.mep.gov.cn/gkml/hbb/qt/200910/t20091023_179819.htm [Accessed 14 May 2012].

Ministry of Environmental Protection of the People's Republic of China and Ministry of Land and Resources of the People's Republic of China (2014). *2014 National Survey of Soil Pollution Bulletin*, Beijing.

Ministry of Transport of the People's Republic of China (2011). *China Transport Statistical Yearbook 2010*, China Statistics Press, Beijing.

Ministry of Environmental Protection of the People's Republic of China, National Committee of Standardization (2002). *The Surface Water Environmental Quality Standard of the People's Republic of China, GB3838-2002*, MEPC, Beijing.

Ministry of Environmental Protection of the People's Republic of China, National Committee of Standardization (2012). *Maximum Levels of Contaminants in Foods, GB2762-2012*, MEPC, Beijing.

National Bureau of Statistics (1996). *China Statistical Year Book 1995*, China Statistics Press, Beijing.

National Bureau of Statistics (2001). *China Statistical Year Book 2000*, China Statistics Press, Beijing.

National Bureau of Statistics (2013). *China Statistical Year Book 2012*, China Statistics Press, Beijing.

National Bureau of Statistics (2014). *China Statistical Year Book 2013*, China Statistics Press, Beijing.

National Bureau of Statistics (2015). *China Statistical Year Book 2014*, China Statistics Press, Beijing.

Ni, J.Z., Chen, W.F., Yang, H.Y., *et al.* (2012). Concentrations and Sources of Soil PAHs in Various Functional Zones of Fuzhou City, *Chinese Journal of Environmental Science* **5**: 921–926.

Peng, C., Wang, M.E. and Liao, X.L. (2010). Distribution and Risk Assessment of Polycyclic Aromatic Hydrocarbons in Urban Soils: A Review, *Chinese Journal of Applied Ecology* **2**: 514–522.

Peng, C., Wang, M.E., Ouyang, Z.Y., *et al.* (2012). Characterization and Potential Risks of Polycyclic Aromatic Hydrocarbons in Green Space Soils of Educational Areas in Beijing, *Environmental Science* **2**: 592–598 (in Chinese).

Qiu, B.X. (2006). Urban Water Environmental Situation, Policies and Challenges, *Beijing Water Affairs* **1**: 2–4.

Ren, C.Y., Wu, D.T. and Dong, S.C. (2006). The Influence of Urbanization on the Urban Climate Environment in Northwest China, *Geographical Research* **25**(2): 233–241.

Rom, W.N. and Samet, J.M. (2006). Small Particles with Big Effects, *American Journal of Respiratory and Critical Care Medicine* **173**(4): 365–366.

Shang, Y., Sun, Z., Cao, J., *et al.* (2013). Systematic Review of Chinese Studies of Short-Term Exposure to Air Pollution and Daily Mortality, *Environment International* **54**: 100–111.

Simkhovich, B.Z., Kleinman, M.T. and Kloner, R.A. (2008). Air Pollution and Cardiovascular Injury, Epidemiology, Toxicology, and Mechanisms, *Journal of the American College of Cardiology* **52**(9): 719–726.

State Environmental Protection Administration of China (1995). *Environmental Quality Standard for Soils (GB 15618–1995)*, SEPA, Beijing.

Straif, K., Baan, R., Grosse, Y., *et al.* on behalf of the WHO International Agency for Research on Cancer Monograph Working Group. (2005). Carcinogenicity of Polycyclic Aromatic Hydrocarbons, *The Lancet Oncology* **6**: 931–932.

Sun, C., Chen, Z.L., Bi, C.J., *et al.* (2010). Risk Assessment Arsenic Concentrations of Vegetables and Vegetable Soil in Chongming Island, Shanghai, *European Journal of Soil Science* **5**: 1226–1230.

Tao, H., Tong, J.Y., Shen, Y.H., *et al.* (2011). Association between Daily Mean Air Temperature and Mortality of Respiratory Diseases in Beijing: a Case-Crossover Study, *Journal of Environmental Health* **28**(7): 569–573.

Tao, Y.Q., Zhang, S.Z. and Xue, B. (2010). Bioavailability of Polycyclic Aromatic Hydrocarbons in Soils and its Evaluation Method, *Journal of the Graduate School of the Chinese Academy of Sciences* **4**: 568–576.

The Central People's Government of People's Republic of China (CPGPRC) (2014). *The New Urbanization State Plan* (2014–2020). Available at http://www.gov.cn/gongbao/content/2014/content_2644805.htm (2014.3.17) [Accessed 22 March 2014].

The World Bank (2007). *Cost of Pollution in China: Economic Estimates of Physical Damages.* Available at http://documents.worldbank.org/curated/en/2007/02/7503894/cost-pollution-china-economic-estimates-physical-damages [Accessed 22 March 2014].

Tsuji, J.S., Benson, R., Schoof, R. A., *et al.* (2004). Health effect Levels for Risk Assessment of Childhood Exposure to Arsenic, *Regulatory Toxicology and Pharmacology* **39**(2): 99–110.

Wang, B., Cheng, X. and Zhou, S.N. (2005). The Analysis of Drinking Water Pollution Accidents in Anshan City from 1983 to 2003, *Occupation and Health* **21**(11): 1752–1753.

Wang, J.J. (2006). Status of Domestic River Pollution and Relevant Countermeasures, Liaoning Urban and Rural, *Environmental Science and Technology* **6**. 13–15.

Wang, P.J., Liu L., Li, F.S., *et al.* (2011). Characteristic Distribution of Typical Contaminants in the Soil of a Coking Plant Site in the Southwest of China, *Journal of China Coal Society* **9**: 1587–1592.

Wang, Q., Zhao, Y.C., Qu, W.D., *et al.* (2010). Investigation of Drinking Water Contamination Incidents in China during 1996–2006, *Journal of Environment and Health* **4**(27): 328–331.

Wang, W.Y., Wang, H.Y., Zhang, Z.G., *et al.* (2009). Time-Series Analysis on the Association between Ambient PM10 and Daily Hospital Services, *Journal of Environment and Health* **26**(12): 1069–1072.

Wang, X., Deng, F.R., Lyu, H.B., *et al.* (2011). Long-Term Effects of Air Pollution on the Occurrence of Respiratory Symptoms in Adults of Beijing, *Journal of Peking University (Health Sciences)* **43**(3): 356–359.

Wang, Y.S., Yao, L., Liu, Z.R., *et al.* (2013). Formation of Haze Pollution in Beijing-Tianjin-Hebei Region and Their Control Strategies, *Bulletin of Chinese Academy of Sciences* **3**: 353–363.

Xie, Z.Q., Du, Y., Zeng, Y., *et al.* (2007). Impact of Urbanization on Regional Temperature Change in the Yangtze River Delta, *ACTA Geographica Sinica* **62**(7): 717–727.

Xu, Y.S. (2002). *In-Situ* Remediation of Contaminated Soils for Former Manufactured Gas Plant, *Gas & Heat* **1**: 60–62.

Yang, G., Wang, Y., Zeng, Y., *et al.* (2013). Rapid Health Transition in China, 1990–2010: Findings from the Global Burden of Disease Study 2010, *The Lancet* **381**(9882): 1987–2015.

Yang, H., Zhong, G.M., Tang, Z.Z., *et al.* (2006). Investigation on drinking water polluting status and its influence factors of middle boarding schools and primary boarding schools in urban and rural region of Guangxi, *Journal of Applied Preventive Medicine* **12**(6): 341–344.

Yang, M.J. and Pan, X.C. (2008). Time-Series Analysis of Air Pollution and Cardiovascular Mortality in Beijing, China, *Journal of Environmental Health* **25**(4): 294–297.

Yang, T., Zhang, Y., Mai, H., *et al.* (2008). An Investigation and Analysis of Paratyphoid Outbreak in a School Caused by the Water Source Pollution, *Journal of Community Medicine* **6**(11): 37–38.

Yang, Y., Li, R., Li, W., *et al.* (2013). The Association between Ambient Air Pollution and Daily Mortality in Beijing after the 2008 Olympics: A Time Series Study, *PlOS One* **8**(10): e76759.

Yu, G.G., Zhang, Z.H., Ye, X.Z., *et al.* (2009). PAHs in Topsoil of Hangzhou Suburb, *Ecology and Environmental Sciences* **18**(3): 925–928.

Zhang, G.Q., Wang, N., Wang, T., *et al.* (2009). Influence of Tobacco Consumption and Air Pollution on Lung Cancer Mortality of Permanent Residents in Beijing Urban Area, *Journal of Environment and Health* **26**(8): 666–669.

Zhang, H.J., Du, Z.C., Li, Z.X., *et al.* (2002). Hazard Compounds and Elements of Dusts from Handan City, *Journal of Hebei Institute of Architectural Science and Technology* **1**: 1–4.

Zhang, H.Y., Gao, R.T., Jiang, S.R. *et al.* (2006). Spatial Variability of Organochlorine Pesticides (DDTs and HCHs) in Surface Soils of Farmland in Beijing, China, *Scientia Agricultura Sinica* **397**: 1403–1410.

Zhang, Y., Tao, S., Shen, H., *et al.* (2009). Inhalation Exposure to Ambient Polycyclic Aromatic Hydrocarbons and Lung Cancer Risk of Chinese Population, *Proceedings of the National Academy of Sciences* **106**(50): 21063–21067.

Zhang, Y.C., Yu, L.H., Wang, P.J., *et al.* (2012). Vertical Distribution of Typical Contaminants at a Coking Plant Site in China, *Journal of China Coal Society* 7: 1211–1218.

Zhao, K., Cao, J.J., and Wen, X.M. (2011). Correlation between PM2.5 Pollution in Air and Mortality of Residents in Urban Area, Xi'an, *Journal of Preventive Medicine Information* **27**(4): 257–262.

Zhao, L.R, Sun, S.L. and Ke, S. (2012). Characteristics and Sources of Polysyclic Aromatic Hydrocarbons in Soils Different in Land Use in Zhanjiang City, *Acta Pedologica Sinica* **4**: 830–834.

Zhao, Y., Zang, Z.Y., Shen, K., *et al.* (2012). Health Risk Assessment on the Site Contaminated by Organochlorine Pesticide, *Journal of Hebei University (Natural Science Edition)* **1**: 33–41.

Zheng, Y., Pan, J.H., Zheng, Z.F., *et al.* (2006). Co-Integration Analysis of Urbanization and Urban Warming in Beijing, *China Population Resources and Environment* **16**(2): 63–69.

Zhi, H.M. (2005). Coking Industry and Environmental Protection, *Sci-Tech Information Development & Economy* **15**(24): 119–121.

Zhou, F.L., Jiang, Q.Y., and Yang, J.Z. (2004). Survey of Water Source Pollution the Waterworks in the Western Suburbs of Guiyang and Infectious Diseases of Residents Surrounding, *Literature and Information of Preventive Medicine* **10**(3): 287–288.

Zhou, H.C. and Li, X. (2010). Research on China's Urbanization and its Environmental Sustainability, *Journal of Nanjing University (Philosophy, Humanities and Social Sciences)* **47**(4): 66–75.

Zou, D. (2004). Viewpoints Concerned with the Urbanization of China's Countryside Towns, *Urban Planning Forum* **3**: 3–5 (in Chinese).

Chapter Twelve

Case Study: Improving Population Health in a Rapidly Urbanizing World: Are Older Chinese People Ready to Adapt to Climate Change?

Ying Zhang, Jin Na Wang, Wei Ma, Monika Nitschke, Alana Hansen, Peng Bi and Bao Fa Jiang

Abstract

Climate change has been called the biggest global health challenge in the 21st century. The latest Assessment Report from the Intergovernmental Panel on Climate Change has once again confirmed the increasing trend in global temperatures, and it is very likely that heatwaves will occur more frequently and with more severe impacts (IPCC, 2013). Another fact of the 21st century is that populations are aging, and it is the aged who are the most vulnerable during extreme heat events. Moreover, rapid urban development may significantly increase the exposure to climate change and the health impact of heatwaves on older people. This chapter, based on our quantitative and qualitative research on climate change adaptation among older people in rural and urban regions in China, explores older people's perceptions and behavior changes in response to climate change and extreme heat. We have also engaged stakeholders relevant to aging health to identify barriers to better climate change adaptation. It aims to assist policy and decision-making to improve the quality of life for older people living within the changing environment. Implications and recommendations are summarized at the end of the chapter.

12.1 Rationale

This chapter addresses two of the biggest public health issues of the 21st century, climate change and healthy aging, in the context of urbanization. A higher speed of economic development in China comes with a huge cost to the environment and health. Current development patterns and human activities are creating a range of new challenges to public health. Many of the most important cases are related to environmental change. Climate change and urbanization are two clear examples.

There is consensus in the scientific community that the climate has been changing and will continue to change. In the newly released Intergovernmental Panel on Climate Change (IPCC) Fifth Assessment Report confirms the global warming trend, and, if no fundamental mitigation to greenhouse gas emissions is achieved, the global average temperature may increase 3° to 4°C by 2100 (IPCC, 2013). Urbanization can affect climate through the emission of atmosphere pollutants, the heat island effect and changes in land use (Ding and Qian, 2011). Significant urbanization effects on climate have been evident in previous research. Zhou *et al.* (2004) reported that warming of mean surface temperature of 0.05°C per decade could be attributable to urbanization in China. Zhan *et al.*, (2013) provides strong current evidence that urbanization has had a significant impact on the regional climate of the Beijing–Tianjin–Tangshan Metropolitan area.

With its unprecedented economic growth, China has been witnessing a dramatic growth in urbanization since 1978 when economic reform began. Statistics from the Ministry of Construction of China show that urbanization increased from 17.9% in 1978 to 53.7% in

2013, demonstrating a growth rate twice as fast as the rest of the world (Ministry of Land and Resources of China, 2014). Accelerated urbanization and economic growth have further increased the shortage of agricultural land over the last two decades. Since 1978, there has been a massive transfer of agricultural land to various uses in southeast China due to the rapid urban sprawl. China is facing a serious challenge from the poor soil quality of its arable land. Growing urbanization may further threaten food security, soil diversity, and sustainability. This situation could be worsened by climate change and other environmental degradation in China.

Human health ultimately depends upon the ecosystem's products and services, including clean water, fresh air and sufficient food to support more than seven billion people living on Earth. Climate change will have the greatest effect on health in societies that are already vulnerable due to a lack of resources, little technology, and poor infrastructure (Kjellstrom and McMichael, 2013). The most vulnerable are in developing countries. Climate change would exacerbate inequalities between and within countries. The adverse health outcomes from warming temperature and extreme heat may include conditions that are directly related to higher temperature, for example heat exhaustion and heat stroke, as well as diseases without a heat-related diagnosis but which can be exacerbated by extreme heat, such as ischemic heart disease and renal failure.

Another fact of the 21st century is that populations are aging. China is the only country with more than 100 million older people (60 years or older) and is the world's fastest aging country. In 2050, it is projected there will be 440 million older people in China (one in three). However, China is not ready to be an aging society, having as it does, a very low proportion of pension funds (2% of GDP) allocated to the support of older people (CEPAR, 2013). The elderly are among the most affected by a changing climate. There is notable consistency in the findings of previous research that older people are at a greater risk during extreme heat events (Astrom *et al.*, 2011; Kovats and Hajat, 2008). For example, significantly elevated risks of hospitalization due to heat-related illnesses were observed in the older population during the 2006 California heatwave (Knowlton *et al.*,

2009). In China, the 2003 heatwave in Shanghai caused a 19% increase in cardiovascular mortality, mainly in the older population (Huang *et al.*, 2010). Contributing factors to heat intolerance in the aged may include not only an age-related decline in general health status but also other physiological, socio–economic, and environmental factors, for example multiple pre-existing conditions, medication use, poor living conditions and insufficient social support (Hansen *et al.*, 2011a).

Adaptation and mitigation are two important strategies for responding to climate change, as highlighted in the latest IPCC Assessment Report (IPCC, 2013). Mitigation is used to 'avoid the unmanageable'. It aims to reduce greenhouse gases (GHS) in the atmosphere, either by reducing their sources or increasing their sinks. The long-term importance of mitigation is critical as the degree to which global climatic conditions will change is subject to the mitigation efforts that can be made in the near future. Some mitigation measures include policies and legislation to reduce GHS emissions, for example, carbon pricing in many countries and the adoption of new technologies, such as renewable energy. There are some co-benefits from climate change mitigation activities in addition to the benefit of reducing carbon emissions. For example, planning to replace the use of private cars in urban areas with active travel modes, such as walking and cycling, will result in the co-benefits of improving air quality and reducing obesity, thus improving health overall.

However, even in the most optimistic mitigation scenarios, there are projections for significant changes to climatic conditions, particularly over the next 50 to 100 years. This means that mitigation will not reverse existing global warming. Individuals and communities will need to adapt to these changes to avoid adverse consequences. Adaptation is used to 'manage the unavoidable'. There are different types of adaptations, for example active and passive adaptations. It is recognized that collective efforts from government at all levels, communities and individuals are essential to better adapt to climate change. In the health sector, better adaptation means reducing adverse health outcomes caused by climate and environmental change. The aim of adaptation is to reduce vulnerability. The IPCC describes vulnerability to climate change as being determined by three factors: exposure to risks, sensitivity to those risks, and the capacity to adapt to those risks (IPCC, 2013). Adaptation measures can help reduce vulnerability by lowering sensitivity or building up adaptive capacity in the community. Better adaptation means increasing the ability to adjust, to take opportunities and to cope with the consequences faster and more effectively. The interactions among climate change mitigation, adaptation, and disaster risk management may have significant influence on resilient and sustainable pathways. In addition, as pointed out in the IPCC report, interactions between the goals of mitigation and adaptation will play out locally, but have global consequences.

The health impact of heatwaves on the elderly could be reduced if there is better adaptation, for example, recognizing the risks and adopting healthy behaviors during a heatwave (Bassil and Cole, 2010). However, even with increased resilience, substantial risks of heat-related mortality remain, due to more extreme heat exposures (Bobb *et al.*, 2014). Adaptive strategies from stakeholders and sufficient support from carers may help reduce potential risks of extreme temperatures, including excess deaths and hospitalizations. However, there is insufficient research on barriers to better adaptation of the elderly in China.

In China, although there is a national committee to coordinate climate change actions, little attention has been paid to the health consequences of extreme heat or to the exploration of relevant adaptive strategies. Our study aims to examine both the barriers to and enablers of adaptation to extreme heat events, by engaging stakeholders and older persons in both rural and urban areas in China in order to gain a better understanding of their perceptions of the relationship between heatwaves and health, and to document changes in their behavior during heatwaves.

12.2 Procedure

We conducted a cross-sectional survey, using both qualitative and quantitative methods, in rural and urban areas in Shandong Province, China. Located in northern China, Shandong is the province with the largest elderly population in China, having more than 15 million residents over 60 years of age, accounting for 14.3% of its total population

(National Bureau of Statistics of China, 2011). It is projected that this figure will increase to 22%, that is, 22 million by 2050 (Hansen *et al.*, 2011b). The province also has very high maximum and minimum temperatures during summer, and is frequently hit by heatwaves, particularly in the selected study sites as described below.

12.2.1 *Quantitative study*

12.2.1.1 *Sampling of subjects*

The selected study areas in Shandong Province all have a temperate climate with four distinct seasons. The summers are very hot with the average maximum temperatures above 32°C between June and August, with frequent heatwaves. In winter, it snows with the average minimum temperature below — 2°C between December and February. A heat wave is defined in this study as having three or more consecutive days with a maximum temperature above the 95 percentile of the average maximum temperature over the last 10 years, based on meteorological data from the local Bureau of Meteorology. All selected locations were in the inland areas of Shandong Province because the peninsula areas do not usually have heatwaves. The study sites included urban and rural areas. Over the last decades, there has been a clear increasing trend in the frequency, duration and intensity of the heatwaves in the study sites. The total number of heatwaves in the last 10 summers in Jinan city, the capital city of Shandong Province was 34, with half of these occurring during the last three years. The occurrence of heatwaves in the rural areas followed a similar trend. In addition, heatwaves have occurred more often in the early part of summer, with a longer duration and record-breaking maximum temperatures in prolonged extreme heat events. For example, in the urban area of Jinan, the summer in 2010 was dramatic, with four heatwaves identified, resulting in excess deaths and hospitalizations due to heat stroke. The urban sample in this study covers all four districts in the metropolitan area of Jinan. The rural areas are the villages of Binzhou, Laiwu, Jining, and Weifang, as shown in Figure 12.1.

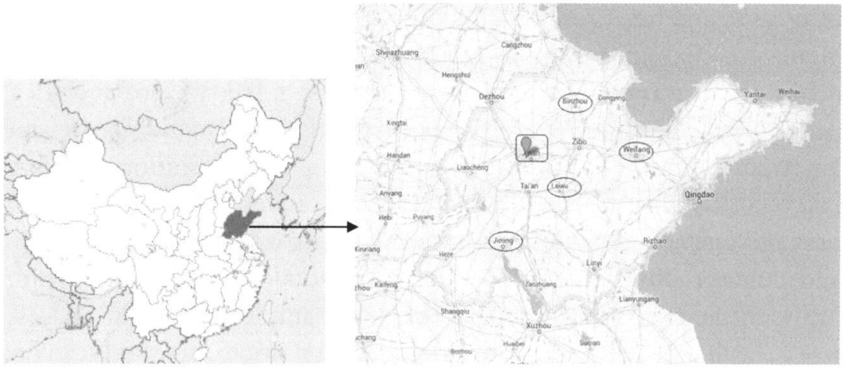

Figure 12.1 Map of study locations in urban and rural areas in Shandong Province (indicated in the left map), China.[1]

[1]In the map on the right, the square indicates the location of Jinan city. The other four circled areas are the four villages in the rural sample.

The participants were randomly selected using a two-stage cluster sampling method at the municipal and the county levels. To recruit eligible participants, interviewers were stationed at seven study sites in the four districts of Jinan city and one study site in each village of the four counties (11 study sites in total). Those who had lived in the study regions for less than one year were not included. The study population were the residents of the selected urban and rural areas who were aged 60 years and over at the time of the survey.

12.2.1.2 *Data collection*

Face-to-face questionnaire-based interviews were conducted in the late summer of 2012. The interviewers were postgraduate epidemiology students who were trained before the field survey for consistency in urban and rural data collection. The questionnaire used was a modified Chinese version of a questionnaire previously used for a similar survey conducted by the research team in Australia, and was designed based on stakeholder engagement (Hansen *et al.*, 2011a). Questions regarding older people's perceptions and attitudes towards heatwaves and health, their behaviors during heatwaves and their willingness to change (for example, to call for help during heatwaves and hence have a higher likelihood of receiving help) were included. Additionally, questions related to contributing factors to heat-related illnesses, including symptoms during heatwaves, medication use, general health status, social activities (defined as regular leisure, recreation and cultural activities and regular contact with friends and family) and demographic information, were included in the questionnaire. No identified personal information, for example name and address, was collected for this quantitative study. All participants signed a consent form before the interview started. A small gift was given to each participant following a completed survey.

12.2.1.3 *Statistical analysis*

The characteristics of the participants were stratified by urban and rural areas respectively. Chi square tests were used to examine the significance of the comparison between the two areas in terms of their characteristics. Logistic regressions were applied to test the difference in perceptions and behaviors between the groups, controlling for identified confounders. Stepwise backward logistic regressions were also applied to quantify contributing factors for having at least one of the self-reported symptoms (anxiety, loss of balance/dizziness, a fall, headache, shortness of breath, heat stress, heart condition, renal condition, or other health issues that the participant thought were related to heat) during heatwaves in urban and rural areas, respectively. All analyses were performed using STATA v11.0 (Stata Corp LP, College Station, TX).

12.2.2 *Qualitative study*

Theoretical sampling was applied according to the method of Draucker *et al.*, (2007). Participants in the survey were asked if they would be willing to participate in an interview after completing the questionnaire. Respondents from the community who agreed to participate included 20 individuals over 60 years of age with diverse socio–economic backgrounds. Stakeholders included a doctor and a nurse from a private nursing home and a public nursing home, a government officer from the local Committee of Aging, and three public health practitioners from the local Centers for Disease Prevention and Control (CDC). Face-to-face in-depth interviews were conducted with each participant. Recruitment ceased when no new themes could be identified. Conversations were recorded with informed consent. Recorded data were transcribed into texts and then translated into English. Data were analyzed by text-based thematic qualitative method, aided by Nvivo9 (QRS International).

12.2.3 *Ethical statement*

The study, including both quantitative and qualitative components, was approved by the Human Research Ethical Committee at the University of Adelaide in Australia and the School of Public Health at Shandong University in China.

12.3 Findings

12.3.1 *The quantitative survey*

To reach the target sample size of the survey with a 5% margin of error, a 95% confidence level and at least a 70% response rate, it was estimated that 1200 participants would be required, with half being from rural areas. Consequently, there was in total 1208 valid questionnaires collected with 600 of the participants from the rural areas, with a participation rate of 90%. The characteristics of the study population were very different in many aspects between the rural and urban groups.

The rural group was older than the urban group (12% over 80 years vs. 8% $p < 0.001$), comprised fewer females (50% vs. 57%, $p < 0.05$), and had a lower annual household income (63% $<$ 12000 RMB vs. 10%, $p < 0.001$). The rural group had poorer self-reported health status than the urban group (45% fair/poor vs. 32%, $p < 0.001$), a lower education level (52% had no schooling vs. 9%, $p < 0.001$), more lived alone (20% vs. 7%, $p < 0.001$), and fewer had air-conditioning at home (5% vs. 84%, $p < 0.001$). Additionally, fewer rural respondents reported taking medicines and had significantly fewer social contacts during the week prior to the survey (Table 12.1). These factors were controlled for in the further comparison between the two groups.

Table 12.1 Characteristics of the study populations and the comparison between the urban and rural areas

	Urban % (95% CI)	Rural % (95% CI)	*P*
Age			
60–69 years	68.59(64.89,72.28)	57.83(53.87,61.79)	<0.001
70–79 years	23.03(19.67,26.38)	30.00(26.33,33.67)	
80+ years	8.39(6.18,10.60)	12.17(9.55,14.79)	
Gender (female)	56.79(52.83,60.75)	49.42(45.40,53.43)	0.010
Annual household income (RMB)			
<12,000	9.74 (7.03,12.45)	62.71(58.78,66.65)	<0.001
12,001–30,000	16.23(12.86,19.60)	30.76(27.00,34.51)	
30,001–50,000	33.33(29.03,37.64)	5.33(3.50,7.15)	
50,001–80,000	29.44(25.27,33.60)	0.86(0.18,1.61)	
>80,000	11.26(8.37,14.14)	0.34(0,0.82)	
Self-reported health status			
Excellent, very good or good	68.09(64.38,71.80)	55.00(51.01,58.99)	<0.001
Fair or poor	31.91(28.20,35.62)	45.00(41.01,48.99)	
Highest education level			
No school	8.55(6.33,10.78)	51.83(47.83,55.84)	<0.001
Primary school	12.83(10.17,15.49)	29.67(26.00,36.33)	
Secondary school	60.86(56.97,64.74)	18.17(15.08,21.26)	
Tertiary education	17.76(14.72,20.81)	0.33(0,0.80)	

(*Continued*)

Table 12.1 (*Continued*)

	Urban % (95% CI)	Rural % (95% CI)	*P*
Living status			
Lives alone	7.469(5.33,9.58)	19.43(16.25,22.61)	<0.001
Air-conditioning at home	83.8(80.86,86.74)	5.03(3.27,6.78)	<0.001
Medication taken for:			
Diabetes	8.55(6.33,10.78)	3.33(1.89,4.77)	<0.001
Heart diseases	11.68(9.12,14.24)	7.67(5.53,9.80)	0.018
Respiratory diseases	1.64(0.63,2.66)	4.83(3.11,6.55)	0.002
Social contacts during the last week			
No phone calls	18.09(15.27,21.16)	37.00(33.13,40.87)	<0.001
No visits	3.5(2.03,4.97)	8.55(6.33,10.78)	<0.001
No going out	1.32(0.41,2.22)	11.67(9.09,14.24)	<0.001

When asked how much they were concerned about their own health during heatwaves, 73% from the rural group and 63% from the urban group reported having little or no concern at all ($p > 0.05$). Their main concerns during heatwaves were the health of their family members, with differences identified between the rural and urban areas. There was a significantly higher proportion of rural older people worried about their own health, how to cope, pets, plants, inconvenience, and duration of heat, while more urban older people worried about the related extra costs and about water use restrictions during heatwaves (Figure 12.2).

The majority of the participants reported that they changed behaviors in order to respond to extreme heat, and the most commonly adopted adaptive behaviors for rural older people were wearing light clothes (93%), reducing time outdoors (73%) and staying indoors (72%); for urban older people these were staying indoors (84%), wearing light clothes (79%), and reducing physical activities (58%). In addition, there were some significant differences in the proportion of

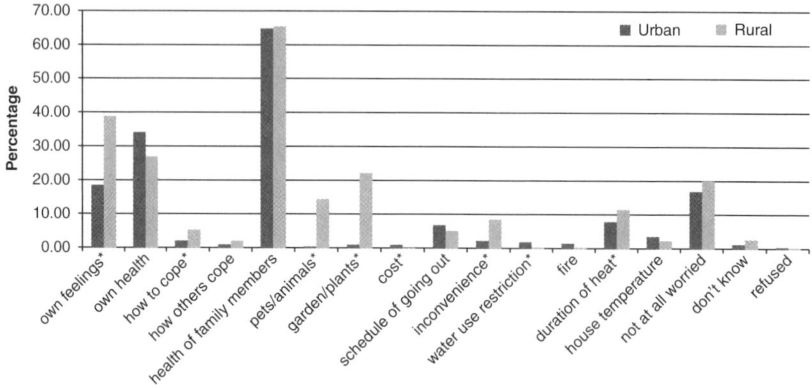

Figure 12.2 Concerns during heatwaves in older people and the comparison between the urban and rural areas.

*Comparison between rural and urban areas with $p < 0.05$.

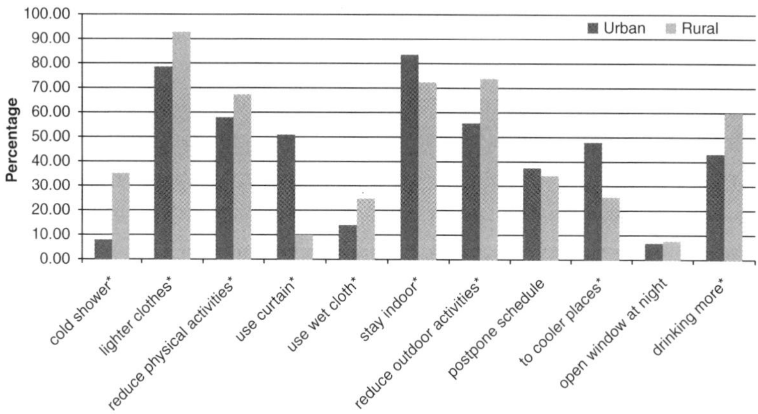

Figure 12.3 Self-reported behaviors adopted most of the time during heatwaves by older people and comparison between the urban and rural areas.

*Comparison between rural and urban areas with $p < 0.05$.

people undertaking any of the adaptive behaviors listed in Figure 12.3. This shows that during a heatwave, older people in the rural areas were more likely to undertake more adaptive behaviors than their urban counterparts.

As shown in Table 12.2, there was significantly less support for the rural older population. A higher proportion of the rural elderly received no phone calls compared to their urban counterparts (52% vs. 30%, $p < 0.001$) and no visits (59% vs. 48%, $p < 0.001$) during heatwaves. The majority of the urban and rural older population indicated that they were willing to call for help during heatwaves, particularly

Table 12.2 Responses to questions about support and resources received regarding heatwaves and health, and comparison between the urban and rural areas

	Urban % (95% CI)	Rural % (95% CI)	*P*
Support			
No phone calls during heatwaves	29.61(25.97,33.24)	52(48,56)	<0.001
No visits during heatwaves	47.87(43.82,51.92)	58.78(54.81,62.76)	<0.001
Willingness to call for help	84.05(81.13,86.96)	69(65.29,72.71)	<0.001
Whom to call for help			
Spouse	65.95(62.18,69.73)	60.33(56.41,64.25)	0.043
Other family members	64.80(61.00,68.61)	65.33(61.52,69.15)	0.847
Doctor/hospital	6.41(4.46,8.37)	31.17(27.45,34.88)	<0.001
Friend	4.77(3.07,6.47)	1.00(0.2,1.8)	<0.001
Neighbor	2.47(1.23,3.70)	5.00(3.25,6.75)	0.002
Unsure	3.62(2.13,5.11)	1.17(3.06,2.03)	0.005
Warnings			
Recalled heatwave messages/warnings	58.04(54.10,61.99)	37.71(33.29,41.04)	<0.001
At least some recall of the messages about how to maintain good health in the heat	46.05(42.08,50.02)	29.17(25.52,32.81)	<0.001
Where were the messages received			
Television	91.53(88.61,94.44)	92.89(89.52,96.26)	0.554
Radio	32.77(27.86,37.68)	16.89(11.97,21.81)	<0.001
Newspaper	22.32(17.96,26.66)	0.89(0,2.12)	<0.001

(*Continued*)

Table 12.2 (*Continued*)

	Urban % (95% CI)	Rural % (95% CI)	*P*
Family/friends	8.47(5.56,11.39)	35.11(28.85,41.37)	<0.001
Mobile service/SMS	7.06(4.38,9.74)	0.89(0,2.12)	0.001
Internet	3.11(1.29,4.92)	0	0.008
Willingness to change behaviors according to warnings			
No	12.99(10.14,15.83)	18.46(15.31,21.61)	<0.001
Sometimes	46.75(42.53,50.97)	37.26(33.34,41.19)	
Yes	39.70(35.56,43.84)	34.19(30.34,38.04)	
Don't know	0	10.09(7.64,12.53)	
Best means of receiving heat-health information			
Television	81.68(78.60,84.77)	93.37(91.35,95.38)	<0.001
Radio	2.97(1.62,4.32)	3.74(2.20,5.28)	
Newspaper	1.16(0.30,2.01)	0	
Mails	0	0	
Internet	0.99(0.20,1.78)	0.17(0,0,50)	
SMS	10.23(7.81,12.65)	1.53(0.54,2.52)	

from their family members. However, there was a significantly higher proportion of rural older people indicating that they were likely to call a doctor and a hospital compared to the urban group (31% vs. 6%, $p < 0.001$). In terms of the messages regarding heatwave and health, TV was the major and preferred means to receive relevant information for both rural and urban groups. Significantly, fewer older people from the rural areas could recall messages about heatwaves and health, and fewer rural older people indicated that they were willing to make changes according to the messages.

Logistic regression models in Table 12.3 show that for the urban older people, taking no medication, using a fan, being willing to call for help and having social activities, could significantly reduce the reported symptoms during heatwaves by 66% (51–76%), 27%

Table 12.3 Logistic regression results showing significant factors contributing to having any symptom during heatwaves

	Odds Ratio	SE	95% CI
Urban			
Taking no medication	0.34	0.63	(0.24,0.49)
Fan use	0.73	0.08	(0.59,0.90)
Willingness to call for help	0.76	0.58	(0.65,0.88)
Having social activities	0.51	0.14	(0.29,0.88)
Rural			
Taking no medication	0.34	0.07	(0.23,0.51)
Poor health status	1.85	0.38	(1.24,2.76)
Go to cooler places in heatwaves	0.57	0.11	(0.38,0.83)
No phone calls in heatwaves	3.83	2.00	(1.37,10.66)
Having concerns about heatwaves	0.41	0.10	(0.25,0.67)
Having social activities	0.13	0.11	(0.025,0.67)

(10–41%), 24% (12–35%) and 49% (12–71%), respectively. For the rural older people, poor health status and receiving no phone calls during the heat may increase morbidity by 85% (24–176%) and 280% (37–970%) respectively. However, people taking no medication, going to cooler places, having concerns about heatwave or having social activities had a reduction in the likelihood of heat-related symptoms of 66% (49–77%), 43% (17–62%), 59% (33–75%) and 87% (33–97%) respectively. Other factors, for example the level of education and income, self-reported health status and medication-indicated co-morbidities were not significantly included in the final models for both groups.

12.3.2 *The qualitative interviews*

The mean age of the participating elderly from the urban and rural regions was 72 (range 65–86): 47% were female, 47% had education levels lower than middle school, and 53% had been local residents for more than 30 years. The barriers identified from the individual older people and the stakeholders, as well as some selected typical quotes from the interviews, are summarized in Table 12.4.

Table 12.4 Barriers for the Chinese elderly to better adaptation to extreme heat, identified from the qualitative interview

Themes	Sub-themes	Example quotes from participants
Barriers identified from the individual elderly		
Lack of concern	Believe climate is getting warmer (mainly based on personal experiences) but not concerned very much about their own health for various reasons	"The climate has definitely changed as I don't need to wear very thick cotton-padded coat like in old days." — F, 75, Rural "I used to believe global warming because last year's summer was very hot but now I am not sure because this year's winter is too cold". — F, 68, Rural "We are all much affected and I am not particularly weaker than others."—M, 70, Rural "I don't think I will be affected by the heat as I have air-conditioning at home, although I try to avoid turning it on." — F, 72, Urban "I have a better economic situation than the average so that I am not worry about myself during the heat." — M, 73, Urban "I am not worried about myself in hot days and don't need any help." — M, 73, Rural
	A high level of concern about other relevant issues even if they don't know they may be related to climate change	"There are many other things far more important than climate change and heat, such as environmental pollution, more cars on the road, crowd buses." — F, 67, Urban "If you ask me about food safety, I can tell you more." — F, 62, Urban "I believe that using more solar panels will solve lots of environmental problems." — M, 76, Urban "I care about my animals and crops when the weather is getting crazy." — M, 70, Rural

(*Continued*)

Table 12.4 (*Continued*)

Themes	Sub-themes	Example quotes from participants
Lack of knowledge	The understanding of climate change/heatwaves and their health impacts is very limited	"I have never heard about 'heatwave' … Is it a wave from the sea? I know nothing about its impact.""— F, 69, Urban; and many other participants "A heatwave is a wave from the sea and I guess only those live along the beach can be affected" — F, 72, Rural; F, 75, Urban; M, 68, Rural "I've heard about climate change but it seems not relevant to me and my life at all." — M, 70, Urban
	Do have some behavior changes for adaptation without understanding the association with reducing health risks	"I will go to the market in early morning if it is going to be very hot." — F, 65, Urban "I will take a cold shower if weather is very hot." — M, 73, Rural "I will reduce the outdoor activities and stay in the room if it is too hot out there." — F, 64, Urban "I always take a bottle of water for me and my grandson when we go out on hot days." — M, 75, Urban
Lack of support	Lack of sufficient and appropriate information for adaptation, particularly in rural regions	"I watch weather forecast every day on TV and sometimes it tells me what to wear."— F, 70, Urban "I have not received any information about health and climate change at all."— F, 65, Rural "We rural older people are used to the hot weather and don't need any extra help. We can look after ourselves." — M, 69, Rural
	Lack of support from family members, neighbours and local community	"My children are all very busy and only come back home once a year." — M, 67, Rural "I don't know who else is living in this building and I shall not talk too much to my neighbours." — F, 65, Urban "No one would find me if I die at home … and I can't think about it."— F, 77, Urban

(*Continued*)

Table 12.4 (*Continued*)

Themes	Sub-themes	Example quotes from participants
		"My daughter paid my mobile phone but I don't know how to use it." — F, 78, Rural "In my village, many young people are working in cities left many 'empty nest' elderly." — F, 62, Rural
	Lack of support from government and health professionals	"I have never ever heard about doctors talking about climate change and heat when I was seeing them."— M, 73, Urban "No one from the government would think of older people like me." — M, 75, Rural "I can't contribute to any policies that are relevant to older people … They would never ask me (laugh)." — F, 72, Urban "No one told me what steps I should take in an emergency." — F, 77, Rural
Lack of trust	Recognising the challenges in response to climate change/ extreme heat	"It would be very difficult for the government to do anything like other things the government faces." — M, 65, Urban "Shared responsibility between transportation, health, weather bauera, etc, is necessary … this is what I heard from the media." — M, 65, Urban "More reforms may be needed, more than what they (government) said." — M, 65, Urban
	The *dilemma*: very low trust for the government but with high expectations	"Increase public awareness of both ageing society and climate change is the responsibility of government." — F, 65, Urban "Only the government has the will to do something, we may achieve some outcomes." — F, 82, Urban "I doubt the government will do anything serious about climate change as it will affect our economic development … look at the bad air quality we still have regardless what the government says" — M, 73, Urban

(*Continued*)

Table 12.4 (*Continued*)

Themes	Sub-themes	Example quotes from participants
		"I don't expect the government can do something that will change our life dramatically … Our life is already very tough." — M, 66, Rural
Barriers identified from the stakeholders		
Lack of concern and knowledge	No up-to-date knowledge and no motivation to have a better understanding	"To let the people understand the health impacts from climate change is very challenging … and media plays a major role in disseminating knowledge."— CDC "The public don't understand (environment risks) and they are used to the poor environment condition … my child doesn't know that colour clean sky should appear as she has never seen." — CDC "It is true that some diseases peak at some time of the year, which may be related to short changes of seasons … As for a long-term climate change, there won't be any impact on older people."— A doctor in a public nursing home "I believe climate change but the issue has been overstated at the moment and there are lots of disbelieving discussions." — A doctor "Climate change is a topic that developed country used to hinder the development in developing countries." — Committee of Ageing "We are aware of the health impact of season variations on older people. They are particularly scared of 'cold winter' but not 'hot summer'."— An owner of a private nursing home "I 'should' believe as newspapers said so. But more concerned about changes of seasons." — A nurse of a private nursing home

(*Continued*)

Table 12.4 (*Continued*)

Themes	Sub-themes	Example quotes from participants
No commitment	Not a work priority	"There are more emergent and more important issues to consider for elderly." — Committee of Ageing "NO quality data/evidence to support the association between environmental risks, climate change and NCDs in older population, which is because it is not a major risk factor for NCDs, and our work is focusing on life styles." — CDC "The government did not take his responsibility in aged care." — Committee of Age "Developing countries are actually living with a low carbon life. We don't have enough money to do everything." — Committee of Age
	Short of resources/ staff	"We have a lot of work to do and really no extra funding and time to think about how to response to climate change at present." — CDC "Re public health sector, based on my own experience, there is a lack of concern, due to limited resources."— CDC "We are short of funding even though we really want to do the health promotion. We also need a national project." — A doctor
	No coordination	"Whom we shall work with if we want to do something?" — Committee of Ageing & CDC
No specific strategies	No guidelines, no clear responsibility	"Our institute does not have any relevant policy or action plan to deal with climate change specifically." — CDC "I haven't thought about strategies at a macro-level, but I think health education and providing timely, necessary medical assistance to the elderly is the key." — A doctor

(*Continued*)

Table 12.4 (*Continued*)

Themes	Sub-themes	Example quotes from participants
		"We are at the stage of "complaining", we haven't started doing anything for climate change, which may be a neglect of our duty." — CDC
Lack of preparation	No forward-thinking to be better prepared for climate change and extremes and specifically focused on elderly	"We don't have any particular preparation for summers as we are living in the mountain area and summer is usually not bad for older people here." — An owner of a private nursing home "Government is always 'bureaucratic' and gives 'lip services', regardless what kind of health promotion projects has been announced."— A doctor "We do have projects for elderly's health promotion. We don't have projects for climate change and not linked them together." — Committee of Ageing. "But health sector has not paid enough attention to this environmental issue, even though more frequent weather extremes are experienced locally." — CDC

The barriers identified at an individual level mainly included: firstly a lack of concern, that is not being concerned about their health even though they believed the climate was getting warmer and more concerned about other issues, for example air pollution and food safety; secondly a lack of knowledge, that is limited understanding of climate change and heatwaves and their health impact and adopting behavior changes without knowing the underlying reasons; thirdly a lack of support from family, local community, health professionals and government, particularly in rural areas; and finally a lack of trust in, and a higher expectation of, the government.

The main barriers to adaptation identified by stakeholders from institutions/organizations included: firstly a lack of concern and knowledge, and no motivation to change; secondly insufficient government commitment and a lack of resources and collaboration; thirdly no existing adaptive strategies, policies or action plans specifically for heat/climate-health response in relevant organizations; and finally a lack of preparation for emergency response during extreme weather events related to climate change.

12.4 Implications

The perceptions of health risks from extreme heat in older people have been examined in only very limited studies and mainly in developed countries, even though evidence shows the elderly are the most affected and vulnerable groups during heatwaves (Sheridan, 2007; Abrahamson *et al.*, 2009). There have been very few studies on adaptation to extreme heat especially among the elderly in a Chinese setting. This study has, for the first time, investigated older people's perceptions of heatwaves and health and their behaviors during heatwaves in urban and rural areas of northern China. Moreover, qualitative interviews with local stakeholders complete the study by adding more insights on potential barriers to better adaptation.

A very low risk perception of heatwaves and health has been identified in this study among the elderly Chinese living in both rural and urban areas. Our findings are similar to those in western countries in that older people do not perceive themselves at risk from the impact of extreme heat. There are several possible explanations for the low health risk perception in our study. Firstly, it is highly likely that there are other more important risks perceived by the Chinese people. In an earlier urban survey in two Chinese cities in 1996, there were many other risks perceived by the urban Chinese people, for example low income and poor quality of products, although this study could not answer how the perceptions were shaped (Xie *et al.*, 2003). This is actually further proved by findings from our qualitative interviews. Secondly, extreme heat or climate change has been perceived by many people as only having impacts on 'geographically and temporally distant' people and places (Leiserowitz, 2005). Thirdly, compared with more developed countries, the greater apparent risk tolerance may be simply due to a lack of sufficient information about potential risks

(Zhai and Suzuki, 2009). Lastly, when approaching risk perception from the psychometric, sociological and cultural paradigm, it seems to be formed by many factors, including the concept and the meaning of risks and the perceived distinction between reality and possibility (Renn and Rohrmann, 2000). Additionally, it is acknowledged that humidity could affect the perception of the heat and associated health outcomes. The study region was in northern China, where summers are usually humid, which would exacerbate the health impact from heat because a higher humidity would hamper the evaporation of sweat, the only available mechanism for reducing the core body temperature when the surrounding temperature is higher than the skin temperature. The inability to lose heat can lead to an increase in core body temperature that could be fatal.

In spite of the low heat-health risk perception, the majority of the elderly reportedly undertake adaptive behaviors in response to extreme heat, in both rural and urban areas. A review of general environmental perception/attitude/values of Chinese people reported that they may not necessarily be related to environmental behaviors (Harris, 2006). Studies in the USA indicate that public responses to climate change are influenced by both psychological and socio–cultural factors (Leiserowitz, 2006). Adaptive behavior models for heatwaves can be affected by many factors, such as education level and perceived benefits from behavior changes (Akompab *et al.*, 2013). Our results suggest that adaptive behaviors may be undertaken without a perception of risks or an understanding of the association between behavior change and risk reduction (based on the qualitative interviews). In our study, many of the participants reported behavior changes during extreme heat, for example staying indoors, wearing light clothes, and reducing outdoor activities. These behavior changes can benefit adaptation, leading to a reduction in heat related morbidity and mortality, directly and indirectly. Older people's experience of extreme weather conditions in the past may help them to adapt during extremely hot weather. However, it should be noted that given projected more intense, frequent and longer heatwaves, insufficient knowledge and support and a low risk perception could be potential barriers to maintaining a good health status in the heat, for both direct heat-related and indirect heat-related conditions. For example, less than half of the urban group reported they would drink more fluids during heat, indicating many may potentially be at risk of dehydration during heatwaves, leading to heat stroke and/or exacerbation of ischemic heart disease due to reduced cardiac output and reduced blood circulation.

There are significant differences between rural and urban older people in perceptions, behavior changes and support received from community and government. We observed a higher level of health concern during heatwaves among the rural older people. Adaptive behaviors varied between the rural and urban groups. Some of the variations in behavior changes during heat could be explained by the difference in lifestyles between urban and rural China (for example, rarely having curtains and only cold showers being available in the rural areas), limited resources and facilities in rural areas (for example, no air conditioners or big shopping malls in which to cool down), and a higher cost of living in urban areas (for example, higher water and electricity bills). The implication is that in order to have successful intervention programs, the importance of the various adaptive behaviors in different areas should be understood and focused on in order to achieve the largest reductions in the heat-related health burden on the older Chinese population. This supports the view of Cooney (2010) on some of the successful experiences in the USA in response to climate change, indicating that in order to achieve individual changes to mitigate or adapt to climate change, multi-faceted policies and measures for various targeted populations should be adopted.

A lack of support is a significant barrier identified. It was originally expected that individual characteristics, for example, education and income levels might play a role in reducing adverse health outcomes in heat. However, the regression analyses indicate that these are not influencing factors. In the final multivariate regression models for both rural and urban areas, after controlling for confounders, it was shown that having regular social activities significantly reduced the likelihood of morbidity associated with extreme heat. The rural older people reported a lower level of support from family, community, health professionals or government regarding how to reduce health risks during heatwaves compared with their urban counterparts, although this is a common problem for the elderly in both regions. In particular, the model indicates that 'receiving no phone calls in heat wave', an indicator of insufficient support/connection, may significantly increase morbidity 3.8 times in rural older people. There are some obvious reasons for the beneficial outcome from having connections with both family members and the community. For example, a phone call before and during excessive heat to check out older people may increase the likelihood of their receiving timely messages and being monitored or experiencing intervention, which could result in better adaptation.

The multiple regression models also indicate that taking no medication could be a protective factor in reducing morbidity in extreme heat. Taking no medication does not necessarily mean a healthier status, and this study could not address the question whether a lower proportion of medication usage among rural older people is due to a lower prevalence of disease, under-diagnosis, or their reduced ability to afford medicines. However, previous studies suggest that some medication, for example, cardiovascular or diabetes medicine may interfere with the body's core temperature control, particularly in older people, leading to morbidity and mortality in periods of high heat (Hansen *et al.*, 2011b). Poor thermoregulation among older people may exacerbate cardiovascular disease events during heat (Pan *et al.*, 1995; Tam *et al.*, 2009). Therefore, taking no medication may reduce the risk of medication-related morbidity during heat events.

Our study has also identified other individual barriers to better adaptation to heatwaves and reducing heat-health illnesses in older people. For example, the unwillingness to change behaviors following health warnings (if there are any), may be related to perceived uncertainty of the risks (Fortner *et al.*, 2000), lack of adaptive capacity (Grothmann and Patt, 2005), lack of knowledge and understanding of the exposure and risks, and a lack of trust in government may all result in challenges in adapting to the warming climate. Additionally, poor air quality has become a prominent public health issue in China in recent years. Although the Chinese government has claimed to curb the worsening air pollution in urban areas, no significant improvement has occurred. This environmental issue was also found to concern the participants.

Four domains of barriers were identified by stakeholders from local government, health organizations, and service providers for the first time in this study. These include a lack of knowledge, concern and commitment by staff, limited resources, a lack of strategies and cross-sectional co-ordination, and a lack of forward-thinking systems for better preparedness for climate-related emergencies. Typical comments received from the qualitative interviews include the need for more reform to reduce government bureaucracy and the desire for more resources to do the work, which shows a willingness to contribute if conditions were to improve. Some of the barriers are consistent with those identified at the individual level, for example a low level of awareness, concern, and knowledge. Perceptions of staff and government leaders may influence the allocation of limited resources and the outcomes of adaptation and resilience. It is noted that health-warning messages regarding heatwaves are very limited in the study region. Only general information about temperatures may be available to the general public from the Bureau of Meteorology. There is no specific information provided to older people on how to reduce health risks during extreme heat events and even less information is available in the rural areas.

Some of the comments were similar across sectors, for example heat is not a priority and there is a shortage of funds and staff. Other comments were quite specific from various sectors, for example, whilst the Committee of Aging focuses on issues relevant to older people, and private nursing homes are more concerned about family support, the priority of CDC staff is the control of infectious and non-communicable diseases. Although their work has some degree of overlap, there is no evident collaboration between participating stakeholders from the different sectors.

Given the rapid population aging in Chinese society and associated social and economic consequences, the implication of the study could go beyond the adaptation to climate change and broadened to health services for the older population in the future, considering the extra economic and social burden brought by the changing environment and poor adaptation. In Chapter Two of this volume, the implication of population aging in China has been thoroughly illustrated, for example the expected need for more long-term health care. Unfortunately, the situation may be exacerbated by the adverse health impacts on China's older population from climate change in a rapidly urbanizing context. Therefore, it is essential for the health system to be ready to respond effectively to potential public health emergencies and extra health burdens associated with the changing climate and environment. The inequity between older people in urban and rural regions should be afforded particular attention in order to achieve healthy aging in a changing environment.

The study has several limitations. Firstly, the most vulnerable in the older population, such as the very frail and those with physical or cognitive impairments were not included in our study. This may undermine the ability of the study to identify other significant barriers to adaptation to heatwaves in older people. Secondly, in order to deal with the problems encountered at an institutional level, it would be useful to include more stakeholders who deal with the elderly. Lastly, the generalization of our study to other ethnic minority groups or regions in different climatic zones (particularly those regions currently without extreme heat events) in China should be interpreted with caution.

In conclusion, according to our findings, it is essential to increase older people's awareness of the health risks associated with extreme heat and climate change in order to reduce barriers to adaptation. Capacity building at both individual and institutional levels is necessary to build climate resilient communities, including developing strategies and emergency response plans, generating local government leadership promoting effective co-ordination across sectors, and providing extra support for older populations in rural regions of China.

12.5 Recommendations

Some strategies for better adaptation to climate change in older people in China are recommended, based on findings from the case study.

Firstly, it is recommended that government efforts towards a better environment can be integrated with climate change and air quality control programs in urbanizing China. Given the co-benefits that can be achieved from climate change mitigation and adaptation, holistic approaches that encompass a range of environmental issues, including climate change, urbanization, air pollution and sustainability, should be and can be adopted by policy and decision makers.

Secondly, given the fact that the rural older population may have relatively few social interactions, often receiving insufficient health messages and services, and having a poorer self-reported general health status together with a lower income and education level, the implications of our study are significant. They highlight the need for targeted programs and intervention strategies that address the needs of the most vulnerable elderly with the least available resources in climate change adaptation. There is a need for innovation in developing these programs in order to reach older people living in remote regions of China, where there is no effective and timely communication system available.

Furthermore, it is recommended that effective heat-health warning and response systems should be developed with specific messages targeted at various vulnerable groups, including older people. The effective Very Hot Weather Warning system in Hong Kong has significantly reduced deaths from ischemic heart disease and stroke among older people (Chau *et al.*, 2009). Examples from the early warning system developed for Shanghai City regarding heat and health could also be expanded to other mega-cities in China (Tan *et al.*, 2004).

Last but not least, for researchers in public health or environmental science, future studies that examine the interaction of urbanization and climate change on population health are essential to support evidence-based policy-making at various levels. This requires that organizations and institutions work across boundaries to achieve expected outcomes. It is acknowledged that these outcomes will require long-term effort.

References

Abrahamson, V., Wolf, J., Lorenzon, I., *et al.* (2009). Perceptions of Heatwave Risks to Health: Interview-based Study of Older People in London and Norwich, UK, *Journal of Public Health* **31**: 119–126.

Akompab, D., Bi, P., Williams, S., *et al.* (2013). Heat Waves and Climate Change: Applying the Health Belief Model to Identify Predictors of Risk Rerception and Adaptive Behaviours in Adelaide, Australia, *International Journal of Environmental Research and Public Health* **10**: 2164–2184.

Åström, D., Bertil, F. and Joacim, R. (2011). Heat Wave Impact on Morbidity and Mortality in the Elderly Population: A Review of Recent Studies, *Maturitas* **69**: 99–105.

Bassil, K.L. and Cole, D.C. (2010). Effectiveness of Public Health Interventions in Reducing Morbidity and Mortality During Heat Episodes: A Structured Review, *International Journal of Environmental Research and Public Health* 7: 991–1001.

Bobb, J., Peng, R., Bell, M., *et al.* (2014). Heat-related Mortality and Adaptation to Heat in the United States, *Environmental Health Perspectives* **122**: 811–816.

CEPAR (2013). Asia in the ageing century — Part II Retirement income. CEPAR Research Brief 2013/02. Available at http://cepar.edu.au/media/113805/asia_in_the_ageing_century_-_part_ii_-_pensions.pdf [Accessed September 2014].

Chau, P.H., Chan, K.C. and Woo, J. (2009). Hot Weather Warning Might Help to Reduce Elderly Mortality in Hong Kong, *International Journal of Biometeorology* **53**:461–468.

Cooney, C. (2010). The Perception Factor: Climate Change Gets Personal, *Environmental Health Perspectives* **118**: A485–A488.

Ding, T. and Qian, W. (2011). Geographical Patterns and Temporal Variations of Regional Dry and Wet Heatwave Events in China During 1960–2008, *Advances in Atmospheric Sciences* **8**: 322–337.

Draucker, C.B., Martsolf, D.S., Ross, R., *et al.* (2007). Theoretical Sampling and Category Development in Grounded Theory, *Qualitative Health Research* **17**: 1137–1148.

Fortner, R., Lee, J., Corney, J., *et al.* (2000). Public Understanding of Climate Change: Certainty and Willingness to Act, *Environmental Education Research* **6**: 127–141.

Grothmann, T. and Patt, A. (2005). Adaptive Capacity and Human Cognition: The Process of Individual Adaptation to Climate Change, *Global Environmental Change* **15**: 199–213.

Hansen, A., Bi, P., Nitschke, M., *et al.* (2011a). Perceptions of Heat-Susceptibility in Older Persons: Barriers to Adaptation, *International Journal of Environmental Research and Public Health* **8**: 4714–4728.

Hansen, A., Bi, P., Nitschke, M., *et al.* (2011b). Older Persons and Heat-Susceptibility: The Role of Health Promotion in a Changing Climate, *Health Promotion Journal of Australia* **22**: 17–20.

Harris, P. (2006). Environmental Perspectives and Behavior in China: Synopsis and Bibliography, *Environment and Behavior* **38**: DOI: 10.1177/0013916505280087.

Huang, W., Kan, H. and Kovats, S. (2010). The Impact of the 2003 Heat Wave on Mortality in Shanghai, China, *Science of the Total Environment* **408**: 2418–2420.

IPCC (2013). *The Fifth Assessment Report*, IPCC, Stockholm, Sweden.

Kjellstrom, T. and McMichael, A.J. (2013). Climate Change Threats to Population Health and Well-being: The Imperative of Protective Solutions That Will Last, *Global Health Action*, DOI: http://dx.doi.org/10.3402/gha.v6i0.20816.

Knowlton, K., Rotkin-Ellman, M., King, G., *et al.* (2009). The 2006 California Heat Wave: Impacts on Hospitalizations and Emergency Department Visits, *Environmental Health Perspectives* **117**: 61–67.

Kovats, R.S. and Hajat, S. (2008). Heat Stress and Public Health: A Critical Review, *Annual Review Public Health* **29**: 41–55.

Leiserowitz, A. (2005). American Risk Perceptions: Is Climate Change Dangerous?, *Risk Analysis Journal China* **25**: 1433–1442.

Leiserowitz, A. (2006). Climate Change Risk Perception and Policy Preferences: The Role of Affect, Imagery, and Values, *Climatic Change* 77: 45–72.

Ministry of Land and Resources of China (2014). *Land Resources.* Available at http://www.mlr.gov.cn/tdzt/ [Accessed 20 February 2015].

National Bureau of Statistics of China (2011). The sixth national census data bulletin 12, China Statistics Press, Beijing.

Pan, W., Li, L. and Tsa, M. (1995). Temperature Extremes and Mortality From Coronary Heart Disease and Cerebral Infarction in Elderly Chinese, *The Lancet* **345**: 353–355.

QSR International Pty Ltd. (2010). NVivo qualitative data analysis software, version 9.

Renn, O. and Rohrmann, B. (eds.) (2000). *Cross-Cultural Risk Perception: A Survey of Empirical Studies*, Kluwer Academic Publishers, The Netherlands.

Sheridan, S. (2007). A Survey of Public Perception and Response to Heat Warnings Across Four North American Cities: An Evaluation of Muni-Cipal Effectiveness, *International Journal of Biometeorology* **52**: 3–15.

Tam, W., Wong, T., Chair, S., *et al.* (2009). Diurnal Temperature Range and Daily Cardiovascular Mortalities Among the Elderly in Hong Kong, *Archives of Environmental and Occupational Health Journals* **64**(3): 202–6.

Tan, J.G., Kalkstein, L.S., Huang, J.X., *et al.* (2004). An Operational Heat/Health Warning System in Shanghai, *International Journal of Biometeorology* **48**: 157–162.

United Nations. World Population Prospects: The 2012 Revision. 2013.

Xie, X., Wang, M. and Xu, L. (2003). What Risks are Chinese People Concerned About? *Risk Analysis* **23**: 685–95.

Zhai, G. and Suzuki, T. (2009). Risk perception in Northeast Asia, *Environmental Monitoring and Assessment* **157**: 151–167.

Zhan, J., Huang, J, Zhao, T., *et al.* (2013). Modeling the Impacts of Urbanization on Regional Climate Change: A Case Study in the Beijing-Tianjin-Tangshan Metropolitan Area, *Advances in Meteorology* **849479**: 1–8.

Zhou, L., Dickinson, R., Tian, Y., *et al.* (2004). Evidence for a significant urbanization effect on climate in China, *Proceedings of the National Academy of Sciences* **101**: 9540–9544.

Chapter Thirteen

Promoting Active Transportation: Lessons for China from International Studies

Li Ming Wen and Hui Lan Xu

Abstract

Over the past two to three decades, rapid urbanization has been accompanied by a dramatic increase in the number of motor vehicles on the road in China. The increasing reliance on private motor vehicles has led to traffic congestion and air pollution as well as an increasingly inactive lifestyle. In contrast, active transportation, which means less reliance on the use of cars, and more on alternative modes of transport such as walking and cycling can potentially not only lead to a cleaner environment, but also a healthier population. Public transport can also be considered as active transportation in contexts where the distance travelled from the nearest public transport interchange to the destination can make a significant contribution to daily physical activity and health, for example, a 10 minute walk each way.

Evidence linking active transportation directly to health outcomes has been documented internationally, but it has not been examined extensively in China. More research is needed to better understand the important correlations between active transportation and population health, and to develop effective strategies to promote active transportation, both in China and more broadly. In 2007, the Chinese government launched a nationwide program for promoting a healthier lifestyle, of which active transportation is an integral part (China Healthy Lifestyle for All, 2007). In this chapter evidence of the health benefits associated with active transportation and potential strategies to promote active transportation among various communities is presented for informing the development of active transportation promotion in China based on lessons from international studies.

13.1 Health Benefits of Promoting Active Transportation

In 1999, the World Health Organization (WHO) identified motor vehicle transport as the main cause of air pollution, the key factor in road accidents, and a major contributor to sedentary lifestyles (WHO Regional Office for Europe, 1999). Driving instead of walking or cycling contributes not only to an unhealthy environment but also to an increasingly sedentary lifestyle. Active transportation is defined as any form of transportation that involves incidental physical activity, such as walking, cycling and traveling by public transport (Davis, 1999). There is emerging and consistent evidence that active transportation increases the level of physical activity (Faulkner *et al.*, 2009; Lee *et al.*, 2008, Ogilvie *et al.*, 2007; Rissel *et al.*, 2012, van Sluijs *et al.*, 2009). The benefits of increased physical activity are broad — reduced morbidity and mortality rates from cardiovascular disease (CVD), hypertension, obesity, diabetes, respiratory disease, certain cancers, and musculoskeletal and mental health problems ('At least five a week', 2004; Nocon *et al.*, 2008; Sofi *et al.*, 2008; Wendel-Vos *et al.*, 2004). However, little such evidence has been generated from the Chinese context.

13.1.1 *Cardiovascular health benefits*

The evidence linking active transportation and better cardiovascular health is consistent and strong internationally. For example, in a longitudinal study from Denmark on cycling to school and cardiovascular risk factors, a consistent pattern was found of a better risk factor profile for cardiovascular disease (CVD) in commuter cyclists compared with students using other means of transport. Even students, who did not cycle to school at baseline, and who had changed to cycling at follow up, were fitter, had better cholesterol/HDL ratio, better glucose metabolism, and a lower composite CVD risk factor score than those who did not cycle at either time point (Andersen *et al.*, 2011).

There have also been two systematic reviews supporting this evidence. In one review of international prospective epidemiological studies of commuting activity and cardiovascular risk, the evidence suggests that active transportation that incorporates walking and cycling is associated with an overall 11% reduction in cardiovascular risk, and is more robust among women than men (Hamer and Chida, 2008). The more recent 2013 systematic review examining the relationship between active transport to work or school and cardiovascular health also concludes that the evidence linking active transportation and cardiovascular health is moderate to strong (Xu *et al.*, 2013).

However, the results from a population-based cross-sectional study conducted in Jiansu Province, China with 8,400 community residents aged 18 or above contradict findings elsewhere: people engaged in active transportation (walking or cycling) had a higher prevalence of elevated cholesterol and a higher risk of diabetes (Lu *et al.*, 2013).

13.1.2 *Healthy body weight*

Most published studies relate to school-aged children commuting to and from school in developed countries. The evidence linking active transportation and healthy body weight is mixed. A systematic review of active school transportation, physical activity levels and body weight of children and youths include 13 studies, most of which explicitly sample in urban, suburban or rural areas (Faulkner *et al.*, 2009). Of these, nine studies demonstrate that children who actively commute to school accumulate significantly more physical activity; and two studies report that they expend significantly more energy in terms of kilocalories burned per day. Where studies examine body weight (n=10), only one reports active commuters having lower body weight compared with passive commuters. The review concludes that active school commuters tend to be more physically active overall than passive commuters; however, the evidence related to healthy body weights for children and youths is not compelling. Similarly, the review by Lee and co-authors (Lee *et al.*, 2008) finds a positive association between active commuting and overall physical activity levels, with an average of approximately 28 minutes difference in overall physical activity between active and passive commuters. However, only a few studies (3 of 18) suggest a weak association between active commuting and reduced body weight or body mass index (BMI). As most studies included in this review are cross-sectional studies, a causal relationship is difficult to conclude. Because of the heterogeneity of studies included, the type of study designs, and the crudeness of measurements for active transportation and physical activity, the results of active transport, physical activity, and body weight in adults are also mixed and inconclusive (Wanner *et al.*, 2012).

There is some evidence emerging from China on links between ways of commuting and overweight and obesity. A national survey of a total of 6826 children aged from 7 to 17 years reveals that whether a child walks to and from school is one of two main determinants of childhood overweight and obesity in China, after adjustment for parental body weight status and socio–economic status (Li *et al.*, 2007). Interestingly, the other main determinant of childhood overweight and obesity is cooking oil consumption. In a longitudinal study examining the association between vehicle ownership and obesity, and the impact of vehicle acquisition on the risk of becoming obese, conducted in eight provinces including both rural and urban areas, it was found that the household ownership of motorized transportation, indicating reduced active transportation is indirectly associated with obesity in men and women. Further, the acquisition of a motorized vehicle increases the risk of obesity in men (Bell *et al.*, 2002).

It is clear that more rigorously designed research is needed in order to gather unequivocal evidence concerning the benefit of commuting-related physical activity and healthy body weight in different age groups.

13.1.3 *Other health outcomes*

Various other health benefits from active transportation have been reported in China and internationally. For example, a study on commuting-related physical activity and risk of colon cancer in Shanghai, China found that colon cancer risk is significantly reduced among people engaged in commuting-related physical activity, particularly among those who had a high level of physical activity from active commuting for at least 35 years (Hou *et al.*, 2004). Further, commuting-related physical activity can significantly modify the risk conferred by high BMI, with the highest risk observed among those at the highest quintile of BMI and the lowest activity level. A Shanghai study also found that walking as the main mode of transportation significantly reduces risk of endometrial cancer among women (Matthews *et al.*, 2005).

A review was undertaken by Shephard (2008) of studies that look at the effect of active transport on mortality in China, Finland, and Denmark. The Chinese study shows that among active commuters there is a stronger association between all-cause mortality with cycling than with walking. This means cycling is more likely associated with lower all-cause mortality. The Finnish study shows that spending ≥15 minutes per day walking or cycling to work is associated with reduced all-cause and cardiovascular mortality in women but not in men. The Danish study notes that all-cause mortality is 40% lower in cyclists than in other commuters after adjusting for self-reported leisure-time activities.

In conclusion, there is solid evidence of cardiovascular health benefits from active transportation. However, few studies have been conducted to examine the association between active transportation and a range of other health outcomes, including mental health, certain cancers, diabetes, and commuting-related injury, which require further investigation with stronger research design and rigorous evaluation.

13.2 Urbanization and Physical Activity in China

China has been experiencing rapid urbanization over the past three decades. In 2011, the proportion of urban residents reached 51.3%. Urban residents surpassed rural residents in number for the first time in China's history (China Development Research Foundation, 2014). The rapid urbanization involving changes in people's working and living conditions has had a significant impact on people's health. For example, an inactive lifestyle, one of the unwelcome consequences of urbanization, is closely related to obesity, which is a risk factor for many non-communicable diseases (NCDs). According to the China Health and Nutrition Survey, the average weekly rate of physical activity dropped approximately 32% among adults between 1991 and 2006 (Ng *et al.*, 2009). James (2008) estimates that, because of urbanization, the energy expenditure may be reduced by about 400–800 kilocalories (kcal) per day for each Chinese adult. Of the reduced energy expenditure, about 200 kcal energy expenditure reduction is the result of changing the mode of transport to work from walking or cycling to driving a car.

Nevertheless, commuting-related physical activity is still the main form of physical activity for many urban residents. In 1996, a survey (Hu *et al.*, 2001) of 3976 residents aged 15–69 years in urban Tianjin Municipality, China, found that most people (67% of females, 61% of males) do not engage in any leisure-time physical activity; physical activity associated with commuting is the major type of physical activity. The average commuting time on foot or by bicycle is 30 minutes per day. Another men's health study in urban Shanghai (Lee *et al.*, 2008) found that approximately 60% of men walk or bicycle for at least 30 minutes each day, five days per week, for transportation or daily living activity; only 26% and 4% of men engage in moderate and vigorous exercise or sports during leisure time, respectively. Similar to the study in Tianjin Municipality, the major proportion of men's physical activity in Shanghai is transportation — for example, walking — or daily living activity-related. Given the fact that China is becoming the world's largest automobile producer and consumer ('Cars in China', 2005), and the roads crowded with motor vehicles making them increasingly dangerous for pedestrians and cyclists, transportation-related physical activity could be squeezed out if active transportation is not advocated and promoted.

13.3 Strategies and Interventions for Promoting Active Transportation

Although physical inactivity is widely recognized as a risk factor for many diseases, only 22% of urban Chinese adults were physically active based on a Chinese national survey conducted in 2000 to 2001; and about 4 in 5 of urban Chinese adults failed to reach a recommended level of physical activity (Muntner *et al.*, 2005). The current recommendation for physical activity states that every adult should accumulate about 30 minutes of moderate physical activity on most days of the week (WHO, 2011). It is also suggested that physical activity can be accumulated in periods as brief as 10 minutes, several times throughout the day.

Potential strategies to promote physical activity and reduce motor vehicle use in China involve encouraging 'lifestyle physical activity' through active transportation. Every day incidental physical activity opportunities arise from the need to travel from place to place, such as going to school, the workplace, markets or shopping centers. Evidence shows that lifestyle activity is less expensive and can be maintained over a longer period than programmed exercise (Dunn *et al.*, 1998).

It is generally agreed that the key strategies for promoting active transportation should include active design in urban areas, supportive policies, and educational intervention programs promoting active transportation in schools, workplaces, and in the wider community. Is there sufficient evidence of success and is there anything more that can be done, or done differently?

13.3.1 *Active transportation to school*

Active transportation to school is a relatively new concept for prompting children's physical activity, and intervention strategies are still in the early stages of development. Internationally, programs have been implemented to encourage children to travel to school actively (walking, cycling or using public transport) (Chillon *et al.*, 2011), and most of them use education as their main strategy. Examples of these programs include Walking School Buses (WSB) in the United States of America (Heelan *et al.*, 2009), and other ways of supervising children walking, although many school communities prefer a more informal approach. The WSB program has increased frequency of walking to school and established a link with increased daily physical activity (Heelan *et al.*, 2009). Although there have been limited evaluations of the effectiveness of the programs such as the Safe Routes to School and the Walking School Buses, evidence suggests that these programs are viewed positively by key stakeholders and have positive effects on children's active commuting to school (Davison *et al.*, 2008). Walking School Bus programs have also been implemented in several other countries, but few evaluation studies have been published in terms of the effectiveness of the interventions.

In New South Wales, Australia, Walk Safely to School Day is an annual event that uses a mass media and public relations approach to encourage parents to walk to school with their primary school-age children on one day of the year. About 28% of primary schools have participated in the event, but its effect on students' regular journeys to school is uncertain (Merom *et al.*, 2005). The Walk Safely to School Day resulted in a moderate short-term change in walking behavior. High levels of in-principle support from parents indicate that greater participation in walking to school is possible, but maintaining changes will require stronger interventions to overcome barriers identified by parents such as safety concerns, lack of walking and cycling paths, and availability of public transport.

In Australia, investigations into factors associated with children who are passive commuters (meaning they are driven to school), indicate that parents' attitudes towards walking to school, and their modes of travel to work influence how their children travel to and from school. The distance between home and school, as well as the number of cars available in the household also influence children's mode of traveling to school (Wen *et al.*, 2008). This is supported by evidence from the 2001 United States of America National Household Travel Survey, which shows that household income, vehicle access, distance between home and school, and residential density are associated with mode of travel to school (McDonald, 2008). Other factors influencing children's active commuting to school — including demographic factors, individual and family factors, school factors (including the immediate area surrounding schools), and social and physical environmental factors — were identified as predictors of children's active commuting behaviors (Davison *et al.*, 2008).

A recent systematic review of intervention studies regarding active transportation to school — up to 2011 — highlights a couple of issues. The studies concentrate on developed countries including the United States of America, Australia, and the United Kingdom; and interventions mainly focus on primary school children. Further, from the study design point of view, almost all the intervention studies (10 out of 14) use quasi-experimental designs. Finally, six out of 14 report that the interventions have not been effective (Chillon *et al.*, 2011). More research with higher quality study designs and rigorous measurements should be conducted to determine the most successful strategies for increasing active transportation to school.

A Chinese population-based longitudinal study found an increase in passive commuting to school over a decade (3.6% in 1997, 14% in 2006); the strongest factor associated with passive commuting in urban areas is that some children attend a school located some distance from their home (Cui *et al.*, 2012). The possible reason that children do not attend local schools in urban China is that parents might be driving their children further to schools with higher educational reputations.

There is a great need for developing effective strategies for promoting active transportation to school, particularly in the context of China's urbanization. For example, one way to address this issue is to develop policies that focus on an equitable distribution of educational resources.

13.3.2 *Active transportation to the workplace*

Active transportation for the journey to work is recognized as a strategy for improving physical activity and the environment. Despite the potential benefits, information on programs and the effectiveness of interventions and policies is limited. A randomized controlled trial at three workplaces in Scotland evaluated the efficacy of an active transport information pack aimed at increasing walking and cycling to work (Mutrie *et al.*, 2002).The trial found a significant increase in the proportion of workers who walked to work in the intervention group, but cycling to work was unaffected. Whilst this study provides the best evidence of the efficacy of active transport promotion because of the comprehensiveness and tailored nature of the intervention, whether it is possible to generalize from its findings is yet to be determined. Another example is the Travel Smart Workplace, a program supporting workplaces in Australia to encourage and enable their employees and clients to use alternative modes of transportation to cars (Travel Smart Workplaces, 2013). There is a lack of information on the evaluation of the program.

The effectiveness of interventions in promoting active transportation to work was examined in a recent systematic review (Scheepersa *et al.*, 2014), which included 19 workplace based interventions, architectural and urban adjustments, population-wide interventions, and bicycle-renting systems. Most of the included studies used more than one intervention tool, and the tools used differed depending on types of interventions. Nearly all studies (16 out of 19) show positive effects of a transport mode shift. However, the quality of the studies is generally low. Another systematic review of the efficacy of behavioral interventions in transport behavior change concluded that there is no evidence for the efficacy of existing behavioral interventions in reducing car trips (Arnott *et al.*, 2014). The evidence for efficacy of behavioral interventions to decrease distance and duration of car journeys is limited and inconclusive. Future research should investigate alternative behavioral interventions informed by existing evidence, theory, and the views of potential users. Further, the design of future intervention studies should also improve scientific rigor, include objective outcome measures, and incorporate a thorough process evaluation as standard.

Recently, there have been some encouraging findings from the United Kingdom 'iConnect Study' in which new walking and cycling routes were built, and increased physical activity was observed in a two year study of 1,796 adult residents in three municipalities (Goodman *et al.*, 2014). This study provides evidence that improved, high quality, traffic-free routes for walking and cycling may help to increase overall physical activity levels in the local population and thereby contribute to the primary prevention of a range of NCDs. This lends support to recent calls to increase the provision of such routes in local communities.

13.4 Lessons for China from International Studies

Over the past two to three decades, the number of vehicles on Chinese roads has increased very rapidly, as part of urbanization in China. For example, in Beijing alone, the number of vehicles increased 10 times, from 0.5 million in 1990 to five million in 2012. In addition, the emission factor (the amount of pollution emitted by one car) in China is much higher than in developed countries as China has much lower emission standards for automobiles (Chinese Academy of Engineering, Chinese Academy of Sciences, National Academy of Engineering, National Research Council, 2005). The increased number of vehicles also significantly affected physical activity levels of urban Chinese (Muntner *et al.*, 2005). In 2008, the Chinese government launched a national program, of which active transportation is an integral part for the purpose of promoting a healthier lifestyle (China Healthy Lifestyle for All, 2007). However, very few programs promoting active transportation have been implemented in China. There is a great need for promoting the concept of active transportation and demonstrating its health benefits, which will, in turn, inform the development of effective strategies in Chinese settings.

The WHO Health Promotion Action can be adopted in promoting active transportation in China (WHO, 1986). Active transportation is seen as a determinant of health and is a positive concept encouraging a reduction in car usage, as well as increased physical activity. Therefore, promoting active transportation should not just be the responsibility of the health sector, but requires a multi-sector partnership approach involving urban planning, construction, transport, health sectors, workplaces, schools, and the entire civil society.

The fundamental conditions for active transportation are transportation infrastructure, government policies, education and community actions, as well as urban structure planning. It is critical to make walking and cycling trips convenient, pleasant and safe. First and foremost, there should be an enabling environment. For example, in new urban development areas a variety of facilities, such as schools and shops, should be built within walking or cycling distance. A traffic network of highly interconnected cycling and walking paths and a coordinated network of streets with bike and pedestrian lanes should be developed. Bicycle storage facilities should be available at public transport stations to enable users to cycle and then connect with public transport.

From a policy development viewpoint, a successful example is the California Safe Routes to School (SR2S) legislation that provided competitive funds for construction projects, such as sidewalks, traffic lights, pedestrian crossing improvements and bicycle paths. The evaluation of SR2S legislation found that these construction projects are very effective in increasing the numbers of children walking or cycling to school (Boarnet *et al.*, 2005). Another program in North Carolina, in the United States of America, also found a strong association between individual-level cycling and transportation-related physical activity and active community environment scores (Aytur *et al.*, 2007). These findings demonstrate the importance of public infrastructure and mixed land use in promoting people's physical activity.

Clear communication of information about active transport options at the workplace is also important. The information should include walking and cycling routes, public transport services, as well as the time required by these means to reach a destination. Organizations should be encouraged to take health promotion action by providing 'active transportation' access guides for their clients. International research has suggested that significant potential benefits can be gained through workplace policies and interventions supporting active commuting by employees, for example providing workplace facilities such as showers and secured bicycle parking spaces. An Australian pilot study conducted in a large health care facility in inner-city Sydney, using social marketing to raise awareness of active transport, and individualized marketing to address barriers to active transport for individual participants, found that there was a reduction in the proportion of participants who drove to work five days per week and a decrease in trips travelled by car on weekends. Staff reporting use of active transport as their usual mode of transport to work, however, was not significantly increased (Wen *et al.*, 2005).

The role of the workplace in developing policies and facilities to encourage employees to use active transportation when traveling to work is relatively unexplored in China. Workplaces can play a significant role in promoting active transportation by making it easy for employees to walk, cycle or use public transport. Developing a workplace travel plan, which details workplace-specific active transportation options, can be a starting point. Workplace travel plans can include behavioral programs to support staff in overcoming personal barriers to walking and cycling to work. Particularly in large cities, increasing awareness of public transport options with clearly signed, safe and direct routes to public transport and stops within a comfortable walking distance, could help employees to plan their travel. Providing appropriate information on travel routes and timetables for public transport could also be helpful. Provision of secure, well-lit and sheltered bicycle parking within, or close to, buildings and providing end-of-trip facilities such as showers, changing and locker facilities would encourage cycling.

In conclusion, successful promotion of active transportation in China, requires more evidence of its benefits. This evidence can then be used in advocating for government leadership and community actions in developing sustainable active transportation interventions. Finally, comprehensive strategies that involve multi-sectors are essential when promoting active transportation in the community. These strategies need to be focused on developing policy, environmental and organizational changes in addition to behavioral changes within the population.

References

Andersen, L.B., Wedderkopp, N., Kristensen, P., *et al.* (2011). Cycling to School and Cardiovascular Risk Factors: A Longitudinal Study, *Journal of Physical Activity and Health* **8**(8): 1025–1033.

Arnott, B., Rehackova, L, Errington, L., *et al.* (2014). Efficacy of Behavioral Interventions for Transport Behavior Change: Systematic Review, Meta-Analysis and Intervention Coding, *International Journal of Behavioral Nutrition and Physical Activity* **11**(1): 133.

'At least five a week' (2004). Department of Health, Physical Activity, Health Improvement and Prevention. Available at http://webarchive.nationalarchives.gov.uk/20130107105354/http:/www.dh.gov.uk/prod_consum_dh/groups/dh_digitalassets/@dh/@en/documents/digitalasset/dh_4080981.pdf [Accessed 30 September 2013].

Aytur, S.A., Rodriguez, D.A., Evenson, K.R., *et al.* (2007). Promoting Active Community Environments Through Land Use and Transportation Planning, *American Journal of Health Promotion* **21**(4 Suppl): 397–407.

Bell, A.C., Ge, K. and Popkin, B.M. (2002). The Road to Obesity or the Path to Prevention: Motorized Transportation and Obesity in China, *Obesity Research* **10**(4): 277–283.

Boarnet, M.G., Anderson, C.L., Day, K., *et al.* (2005). Evaluation of the California Safe Routes to School Legislation: Urban Form Changes and Children's Active Transportation to School, *American Journal of Preventive Medicine* **28**(2 Suppl 2): 134–140.

'Cars in China: Dream machines' (2005). *The Economist*, June 2. Available at http://www.economist.com/node/4032842 [Accessed 2 March 2015].

WHO Regional Office for Europe (1999). Charter on Transport, Environment and Health. Available at http://www.euro.who.int/__data/assets/pdf_file/0006/88575/E69044.pdf [Accessed 8 November 2014].

Chillón, P., Evenson, K.R., Vaughn, A., *et al.* (2011). A Systematic Review of Interventions for Promoting Active Transportation to School, *International Journal of Behavioral Nutrition and Physical Activity* **8**:10. DOI: 10.1186/1479-5868-8-10.

China Development Research Foundation (2014). *Demographic Development in China*. Routledge, USA.

'China Healthy Lifestyle for All' (2007). Available at http://www.jiankang121.cn/FFP.aspx?code=introduce [Accessed 15 November 2014].

Chinese Academy of Engineering, Chinese Academy of Science, National Academy of Engineering, National Research Council (2005). *Urbanization, Energy, and Air Pollution in China: The Challenges Ahead—Proceedings of a Symposium*. National Academies Press, Washington D.C.

Cui, Z., Bauman, A. and Dibley, M.J. (2012). Temporal Trends and Correlates of Passive Commuting to and from School in Children from 9 Provinces in China, *Preventive Medicine* **52**(6): 423–427.

Davis A. (1999). *Active transport: A Guide to the Development of Local Initiatives to Promote Walking and Cycling*. UK Health Education Authority, London.

Davison, K.K., Werder J.L. and Lawson C.T. (2008). Children's Active Commuting to School: Current Knowledge and Future Directions, *Preventing Chronic Disease* **5**(3): A100.

Dunn, A.L., Andreson, R. and Jakicic, J. (1998). Lifestyle Physical Activity Interventions. History, Short- and Long-term Effects, and Recommendations, *American Journal of Preventative Medicine* **15**(4): 398–441.

Faulkner, G.E., Buliung, R.N., Flora, P.K. *et al.* (2009). Active School Transport, Physical Activity Levels and Body Weight of Children and Youth: A Systematic Review, *Preventive Medicine* **48**(1): 3–8.

Goodman, A., Sahlqvist, S., Ogilvie, D. and iConnect Consortium. (2014). New Walking and Cycling Routes and Increased Physical Activity: One- and Two-year Findings from the UK iConnect Study, *American Journal of Public Health* **104**(9): e38–e46.

Hamer, M. and Chida, Y. (2008). Active Commuting and Cardiovascular Risk: A Meta-analytic Review, *Preventive Medicine* **46**(1): 9–13.

Heelan, K.A., Abbey, B.M., Donnelly, J.E., *et al.* (2009). Evaluation of a Walking School Bus for Promoting Physical Activity in Youth, *Journal of Physical Activity and Health* **6**(5): 560–567.

Hou, L., Ji B.T., Blair, A., *et al.* (2004). Commuting Physical Activity and Risk of Colon Cancer in Shanghai, China, *American Journal of Epidemiology* **160**: 860–867.

Hu, G., Pekkarinen, H., Hanninen, O., *et al.* (2001). Physical Activity During Leisure and Commuting in Tianjin, China, *Bulletin of the World Health Organization* **80**: 933–938.

James, W.P. (2008). The Fundamental Drivers of the Obesity Epidemic, *Obesity Reviews* **9**(Suppl 1): 6–13.

Lee, M.C., Orenstein, M.R. and Richardson, M.J. (2008). Systematic Review of Active Commuting to School and Children's Physical Activity and Weight, *Journal of Physical Activity and Health* **5**(6): 930–949.

Li, Y., Zhai, F, Yang, X., *et al.* (2007). Determinants of Childhood Overweight and Obesity in China, *British Journal of Nutrition* **97**(1): 210–215.

Lu, S.R., Su, J., Xiang, Q.Y., *et al.* (2013). Active Transport and Health Outcomes: Findings from a Population Study in Jiangsu, China, *Journal of Environmental Public Health* 624194. DOI: 10.1155/2013/624194.

Matthews, C.E., Xu, W.H., Zheng, W., *et al.* (2005). Physical Activity and Risk of Endometrial Cancer: A Report from the Shanghai Endometrial Cancer Study, *Cancer Epidemiology, Biomarkers and Prevention* **14**(4): 779–785.

McDonald, N.C. (2008). Critical Factors for Active Transportation to School Among Low-income and Minority Students. Evidence from the 2001 National Household Travel Survey, *American Journal of Preventive Medicine* **34**(4):341–344. DOI: 10.1016/j.amepre.2008.01.004.

Merom, D., Rissel, C., Mahmic, A., *et al.* (2005). Process evaluation of the New South Wales Walk Safely to School Day, *Health Promotion Journal of Australia* **16**(2):100–106.

Muntner, P., Gu D. and Wildman, R., *et al.* (2005). Prevalence of Physical Activity Among Chinese Adults: Results from the International Collaborative Study of Cardiovascular Disease in Asia, *American Journal of Public Health* **95**(9): 1631–1636.

Mutrie, N., Carney, C., Blamey, A., *et al.* (2002). "Walk in to Work Out": A Randomised Controlled Trial of a Self Help Intervention to Promote

Active Commuting, *Journal of Epidemiology and Community Health* **56**(6):407–412.

Ng, S.W., Norton, E.C. and Popkin, B.M. (2009). Why Have Physical Activity Levels Declined Among Chinese Adults? Findings from the 1991–2006 China Heath and Nutrition Surveys, *Social Science and Medicine* **68** (7): 1305–1314.

Nocon, M., Hiemann, T., Muller-Riemenschneider, F., *et al.* (2008). Association of Physical Activity with All-Cause and Cardiovascular Mortality: A Systematic Review and Meta-analysis, *European Journal of Cardiovascular Prevention and Rehabilitation* **15**: 239–246.

Ogilvie, D., Foster, C.E. and Rothnie, H., *et al.* (2007). Interventions to Promote Walking: Systematic Review, *BMJ* **334**:1204.

Rissel, C., Curac, N., Greenaway, M., *et al.* (2012). Physical Activity Associated with Public Transport Use: a Review and Modelling of Potential Benefits, *International Journal of Environmental Research and Public Health* **9**: 2454–2478.

Scheepersa, C.E., Wendel-Vosb, G.C.W. and den Broeder, J.M. (2014). Shifting from Car to Active Transport: A Systematic Review of the Effectiveness of Interventions, *Transportation Research Part A: Policy and Practice* **70**: 264–280.

Shephard, R.J. (2008). Is Active Commuting the Answer to Population Health? *Sports Medicine* **38**(9): 751–758.

Sofi, F., Capalbo, A., Cesari, F., *et al.* (2008). Physical Activity During Leisure Time and Primary Prevention of Coronary Heart Disease: An Updated Meta-analysis of Cohort Studies, *European Journal of Cardiovascular Prevention and Rehabilitation* **15**: 247–257.

Travel Smart workplaces (2013). Active Transport. Department of Transport, Western Australia. Available at http://www.transport.wa.gov.au/activetransport/24631.asp [Accessed 2 November 2013].

van Sluijs, E.M.F., Fearne, V.A., Mattocks, C., *et al.* (2009). The Contribution of Active Travel to Children's Physical Activity Levels: Cross-sectional Results from the ALSPAC Study, *Preventive Medicine* **48**: 519–524.

Wanner, M., Götschi, T., Martin-Diener, E., *et al.* (2012). Active Transport, Physical Activity, and Body Weight in Adults: A Systematic Review, *American Journal of Preventive Medicine* **42**(5): 493–502.

Wen, L.M., Fry, D. and Rissel, C. (2008). Factors Associated with Children Being Driven to School: Implications for Walk to School Programs, *Health Education Research* **23**(2), 325–334.

Wen, L.M., Orr, N., Bindon, J., *et al.* (2005). Promoting Active Transport in a Workplace Setting: Evaluation of a Pilot Study in Australia, *Health Promotion International* **20**(2): 123–133.

Wendel-Vos, G.C., Schuit, A.J. and Feskens, E.J. (2004). Physical Activity and Stroke: A Meta-analysis of Observational Data, *International Journal of Epidemiology* **33**: 787–798.

WHO (2011). Global recommendations on physical activity for health. Available at http://www.who.int/dietphysicalactivity/leaflet-physical-activity-recommendations.pdf?ua=1 [Accessed 10 November 2014].

WHO (1986). The Ottawa Charter for Health Promotion. Available at http://www.who.int/healthpromotion/conferences/previous/ottawa/en/ [Accessed 12 November 2014].

Xu, H., Wen, L.M. and Rissel, C. (2013). The Relationships Between Active Transport to Work or School and Cardiovascular Health or Body Weight: A Systematic Review, *Asia Pacific Journal of Public Health* **25**(4):298–315. DOI: 10.1177/1010539513482965.

Chapter Fourteen

Eco-City Development and Urban Health Reform: The Sino-Singapore Tianjin Eco-City as a Model for Chinese and other Cities

Phil McManus

Abstract

An eco-city is a purpose-built city that is more ecologically sustainable than existing urban areas. The Sino-Singapore Tianjin Eco-city in northeast China is widely recognized as one of the world's leading contemporary eco-city developments. This chapter explores the key concepts underpinning this eco-city in relation to urban reform over the last two centuries, and to sustainable urban development principles. It investigates what is being done in practice to achieve urban sustainability goals. The chapter considers whether the Sino-Singapore Tianjin Eco-city is an appropriate model for eco-city development in other Chinese cities, and on a global scale.

14.1 Introduction

There is a tradition of improving urban conditions that, in western countries, can be traced to at least the late 18th century and the urban philanthropists who attempted to address the social and urban environmental issues of their time and place (McManus, 2005; Benton-Short and Short, 2008). Even earlier, the visions of John Evelyn emphasized health concerns in cities (McMichael, 2008), concerns that extend to contemporary eco-city development in the Sino-Singapore Tianjin Eco-city project in China being developed by a consortium led by Keppel Corporation from Singapore.

The Sino-Singapore Tianjin Eco-city along with Masdar in Abu Dhabi in the United Arab Emirates is receiving significant global attention (Whitehead, 2010; McManus, 2012). There have been earlier eco-city proposals in China, such as Dongtan near Shanghai (Chang and Sheppard, 2013), plus earlier eco-town and eco-city initiatives in Japan (Low, 2013) and in India, where programs such as the Eco-city India have been operating for approximately a decade. These initiatives vary in their focus, from industrial ecology in Japanese eco-cities through to Lavasa (near Pune in west India) which is a mix of New Urbanism and biomimicry (Dhanapal, 2011; Lavasa Corporation, 2009).

At the global level, eco-cities have been promoted by various agencies, notably the United Nations (UN), through their 1991 The Sustainable Cities Program to promote environmentally sustainable urban development. The emphasis has changed during various phases of this program. It is, however, an example of international organizations, partly funded by wealthier countries such as the United Kingdom, the Netherlands, Japan, and Denmark, working through an internationally recognized organization to enable developing countries (such as Zambia, Morocco, Cuba, and Ecuador) to improve the environments of their often fast growing cities (McManus, 2012).

In late 2009 the World Bank released its Urban and Local Government Strategy (System of Cites) highlighting the connections between cities, and the links between cities and issues such as climate change. The role of Singapore, in encouraging private and state investment in urban infrastructure, and managing urban environments, was considered crucial by the World Bank as a leading example of what other countries could emulate. The expansion of this model was encouraged by World Bank–Singapore government partnerships to promote investment in countries such as Vietnam and China (McManus, 2012). This international promotion is important in boosting the Sino-Singapore Tianjin Eco-city's development trajectory.

This range of developments in Asian, western and some developing countries raises questions about whether making cities more sustainable is an end in itself, or whether this is a vital step in making our planet sustainable. The quest for sustainable cities is the latest in a long line of ideas to improve cities and the lives of people living in them. It raises questions about the efficacy of various approaches, as well as which people are likely to benefit from such initiatives. This chapter explores these questions by first looking at urban reform in history, then focusing on the notion of eco-cities. The third section of the chapter explores the context, origins, goals, progress and potential future of the Sino-Singapore Tianjin Eco-city. This enables an evaluation of the actual performance of this eco-city in relation to the stated goals, and an analysis of its potential as a model for other Chinese cities, for urban areas in other parts of Asia and as a potential global model for future healthy and sustainable urban development.

14.2 Urban Reform in History

There is a long tradition of urban reform in various parts of the world. In Europe the expansion of cities during the Industrial Revolution was uninhibited by defensive walls, but the reliance on walking as a means of transport meant that workers often lived close to their site of employment. In the booming industrial cities of the 19th century, workers were often housed in buildings that were poorly designed, poorly built, poorly maintained and overcrowded (Engels, 1845). This led to calls for reform and/or revolution. Some wealthier industrialists built new factory towns such as New Lanark (near Glasgow) in Scotland, and Bourneville (near Birmingham), Saltaire (near Bradford) and later Port Sunlight (in the Wirral, across the River Mersey from Liverpool), to provide good quality housing, access to sunlight and recreational opportunities for their workers. These towns catered to the physical and moral health of residents by providing open space, gardens, meeting facilities, a church and were usually characterized by an absence of establishments serving alcohol (McManus, 2005). Similar developments occurred in other European countries, notably near the city of Lodz, which was known as 'Poland's Manchester' (Poplawska and Muthesius, 1986).

The establishment of new towns by wealthy industrialists was accompanied by proposals for new settlements from people who did not have the means to implement this vision. In effect, they relied on the willingness of wealthy industrialists and landowners, or the government, to adopt their visions. Foremost among these reformers were Sir Benjamin Ward Richardson (1828–1896) and Sir Ebenezer Howard (1850–1928).

In 1876, after establishing his reputation as a physician, writer and Fellow of the Royal Society, Richardson wrote *Hygeia, A City of Health*. In this publication Richardson (1876: 17–18) noted "I have projected a city that shall show the lowest mortality. I need not say that no such city exists ...." Richardson then described what a healthy city would look like, with space in this chapter permitting only a summary of six major points that have the most relevance to contemporary sustainable cities and eco-city development.

First, the proposed city of Hygeia had the "advantage of being a new foundation, but it is so built that existing cities might be largely modelled upon it" (Richardson, 1876: 18). This is similar to eco-city development in China, particularly flagship projects such as the Sino-Singapore Tianjin Eco-city. Second, "the population of the city may be placed at 100,000, living in 20,000 houses, built on 4000 acres of land, — an average of 25 persons to an acre" (Richardson, 1876: 18). Richardson (1876: 18–19) was concerned about "the effect of density on vitality", citing what he called the extreme examples of Glasgow and Liverpool as evidence of what happens when density is excessive. This concern about density and overcrowding as having health impacts, both physically and morally, is common to many early reform visions. The answer was to provide more living space, and more green space for residents, whereas contemporary eco-city and sustainable city logic in western countries opposes 'sprawling' cities and generally aims to increase densities (McManus, 2005). Third, there were to be no "tall houses overshadowing the streets, and creating necessity for one entrance to several tenements," (Richardson, 1876: 19), nor should there be "underground cellars, kitchens, or other caves, which ... are even now the loathsome residences of many millions of our domestic and industrial classes. There is not permitted to be one room underground" (Richardson, 1876: 21–22).

In addition to density and concerns about sunlight and fresh air, smoke was a major pollution concern in western cities during the Industrial Revolution, and in contemporary China. The fourth point raised by Richardson (1876: 23) was, "the most radical changes in the houses of our city" which was the chimneys. He proposed that they all be "connected with central shafts, into which the smoke is drawn, and, after being passed through a gas furnace to destroy the free carbon, is discharged colourless into the open air" (Richardson, 1876: 23–24). Richardson (1876: 24) saw the benefits at the household and the city level: "the city, therefore, at the expense of a small smoke rate, is free of raised chimneys and of the intolerable nuisance of smoke". Fifth, similar to developments such as New Lanark and Saltaire, improvements in personal health included "an absence of places for the public sale of spirituous liquors" (Richardson, 1876: 29). Richardson (1876: 29–30) saw alcohol and tobacco as being related problems, with "tobacco by far the most innocent partner in the firm" living a little longer than alcohol, but in Hygeia, the "tobacconist's counter, like the dram counter, has disappeared" (Richardson, 1876: 30). Sixth, building on Richardson's concern for matters of health, there was to be a "model hospital for the sick. To make these institutions the best of their kind, no expense is spared" (Richardson, 1876: 32).

Richardson, however, faced a similar issue to Ebenezer Howard who proposed the idea of Garden Cities, in that, unlike the early philanthropic industrialists, neither author had the means to actually develop their ideal city. While initially a social project that included communally owned land and physical and moral health achieved by people being in touch with nature through working the soil, Howard's inclusion of maps added a dimension lacking in Richardson's text-based proposal for Hygeia. This contributed to the popularity of Howard's ideas, but also to the social emphasis in *To-Morrow: A Peaceful Path to Real Reform* (1898) being overtaken by the physical aspects of his ideas in the re-titled *Garden Cities of To-Morrow* (1902) (McManus,

2005). While Howard's ideas required land and capital, the scale of the projects meant few examples were built in England (Rudlin and Falk, 1999). The concept traveled to other locations, including Japan where government support included publication of these ideas in a book in 1907 (Low, 2013). The key point about these earlier ideas for new urban developments and the relationship to contemporary developments such as eco-cities is that they all propose to address the main economic, social and environmental issues as they are understood at a particular time in a particular place.

In addition to the design of new towns located at a distance from the existing urban centers, in western countries there have been organizations formed to improve the health of the existing cities, something that eventually became a municipal and state responsibility. There was a concentration on improving the health conditions of the poorer parts of cities, understandable given the correlation between poverty and health issues, but as noted above, it wasn't just physical health but also moral health. For example, The Association for Promoting Cleanliness Among the Poor, and the Society for the Improvement of the Conditions of the Laboring Classes, both aimed to improve the physical aspects of the city (baths and dwellings respectively) with a view to improving the health of the most vulnerable residents (Ashton and Ubido, 1991).

The early model towns and cities, especially those built on so-called 'greenfield sites', were the forerunners of many planning attempts to improve the built environment for social, economic, and environmental reasons. Similar to contemporary eco-cities such as the Sino-Singapore Tianjin Eco-city, these early model towns wielded "considerable influence over urban ecological landscapes beyond their own locality" (Chang and Sheppard, 2013: 59), in much the same way that ideas such as Garden Cities flourished in Japan (Low, 2013). In contrast, Le Corbusier's plans were implemented in Chandigarh, northern India through personal involvement (Perera, 2004; Shaw, 2009). However understood, the ability of iconic cities to travel and have import beyond their own locality is part of the story of the Sino-Singapore Tianjin Eco-city. It is important to note, however, that as Chang and Sheppard (2013) demonstrate with Dongtan and Chongming near Shanghai, and Low (2013) argues in relation to Japan and Shaw (2009) in the Indian context, this transnational travel of iconic cities is only part of the story. In other contexts, these cities fit within national and regional histories and geographies, often being an attempt to recreate or build on a historical period that is perceived to have been the golden era of a people and place.

The concepts of sustainable cities and eco-cities also represent a change in thinking by some environmentalists. Whereas cities were previously seen as 'dark satanic mills' (McMichael, 2008), or more recently as parasites (Rees, 1998) and vortices (McManus, 2005), the evolving "urban sustainability policies highlight the role of cities as strategic geographical locales for the emergence, translation, circulation, and realization of sustainability, at all scales" (Chang and Sheppard, 2013: 58). This means that more attention is being given to restructuring cities, with greater recognition that most of the world's people are now urban dwellers. Yanarella and Levine (1992: 772), recognized that "the ecological city in its many versions can serve as a working model whose benefits, lessons and consequences can radiate outwards, touching more and more societies around the world", but saw that in order to "become a genuine model and stimulus to broader restructuring in society and around the globe, the sustainable city must literally find its place or places in the evolving world of contradictory possibilities and risks".

14.3 Eco-Cities

The concept of an eco-city is open to debate. Eco-cities may be existing cities, but the term is often used to indicate new cities. The new cities appear exciting because to seem to start from nothing. To build an entire new city that includes all the latest eco-technology, design and materials, and to not have to engage with the problems of the existing built environment, is an achievement that can be easily demarcated and promoted. In the western context, this type of new settlement has often emphasized "compact, self-sufficient communities with minimal ecological impact, constrained economic growth, orientation toward the locality, community participation, and social equity" (Chang and Sheppard, 2013: 61). According to Chang and Sheppard (2013: 61) "this should not be taken as the norm for an eco-city" and a relational perspective is required, rather than measuring eco-cities in terms of "degrees of deviation from a supposedly paradigmatic norm".

This 'paradigmatic norm' is arguably that of the creator of the term 'eco-cities', Richard Register, who used it in relation to Berkeley (Oakland, California). Register advocated 'bulldozing suburbia' to start again, similar to what Le Corbusier proposed in the early 20th century for the Right Bank of Paris, and to what was implemented in the mid-19th century in Paris under the direction of Baron von Haussmann, when the medieval city was demolished to make way for a city of boulevards (for military control of the city) and to let light into what had been a dense, dark city (Harvey, 2006; McManus, 2005).

According to Ecocity Builders (2010), the organization founded by Richard Register in 1992, an eco-city is defined as:

> A human settlement modeled on the self-sustaining resilient structure and function of natural ecosystems. The eco-city provides healthy abundance to its inhabitants without consuming more (renewable) resources than it produces, without producing more waste than it can assimilate, and without being toxic to itself or neighboring ecosystems. Its inhabitants' ecological impact reflect planetary supportive lifestyles; its social order reflects fundamental principles of fairness, justice and reasonable equity.

Richard Register (1987: 3) defined an eco-city as "an ecologically healthy city", but writes in the next sentence that "no such city exists". This comment is similar to the words of Benjamin Ward Richardson 111 years earlier in relation to a healthy city. What does exist are "bits and pieces of the eco-city scattered about in present-day cities and sprinkled through history" (Register, 1987: 3), and attempts to create eco-cities. Some of these attempts are by community-based organizations operating on bio-regional principles (Downton, 2009), while — using the same terminology — government and industry partnerships are focused on building eco-cities that are both global in their impact and local/regional/national in their *raison d'être* and their identity formation. For example, Chang and Sheppard (2013: 68) situate Dongtan and Chongming in relation to the Chinese desire to avoid 'over-urbanization', such that "whereas the world outside China came to know Dongtan as a model for green settlements in global cities ... in China it is recognized as a model for agricultural towns on the urban fringe". Another example is Masdar, located near Abu Dhabi. It is the collaboration between the government and the British architectural firm Foster + Partners. Masdar is important because it emphasizes commercial viability as part of ecological sustainability and a high quality of life (Whitehead, 2010). The architecture often invokes tradition Arabian architectural themes, but the emphasis is on clean technology, energy reduction and reducing the environmental impact of the city.

The existence of new eco-cities in different geographic locations, embedded in particular cultural contexts, is indicative of the potential of this concept to spread beyond a small part of the world, and to be adapted so that it fits appropriately into various settings. This conforms to what Chang and Sheppard (2013) called 'variegated urban sustainability' and rejects the notion of a paradigmatic norm. The danger with developments such as the Tianjin Eco-city is that they can quickly become the 'new norm'.

The creation of a 'new norm' is, of course, one of the goals of the project, as confirmed by the global engineering consultancy Mott MacDonald (2009: 2) when they wrote that the eco-city will become a "model eco and low carbon city replicable by other cities in China". This view aligns with that of the Government of Singapore (2012) which observes that the 'three abilities' of the eco-city are that it is:

- Practicable — the technologies adopted in the eco-city must be affordable and commercially viable.
- Replicable — the principles and models of the eco-city could be applied to other cities in China and even in other countries.
- Scalable — the principles and models could be adapted for another project or development of a different scale.

Chang and Sheppard (2013: 66), quoting Herbert Giradet (who was a former consultant on the Dongtan project), believe "China will play a key role in the emergence of a world of ecological and economically sustainable human settlements". According to Chang and Sheppard (2013: 67), the "mindset of 'first' and 'biggest' is itself an important feature, looked for by the Chinese government when it picks development projects to support". This view is supported by Hald (2009) who argues that eco-city development reflects China's desire to be at the forefront of green urbanism, and by the existence of over one hundred eco-cities in China as of 2012 (Wu, 2012). In other words, the creation of a city as a paradigmatic norm is advanced by the Chinese state for political advantage. This provides a model for other locations, which may or may not be appropriate, but may also limit the potential for additional variegated urbanism to emerge. The model eco-city that is most advanced in development in China is the Sino-Singapore Tianjin Eco-City.

14.4 The Sino-Singapore Tianjin Eco-City

14.4.1 *Context*

The number of people living in China's cities exceeded those living in rural areas at the end of 2011, according to the National Bureau of Statistics of China (Wines, 2012). At that time there were 690.79 million urban dwellers, accounting for 51.27% of the country's total population. The rapid urbanization of China, which is expected to add 440 million new urban residents between 1990 and 2020 (more than the entire US population) will inevitably produce different types of cities (Heikkila and Xu, 2014; see Zheng and Guo this volume). Much of this population growth and urbanization is concentrated in the east of the country, around coastal locations. For these reasons, the Chinese Government established two criteria to be met in the site selection process for the location of the eco-city: it should be developed on non-arable land and it should be located in an area facing water shortage (Government of Singapore, 2012).

The Sino-Singapore Tianjin Eco-city is a new project situated in the Bohai Rim region of northeast China, close to the port city of

Binhai. It is about 40 kilometers east of Tianjin (often regarded as China's third largest city) and about 150 kilometres south-east of Beijing. Over 240 million people live in the Bohai Rim region, which in 2010 produced over a quarter of China's GDP (in Caprotti, 2014). The rapid urban development of former agricultural land is a major concern of Chinese officials given that, allowing for topography, rainfall and soil conditions, the country has a mere .09 hectares of cultivatable land per person (Cui and Kattumuri, 2010; see also Wang *et al.*, this volume). The eco-city is located in a region of low rainfall, thereby making water management an important part of the city's planning. While it is not the first eco-city project proposed in the world, nor even in China, its scale and its rapid development aimed at making it the first successful eco-city, and therefore a template, are important features of the Sino-Singapore Tainjin Ecocity.

14.4.2 *Origins*

The concept of an eco-city was initiated by the Singaporeans in 2007, following their earlier collaboration in developing Suzhou Industrial Park (Mott MacDonald, 2009). There were four initial sites under consideration; in Baotou (Inner Mongolia), Tangshan (Hebei province), Tianjin municipality and Urumqi (Xinjiang) (Government of Singapore, 2012). By late 2007 the site near Tianjin had been selected because of advantage in the timeframe for completing the start-up area, commercial viability, economic strengths and robustness compared with other candidate cities, and site-specific issues such as accessibility and ease of pollution control. A Draft Master Plan was endorsed by April, 2008 and a ground-breaking ceremony was conducted in September of that year.

The planned area of the eco-city is 30 square kilometres, comprising 16 square kilometres of non-arable land and 14 square kilometres of water. The land was requisitioned by the government from "3 villages, 2 state-owned enterprises and 1 military enterprise within the project area" (Mott MacDonald, 2009: 4). The eco-city is being built in an environment that comprises one-third saline affected land, one-third considered a wasteland, and one-third water. While this may arguably be contentious for coastal environments, it may potentially reduce urban development pressures on an equivalent sized area of agriculturally productive land. It also overcomes some of the site selection problems associated with Dongtan (Chang and Sheppard, 2013: 63), which was "planned on a conservation wetland to host exclusively high-end property" and therefore was seen as "harmful to the ecologically sensitive Yangtze estuary".

14.4.3 *Goals*

The Sino-Singapore Tianjin Eco-city embodies the 'three harmonies', represented by the Government of Singapore (2012), these being:

> People living in harmony with other people, i.e. social harmony; people living in harmony with economic activities, i.e. economic vibrancy; and people living in harmony with the environment, i.e. environmental sustainability.

This is a Chinese cultural representation of what has been presented internationally and in western contexts, as sustainable development, a balance of the social, economic and environmental concerns for current and future generations (McManus, 2005).

The Tianjin Eco-city builds on Singapore's developmental experience and China's experience with eco-cities. In China, the Ministry of Environmental Protection (MEP) and the Ministry of Housing and Urban-Rural Development (MoHURD) have both developed national standards for eco-cities. The approach to sustainability begins at the macro-level with comprehensive master planning integrating land use and transport planning, a planning approach that is in synchrony with contemporary Chinese governance. The planned city will be divided into seven distinct sectors: a Lifescape, an Eco-Valley, a Solarscape, an Urbanscape, a Windscape, an Earthscape and Eco-Corridors. The key performance indicators (KPIs) include energy efficiency and the use of renewable energy, with at least 90% of trips to be by public transport or active transport (cycling, walking), water recycling and all buildings conforming to green building standards. When completed in 2020, the eco-city is anticipated to have a population of 350,000 residents

(Government of Singapore, 2012). In this sense, the eco-city is a response to contemporary problems of traffic congestion, energy security, water quality and availability and the impact of cities on human health.

14.4.4 *Progress*

The first phase of the city (three square kilometres) was to be completed by 2013, with the entire site of over 30 square kilometres developed by 2020. In late October, 2013 the Singapore Government's National Development Minister Khaw Boon Wan said:

> Now, the population is about 6000, (which) seems like a very small number. But the growth rate from now on will be quite rapid. Those of you who went there five years ago, I think you'll be amazed at the transformations" (Ou, 2013).

Not everybody is impressed. Caprotti (2014) contrasted the Tianjin Eco-city with his own transition town of Totnes, in south-west England, with its population of about 23,000 residents. He noted that the Tianjin Eco-city is "built on a structure of large urban residential blocks separated by multi-lane highways" and that "the eco-buildings are significant in size, being mostly over 25 stories in height" (Caprotti, 2014: 12). While there is definitely rapid progress in construction, this is not yet matched by occupation. Caprotti (2014: 13) found a city that:

> Looks remarkably like any other contemporary Chinese residential development: tall residential apartment blocks and a clear focus on the car as a means of getting from area to area and to the newly-constructed commercial 'blocks' housing empty supermarkets and cinemas.

The feeling is of being in a "large but as yet empty city" (Caprotti, 2014: 12). Caprotti (2014: 13) also observed "very little grass — everything here has been uprooted and decontaminated, as this was formed (sic) salt marsh and industrial land". This site selection results in issues such as minimal vegetation, with the two trees that were visible having leaves made of plastic, "stuck carefully on to the branches with tape" (Caprotti, 2014: 13).

The development of Tianjin Eco-city has both attributes and weaknesses from a health perspective. While there are green-energy buses and other initiatives that improve air quality in this particular urban environment, there are also delays in providing appropriate health facilities. The city appears to be slow in providing doctors, although now a doctor is assigned to every 300 to 500 households (Min, 2013). The city's hospital is still under construction, and is expected to open in 2015, at least a year after residents have moved into the eco-city (Jander, 2013; Min, 2013).

14.4.5 *Potential future*

The future of Tianjin Eco-city is promising, despite Caprotti's observations. The location of the city in the booming Bohai Rim region of northeast China, about 40 kilometres east of Tianjin and about 150 kilometres southeast of Beijing, means that it is likely to attract the pan-Asian executive urbanites that Chang and Sheppard (2013) and Caprotti (2014) believe to be the main clientele for these residential developments. The Sino-Singapore Tianjin Eco-City is seen by Caprotti (2014: 15) as being "another example of top-down urban dystopias such as Pruitt-Igoe" (an award-winning 1950s public housing development in St. Louis that was demolished in the early 1970s). Caprotti's observations of the social structure of Tainjin Eco-city accord with the comments of Wu (2012) who observed that the eco-cities are a Chinese version of 'post-suburbia', which is not the location of vegetable gardens (similar to the Japanese suburban "garden cities" in Low, 2013), but are the realm of government support for Chinese land investment corporations working in partnership with foreign development corporations.

14.5 Potential Model for Other Cities

One feature common to Hygeia, the Garden Cities and the eco-cities is that the city serves as a model for other cities in their development.

China will need to build the equivalent of 18.4 cities the size of the Sino-Singapore Tianjin Eco-city each year to accommodate the population growth of 6.44 million people between 2010 and 2011, not allowing for rural-to-urban migration (derived from National Bureau of Statistics, 2012). According to Wu (2012: 169), "more than 100 Chinese municipal governments are proposing to build eco-cities or eco-towns". Although Wu (2012: 170) acknowledges that there "are some doubts about whether some eco-cities are really ecologically sound, and the eco-city movement may be driven by other motivations", he believes that the ecological turn in China is genuine and that it will be perpetuated. There are clear differences between current Chinese eco-cities. For example, the catalyst for the development of Caofeidian in Tangshan was the relocation of a steel company from Beiijng, whereas in the Guangming district of Shenzen in south-west China, the aim is to build an ecological new town based on high-tech industries (Wu, 2012). In any case, aspects of eco-cities such as the Sino-Singapore Tianjin Eco-city will likely be included both in new eco-cities, and in the redevelopment of existing urban areas. In this sense, the Sino-Singapore Tianjin Eco-City is already a role model for other Chinese cities, but this model could be improved by the earlier establishment of appropriate health and medical facilities for the anticipated population.

While the Tianjin Eco-City is situated in an area of rapid population and economic growth around the Bohai Sea, throughout the world new locations for cities may be generated by climate change impacts, notably rising sea levels. These new cities may be very important in reducing the vulnerability, and often multiple vulnerabilities, of poorer people to the impacts of climate change. In this sense, China's recent experience with eco-cities offers lessons not just within China, but for other countries with rapid population growth, vulnerable coastal cities and the likelihood of rural-to-urban migration. One obvious example is India, which is anticipated to overtake China in total population around 2028. In 2011 the proportion of the total Indian population classified as urban was 36.5% (Swerts *et al.*, 2014). The United Nations has focused on the development of the most populous cities in India, but Swerts *et al.* (2014: 51) argue that the United Nations "has a tendency to underestimate the expansion of the whole city-system".

Their population projects, based on United Nations data, shows that by 2050 over 55% of the Indian population is anticipated to be living in urban areas. This would represent more than 925 million people, which is "equivalent to India's entire population in 1993" (Swerts *et al.*, 2014: 51). There is enormous potential, and need, for eco-city development in such a context, and although countries such as India and Japan have experience with their own versions of eco-cities, as shown in this chapter, templates from Chinese eco-cities cannot be simply relocated to other cultural and political–economic contexts.

14.6 Conclusion

China's contemporary experience of eco-cities is part of a long engagement by philanthropic factory owners, health professionals, urban planners, architects and governments that has aimed to improve cities at particular moments in time. Sometimes the ideas for better cities did not get beyond the page or off the map, but in other cases, including the Sino-Singapore Tianjin Eco-city, these ideas are being realised. Throughout the roughly 200 year period covered in this chapter, it is apparent that one area for city improvement is health, with proposals over time variously emphasizing physical, emotional and moral health. In the Sino-Singapore Tianjin Eco-City, health is represented within the three harmonies, with environmental health, social health and economic health (meaning a prosperous and vibrant city) being part of the approach to urban development.

The Sino-Singapore Tianjin Eco-city represents a departure from the concept of eco-cities promoted by Richard Register. As Yanarella and Levine (1992) and Chang and Sheppard (2013) recognized, a variety of approaches are needed given different political, social, cultural and environmental contexts. 'Vernacular models' based on local conditions and needs, and inspired by meaningful actions such as the Sino-Singapore Tianjin Eco-city, are required. Such an approach would conform with Chang and Sheppard's (2013) call for a variegated urbanism in relation to eco-cities, where the Sino-Singapore Tianjin Eco-city is but one of a number of possible eco-city types that promote sustainable urbanism within their local geographic context, and to a wider international audience.

References

Ashton, J. and Ubido, J. (1991). The Healthy City and the Ecological Idea, *Social History of Medicine* **4**(1): 17–180.

Benton-Short, L. and Short, J.R. (2008). *Cities and Nature*, Routledge, London.

Caprotti, F. (2014.) Critical research on eco-cities? A Walk Through the Sino-Singapore Tianjin Eco-City, China, *Cities* **36**: 10–17.

Chang, I-C.C. and Sheppard, E. (2013). China's Eco-Cities Variegated Urban Sustainability: Dongtan Eco-city and Chongming Eco-island, *Journal of Urban Technology* **20**(1): 57–75.

Cui, S. and Kattumuri, R. (2010). 'Cultivated land conversion in China and the potential for food security and sustainability', *Working Paper 35*, Asia Research Centre, London School of Economics and Political Science, London.

Dhanapal, G. (2011) Eco-cities for India. Available at http://india.carbon-outlook.com/content/eco-cities-india [Accessed 13 January, 2012].

Downton, P. F. (2009). *Ecopolis: Architecture and Cities for a Changing Climate*, Springer Science+Business and CSIRO, Dordrecht and Mebourne.

Ecocity Builders (2010). Ecocity Definition. Available at http://www.ecocitybuilders.org/why-ecocities/the-solution/ecocity-definition/ [Accessed 2 March, 2014].

Engels, F. (1845). *The Condition of the Working Class in England in 1844*, Translated by F.K. Wischnewetzky (1892), Reprinted 1952, Allen & Unwin, London.

Government of Singapore (2012). Yianjin Eco-City: A Model for Sustainable Development. Available at http://www.tianjinecocity.gov.sg/bg_intro.htm (updated 28 March, 2012) [Accessed 3 November 2014].

Hald, M. (2009). *Sustainable Urban Development and the Chinese Eco-City: Concepts, Strategies, Policies and Assessments*, Fridtjof Nansens Institute, Oslo.

Harvey, D. (2006) *Paris, Capital of Modernity*, Routledge, New York.

Heikkila, E. and Xu, Y. (2014). Seven Prototypical Chinese Cities, *Journal of Urban Studies* **51**(4): 826–847.

Jander, M. (2013). China-Singapore Eco-City: Slow, but on Track. *UBM's Future Cities*. Available at http://www.ubmfuturecities.com/author.asp?section_id=234&doc_id=526004 [Accessed 3 November 2014].

Lavasa Corporation (2009). Lavasa. Available at http://www.lavasa.com/high/current_status.aspx [Accessed 21 January, 2012].

Low, M. (2013). Eco-Cities in Japan: Past and Future, *Journal of Urban Technology* **20**(1): 7–22.

McManus, P. (2005). *Vortex Cities to Sustainable Cities: Australia's Urban Challenge*, UNSW Press, Sydney.

McManus, P. (2012). 'Ecocities and sustainable urban environments' in Murray, J., Cawthorne, G., Dey, C. and Andrew, C. (eds.), *Enough For All Forever: A Handbook For Learning About Sustainability*, Common Ground Publishing. Champaign, Illinois, pp. 201–214.

McMichael, A. (2008). 'The urban environment and health' in Newton, P.W. (ed.) *Transitions: Pathways towards sustainable development in Australia*. CSIRO, Melbourne, pp.573–584.

Min, Z. (2013). Family healthcare offered to eco-city residents. Available at http://usa.chinadaily.com.cn/china/2013-11/18/content_17111406.htm [Accessed 3 November 2014].

Mott, MacDonald (2009). *Sino-Singapore Tianjin Eco-City Project: Report on Review of Land Acquisition and Resettlement* **2**: RP907, v2.

Ou, J. (2013). Khaw confident on outlook for Tianjin Eco-City, *The Straits Times*, Available at http://business.asiaone.com/news/khaw-confident-outlook-tianjin-eco-city [Accessed 3 March 2014].

Perera, N. (2004). Contesting visions: Hybridity, Liminality and the Authorship of the Chandigarh Plan, *Planning Perspectives* **19**: 175–199.

Poplawska, I. and Muthesius, S. (1986). Poland's Manchester: 19th-Century Industrial and Domestic Architecture in Lodz, *Journal of the Society of Architectural Historians* **45**(2): 148–160.

Register, R. (1987). *Ecocity Berkeley: Building cities for a healthy future*, North Atlantic Books, Berkeley.

Richardson, B.W. (1876). *Hygeia, A City of Health*, MacMillan & Co., London.

Rudlin, D. and Falk, N. (1999). *Building the 21st Century Home: The Sustainable Neighbourhood*, Architectural Press, Oxford.

Shaw, A. (2009). Town Planning in Postcolonial India, 1947–1965: Chandigarh Re-examined. *Urban Geography Journal* **30**(8): 857–878.

Swerts, E., Pumain, D. and Denis, E. (2014). The Future of India's Urbanization, *Futures: The journal of policy, planning and futures studies* **56**: 43–52.

Whitehead, I. (2010). *Models of sustainability? A comparative analysis of ideal city planning in Saltaire and Masdar City.* GEOView.

Wines, M. (2012). Majority of Chinese Now Live in Cities, *The New York Times*, 17th January Available at http://www.nytimes.com/2012/01/18/world/asia/majority-of-chinese-now-live-in-cities.html?_r=0 [Accessed 3 March 2014].

Wu, F. (2012). China's Eco-Cities, *Geoforum* **43**: 169–171.

Yanarella, E.J. and Levine, R.S. (1992) Does Sustainable Development Lead to Sustainability? *Futures: The Journal of Policy, Planning and Futures Studies* **24**(8): 759–774.

Chapter Fifteen

Urbanization, Population Health, and Policy Reforms

Gordon G. Liu, Jay Pan, and Xiao Yu Wu[1]

Abstract

There are intricate connections between urbanization and population health. Through a review of the economic and other relevant literature this chapter presents a mainstream view of how population health is influenced by the urbanization process. From findings of empirical analyses of two large Chinese national studies datasets, the authors postulate the possible mechanisms through which urbanization influences health. The chapter provides insights into and practical recommendations for the ongoing health policy reforms likely to shape the future influence of urbanization on population health in China.

15.1 Introduction

China has experienced rapid urbanization during the past three decades. The percentage of people living in cities increased from 19.4% in 1980 to 51.3% in 2010 (National Bureau of Statistics of China, 2011a).

[1] Xiaoyu Wu thanks the National Natural Science Foundation of China (#71103211) for financial support.

The consequences for individuals of such a rapid urbanization process, such as health status, are important for human capital accumulation and sustainable economic development. In the economic literature, the impact of urbanization on health is complex. On the one hand, cities offer better job opportunities, higher wages, better education, and health services (McDade and Adair, 2001). On the other hand, urbanization is accompanied by a range of increasing health risks, including obesity, chronic diseases, environmental degradation, infectious diseases, stress and mental health issues, and congestion in the consumption of medical services (Moore *et al.*, 2003). The overall effects of urbanization on health, therefore, are mixed.

In this chapter, we present a brief review of both Chinese and international literature on urbanization and its effect on human health. We take people living in urban areas over total population at city level from Census data, and use it as a measure of the degree of urbanization (National Bureau of Statistics of China, 2005, 2010).[2] We then conduct an empirical analysis of the impact of urbanization on population health at the individual level. The focus of our analysis is on the major mechanisms through which population health is influenced by urbanization. Finally, we provide critiques of the health policy reforms related to urbanization and make recommendations for ways forward.

15.2 Urbanization and Population Health

Compared with rural areas, urbanized areas generally provide better public health and medical services (Vlahov *et al.*, 2007). The numbers of hospitals and doctors are higher in urban areas compared with rural areas (Grumbach *et al.*, 1997). Health insurance coverage is positively associated with the degree of urbanization (Liu *et al.*, 2003). During the process of urbanization, more people move to cities and have better access to health related services, which has positive effects on individual health status. For example, Mangyo (2008) found that the

[2] We use the 2005 Inter-Population Census and the 2010 Population Census to construct the measure for the degree of urbanization.

accessibility and safety of drinking water significantly improves the health of adults and children. However, rising population density in urban areas increases congestion in medical consumption. The growth of medical resources is much slower than population growth (Qin *et al.*, 2013). The costs of medical services are higher than in the past.

What is more concerning, is that access to health care for the rural-to-urban migrants is a big challenge. For one thing, they are less likely than local people in urban areas to have local medical insurance. For another, it is not convenient for them to use health services in their origin communities. Thus, the migrants consistently underuse health services, both in their origin communities and destination cities (Gong *et al.*, 2012). For example, a study in Shenzhen City, one of the top destinations for migrant workers in China, showed that 55% of migrants were uninsured, and 62% of migrant workers who reported illness did not visit a doctor (Mou *et al.*, 2009). All these create potential short-term and long-term health problems. Hong *et al.* (2006) found that infant survival rates and health status are lower for migrants than local urban residents. Liu *et al.* (2014) using the national representative household survey data found that migration has had a significantly negative impact on migrant health.

Urbanization is also accompanied by environmental degradation (Zheng and Kahn, 2013; Wang *et al.*, 1999; Brajer and Mead, 2003). Highly concentrated population and industrial production are the major sources of urban pollution (Henderson, 2002). Cole and Neumayer (2004) found that the urbanization rate positively correlates with carbon dioxide (CO_2) and sulfur dioxide (SO_2) emissions. Rapid increases in motor vehicle use (vehicle emissions, including ozone and inhalable particles) and household energy consumption, mainly produced from coal, contribute to air pollution that far exceeds health standards in many cities (Health Effects Institute, 2004). What is worse, the pollution spreads from highly urbanized areas to nearby rural areas (Zhang *et al.*, 2010). The reported negative impacts of air pollution on health are extensive. They include an increase in premature deaths, low birth weight, hospital admissions, asthma, respiratory disease, lung cancer, and cardiovascular diseases (Neidell, 2004; Currie and Neidell, 2004; Chay and Greenstone, 1999; Cohen *et al.*, 2004;

Wang *et al.*, 1997; Alberini and Krupnick, 1998; O'Neill *et al.*, 2003; Vigotti *et al.*, 1996).

Water pollution also increases during urbanization due to a growing volume of industrial wastewater discharge and inadequate investment in water supply and treatment. Ito (2005) found that population size had significantly negative impacts on water quality in Chinese cities. Wastewater treatment systems in urban areas cannot accommodate the population increase. A 2006 survey showed that more than a quarter of public and private water suppliers in China were not complying with water quality requirements (Zhang, 2007). Data from Pearl River Delta Economic Zone in China found a positive correlation between the rapidity of urbanization and the pollution levels of urban river water (Ouyang *et al.*, 2006). Urbanization is proceeding rapidly even though nearly half of China's major cities do not comply with the basic national health standards for drinking water (SEPA, 2006). Water pollution increases the risk of exposure to infectious, parasitic, digestive and vector-borne diseases (Dasgupta, 2004; Ebenstein, 2012; Knudsen and Slooff, 1992; Wu *et al.*, 1999). Shin *et al.* (1997) found that water-borne diseases were the leading cause of child death in developing countries.

Lifestyle and health-related behaviors (patterns of human activity) have changed during urbanization. To begin with, the patterns of diet have changed. People living in urban areas tend to consume more processed foods, which are higher in fat and calories (Popkin and Bisgrove, 1988). Secondly, people engage in less physical activity. Occupation-related physical activity declines with modernization and cities offer more sedentary jobs (Monda *et al.*, 2007). Motorized transport and labor-saving household appliances that are common in urban areas are further causes of the decline in physical activity. These deficits in energy expenditure are unlikely to be compensated for through physical leisure activities (Bauman *et al.*, 2008). Furthermore, physical leisure activities are less common in China than in developed countries (Bell *et al.*, 2001; Fu and Fung, 2004; Hu *et al.*, 2002). Studies show that obesity, hypertension, physical inactivity, and high intake of dietary fat are more prevalent in towns and cities in China, but the urban–rural gap is closing with the recent economic boom in rural areas. Although the drivers of these trends are not well understood, urbanization has led to changes in patterns of human activity, diet, and social structures in China. With these changes, people have become increasingly exposed to a high risk of hypertension and many other non-communicable chronic diseases (Liu *et al.*, 2004; Weng *et al.*, 2007).

Urbanization can also promote neuropsychiatric disorders and injury-related deaths, especially in the rural-to-urban migrant population. Mental disorders are one of the leading health problems in China (Yang *et al.*, 2013), and it is estimated that 17% of the adult population suffers from one or more mental disorders (Phillips *et al.*, 2009). With rapid urbanization, urban environments present psychological and social stressors, particularly to the rural-to-urban migrants. Compared with non-migrant peers, migrants are especially vulnerable to these stressors, and are at higher risk of mental disorders (Chen, 2011). On the one hand, they withstand psychological stressors such as homelessness and social isolation (Krieger and Higgins, 2002). On the other hand, they are vulnerable to the social stressors involving assimilation and acculturation, language acquisition, identity change, social discrimination, income inequality, deprivation of opportunities for upward mobility, and a sense of marginality (Cheung, 2014).

Injury-related deaths are recognized as another public health problem associated with urbanization in China. Over the past decades, traffic-related injuries and occupational accidents have become the most common form of accidents and injuries (Hu *et al.*, 2008; Zhang *et al.*, 2013; Zhangtao, 2010), and are considered an adverse result of rapid urbanization (Li *et al.*, 2012). In 2010, road traffic accidents resulted in 65,225 deaths, and cost over RMB 900 million in direct property losses (Zhang *et al.*, 2013). In urban areas, increasingly crowded roadways are shared by a mix of pedestrians, and motorized and non-motorized vehicles, that compete for road space. The number of motorcycles and other vehicles increased six times more than automobiles during 1985–2005. The increased number of motorcycles may have been a potential risk factor in the increased road-traffic death rate (Hu *et al.*, 2008). Cyclists and pedestrians are especially at risk, and make up 60% of traffic-related deaths (Pucher *et al.*, 2007; Wang *et al.*, 2008). Non-motorized transport is still used for as many as 40–55% of total trips taken in Beijing and Shanghai, and a much higher proportion of journeys than that in smaller cities in China. Since the urban residents of low socio–economic status, especially migrants, mainly depend on these non-motorized vehicles, they are exposed to the high risk of road traffic (Pucher *et al.*, 2007).

Occupational accidents are another source of injuries. The number of people in China exposed to occupational hazards is highest in the world (Yu and Zhou, 2004). The less safe working conditions and longer working hours for migrant workers expose them higher risks of occupational injuries (Chang and Wang, 2009; Gong, 2012).

With respect to the measurement of urbanization, most studies use the dichotomy of rural and urban areas comparison. This method ignores the variation within rural and urban areas, and tends to overlook the impact on health of different degrees of urbanization. Other studies use factor analysis approach and construct an urbanicity index (Dahly and Adair, 2007; McDade and Adair 2001; Van de Poel *et al.*, 2012). The disadvantage of this method is that the urbanicity index can only demonstrate the level of urbanization of the communities under survey, and is not comparable across surveys.

15.3 Empirical Analysis of the Impact of Urbanization on Health

15.3.1 *Evidence from individual level data*

To estimate the impact of urbanization on health, we use two individual-level datasets that contain information on health and socio-economic outcomes. The first dataset is based on the 2005 Inter-Census Population Survey. This survey, conducted by the National Bureau of Statistics of China (2011b), covered 1% of the total population. Data analyzed and presented in this chapter is a sub-sample, that is, one-fifth of randomly selected samples from all surveyed people. We use 'self-reported health outcome' as the indicator for health. Although 'self-reported outcome' is a subjective measure, it can reflect a comprehensive status of health and is an independent predictor of mortality (Idler and Benyamini, 1997). The health indicator equals 1, if people reported a good health status, and equals 0 if not. In our sample set, 93% of the respondents reported a good health status. The fractions of people who are living in urban areas at the prefecture level are used as the index of urbanization.[3] In regression analysis, we looked at three groups, namely the urban residents with a non-agricultural permanent residence registry (*Hukou*), the rural residents, and the rural-to-urban migrants meaning people living in the urban areas but with an agricultural *Hukou*. A description of the basic characteristics of the three groups is presented in Table 15.1. It is clearly shown that the urban residents, including the rural-to-urban migrants, have a better health status, higher income and higher education levels compared with the rural residents.

To complement this study, we used a second dataset, the 2010 Chinese Family Panel Studies (CFPS) (Institute of Social Science Survey, 2010), which includes objective measures of health status. This survey was conducted by the Institute of Social Science Survey at Peking University, China, in collaboration with the Survey Research Center at the University of Michigan, The United States of America. It covered 25 provinces in China, and information on various health indicators, such as whether the respondent was diagnosed with specific chronic diseases, was collected. We used the prefecture level urbanization rate from the 2010 Population Census as the index and matched the rate to the individuals' health data in the 2010 CFPS (Institute of Social Science Survey, 2010). This is also shown in Table 15.1. The average urbanization rate in 2010 reported in this survey was 51.1%, which is consistent with the reported national urbanization level.[4] The self-reported health status equals 1 if the respondents reported their health was good or fine, and equals 0 if they reported their status was somewhat bad, bad or very bad. According to this definition, 83.4% of people report a good health status. The other health indicators that are not shown in this table are whether the respondent was diagnosed with any chronic disease, or whether they were underweight

---

[3] A Prefecture-level city is an administrative division in China. It ranks below a province and above a county.

[4] According to China Statistical Yearbooks, the fraction of people living in urban areas in 2010 is 50% (National Bureau of Statistics of China, 2011b).

Table 15.1 Descriptive statistics

	2005 Inter-census population survey				
	Total sample	Urban residents	Rural residents	Migrants in urban areas	2010 CFPS
Urbanization rate	0.476	0.601	0.383	0.547	0.511
	(0.220)	(0.229)	(0.159)	(0.232)	(0.207)
Self-reported health status	0.930	0.935	0.920	0.947	0.834
	(0.255)	(0.246)	(0.271)	(0.224)	(0.372)
Household annual per capita income	0.432	0.473	0.407	0.441	0.824
	(0.204)	(0.224)	(0.173)	(0.238)	(1.211)
Age	36.58	38.67	36.37	34.52	46.49
	(18.91)	(18.23)	(19.56)	(17.83)	(15.42)
Male	0.499	0.503	0.502	0.489	0.494
	(0.500)	(0.500)	(0.500)	(0.500)	(0.500)
Married	0.625	0.668	0.608	0.613	0.839
	(0.484)	(0.471)	(0.488)	(0.487)	(0.367)
Illiterate	0.099	0.035	0.137	0.084	0.296
	(0.298)	(0.183)	(0.344)	(0.277)	(0.456)
Elementary school	0.332	0.167	0.417	0.326	0.212
	(0.471)	(0.373)	(0.493)	(0.469)	(0.409)
Middle school	0.375	0.306	0.374	0.463	0.290
	(0.484)	(0.461)	(0.484)	(0.499)	(0.454)
High school	0.132	0.283	0.063	0.114	0.128
	(0.338)	(0.450)	(0.242)	(0.317)	(0.334)
College	0.061	0.203	0.008	0.013	0.072
	(0.239)	(0.403)	(0.089)	(0.114)	(0.258)
Master and above	0.002	0.006	0.000	0.000	0.001
	(0.041)	(0.078)	(0.005)	(0.007)	(0.038)
Have any health Insurance	0.516	0.354	0.568	0.589	0.815
	(0.500)	(0.478)	(0.495)	(0.492)	(0.388)
Have access to drinking water	0.550	0.935	0.311	0.659	0.635
	(0.497)	(0.247)	(0.463)	(0.474)	(0.482)
Observations	2,404,319	633,413	1,254,597	516,309	29,171

Source: 2005 Inter-Census Population Survey (National Bureau of Statistics of China, 2005), and 2010 CFPS (Institute of Social Science Survey, 2010).

(BMI < 18.5), overweight (25 < BMI < 30) or obese (BMI > 30).[5] Fifteen percent of the respondents in this survey reported a chronic disease diagnosis in the past six months, 9.8% were underweight, 18% were overweight, and 2.1% were obese.

Regression analysis of the 2005 Inter-Census Population Survey using the linear probability model shows that urbanization has a statistically significant negative effect on population health (Table 15.2). The probability of having a 'good' health status decreases by 0.6 percentage points with every 1 percentage point increase in urbanization rate. Furthermore, urbanization has a negative effect on the health status of urban residents, compared with rural residents.

In addition to what has been highlighted in the literature review, there are several explanations for how urbanization could negatively affect population health. As discussed, urbanization increases population density in cities. As a consequence, medical facilities in cities become more overcrowded. The actual accessibility of medical services decreases, which tends to lead to negative effects on an individual's health status. The urbanization process is also accompanied by industrialization, leading to more industrial wastewater discharge, and more greenhouse emissions from industries and motor vehicles. Environmental pollution might be another major reason for the negative effects of urbanization on population health. The inequity in distribution of medical resources between rural and urban areas might be increased during the urbanization process. Rural residents therefore, would be negatively affected even more by the degree of urbanization.

We also used the 2010 Chinese Family Panel Study to examine the impact of urbanization on more health related indicators (Table 15.3). The first dependent variable is self-reported health outcome. The demonstrated negative effect of urbanization is consistent with findings using the 2005 Inter-Census Population Survey. A higher level of urbanization is associated with a lower level of self-reported health outcome.[6] The second dependent variable is whether the respondent

---

[5] BMI is Body Mass Index, which equals to weight (kg) divided by height (m) square.

[6] Since the definition of self-reported health outcome in 2010 CFPS is different from that in 2005 Inter-Census Population Survey, we cannot directly compare the magnitude of the effect.

Table 15.2 Impact of urbanization on health

	(1) Total sample	(2) Urban residents	(3) Rural residents	(4) Migrants in urban areas
Urbanization rate	–0.006***	–0.009***	–0.010***	–0.002
	(0.001)	(0.002)	(0.002)	(0.002)
Household annual per capita income	0.013***	0.001	0.023***	0.010***
	(0.001)	(0.001)	(0.001)	(0.001)
Age	–0.006***	–0.006***	–0.007***	–0.006***
	(0.000)	(0.000)	(0.000)	(0.000)
Male	0.002***	0.001	0.005***	0.001
	(0.000)	(0.001)	(0.000)	(0.001)
Married	0.132***	0.098***	0.150***	0.118***
	(0.000)	(0.001)	(0.001)	(0.001)
Elementary school	0.122***	0.131***	0.115***	0.121***
	(0.001)	(0.002)	(0.001)	(0.001)
Middle school	0.141***	0.179***	0.129***	0.135***
	(0.001)	(0.002)	(0.001)	(0.002)
High school	0.154***	0.191***	0.144***	0.144***
	(0.001)	(0.002)	(0.001)	(0.001)
College	0.162***	0.198***	0.141***	0.149***
	(0.001)	(0.002)	(0.002)	(0.003)
Master and above	0.171***	0.209***	0.130***	0.147***
	(0.004)	(0.004)	(0.044)	(0.037)
Have any health insurance	0.007***	–0.010***	0.014***	0.010***
	(0.000)	(0.001)	(0.001)	(0.001)
Have access to Drinking water	0.002***	0.006***	0.003***	0.003***
	(0.000)	(0.001)	(0.000)	(0.001)
R-squared	0.250	0.195	0.275	0.250
Observation	2,404,319	633,413	1,254,597	516,309

Standard errors are shown in parenthesis. *significant at 10%; **significant at 5%; ***significant at 1%.

Source: 2005 Inter-Census Population Survey (National Bureau of Statistics of China, 2005).

Table 15.3 Impact of urbanization on health: more indicators

	(1) Self-reported health	(2) Diagnosed with any chronic disease	(3) Underweight	(4) Overweight	(5) Obese
Urbanization rate	–0.038**	0.041**	–0.074***	0.124***	0.023***
	(0.018)	(0.017)	(0.015)	(0.019)	(0.007)
Household annual per capita income	0.018***	0.004**	–0.009***	0.010***	0.001
	(0.002)	(0.002)	(0.002)	(0.002)	(0.001)
Age	–0.005***	0.005***	0.001***	0.001***	–0.000
	(0.000)	(0.000)	(0.000)	(0.000)	(0.000)
Male	0.037***	–0.030***	–0.042***	0.024***	0.007***
	(0.004)	(0.004)	(0.003)	(0.005)	(0.002)
Married	0.020***	–0.004	–0.103***	0.078***	0.010***
	(0.006)	(0.006)	(0.005)	(0.006)	(0.002)
Elementary school	0.062***	0.010***	–0.022***	0.009	0.001
	(0.006)	(0.006)	(0.005)	(0.007)	(0.002)
Middle school	0.097***	–0.004	–0.028***	0.024***	–0.003
	(0.006)	(0.006)	(0.005)	(0.007)	(0.002)
High school	0.097***	0.012	–0.022***	0.020**	–0.000
	(0.008)	(0.007)	(0.006)	(0.008)	(0.003)
College	0.103***	0.018*	–0.004	0.024**	–0.007*
	(0.010)	(0.010)	(0.008)	(0.011)	(0.004)
Master and above	0.119**	0.046	–0.032	0.048	–0.027
	(0.055)	(0.054)	(0.045)	(0.059)	(0.022)
Have any health insurance	–0.003	0.016***	–0.014***	0.001	0.001
	(0.005)	(0.005)	(0.004)	(0.006)	(0.002)
Have access to drinking water	0.020***	–0.000	–0.009**	0.025***	0.000
	(0.005)	(0.004)	(0.004)	(0.005)	(0.002)
R-squared	0.094	0.056	0.045	0.034	0.010
Observation	29,171	29,171	29,171	29,171	29,171

Standard errors are shown in parenthesis. *significant at 10%; **significant at 5%; ***significant at 1%.

***Source*: 2010 CFPS (Institute of Social Science Survey, 2010).**

had been diagnosed with any chronic disease during the past six months. The results indicated that people would be more likely to be diagnosed with chronic diseases if they were living in an area with a higher degree of urbanization. The other dependent variables are weight status, including underweight, overweight and obese. Urbanization significantly increases the probability of being obese and overweight, and decreases the probability of being underweight. During the process of urbanization, household disposable income increases in both rural and urban areas. Families have more resources to improve the nutrition of their family members. The under-nutrition problem has been greatly alleviated. However, at the same time, over-intake of food and consumption of fast food in cities might also induce obesity and increase the probability of chronic diseases such as diabetes and heart disease.

15.3.2 *Main mechanisms of urbanization impact on health*

From the findings of the empirical data analysis we postulate the main mechanisms through which urbanization affects health, focusing on several issues, including income, availability of medical services and pollution.

People receive higher income in more urbanized areas, especially those who migrate from villages to cities. Higher income increases the resource available to be invested in health. In Tables 15.2 and 15.3, annual household income is one of the factors considered. Income is always positively related to self-reported health outcome, which means that a higher income improves an individual's health status. Other control variables related to socio–economic characteristics, such as a higher education level and access to clean water also have positive effects on self-reported health outcome. Results in Table 15.3 also indicate that, although increase in income reduces the probability of being underweight, it increases the probability of being overweight, and being diagnosed with chronic diseases. The results further confirm that as urbanization progresses, people need to pay attention to leading a healthy lifestyle and preventing over-consumption of food and nutrition.

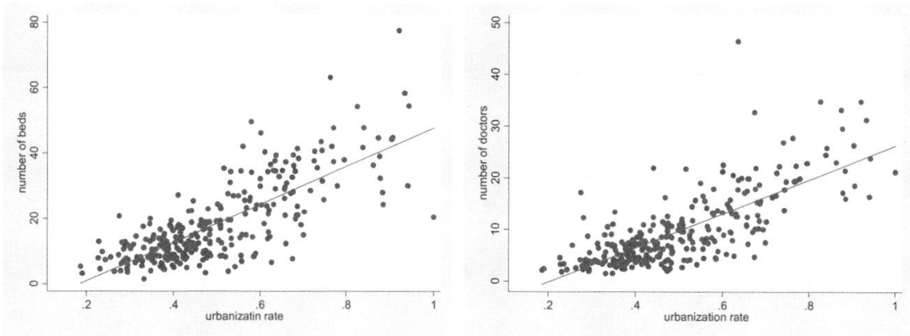

Figure 15.1 Urbanization and medical resources (2010).

Source: 2010 China City Statistical Yearbook (National Bureau of Statistics of China, 2011b).

Urbanized areas provide better public health and medical services compared with rural villages. People who migrate from villages to cities could potentially have better access to advanced medical resources and public health facilities. Figure 15.1 describes the relationship between urbanization and medical resources using data from the 2010 China City Statistical Yearbook. Both number of beds and number of doctors per ten thousand people increases as the urbanization rate increases.

Since urbanization is accompanied by improvement in medical services, it should have a positive effect on health. However, we do not see this result in regression analysis. For rural residents, the negative effect of urbanization on health might come from the increased gap in medical resources between rural and urban areas. Medical resources tend to be more concentrated in cities. Rural residents do not benefit from the improvement in the provision of medical services that comes with urbanization. For urban residents, the congestion in medical consumption and inequity might reduce the actual accessibility of medical services by some residents, for example the rural-to-urban migrants and the laid-off workers. We use the number and expenditure of inpatient services to examine the relationship between urbanization and medical consumption. Figure 15.2 indicates that both the number and the total expenditure on in-patient services increase with the rate of urbanization. On the one hand, people have more access to medical services in a more urbanized area, and as a

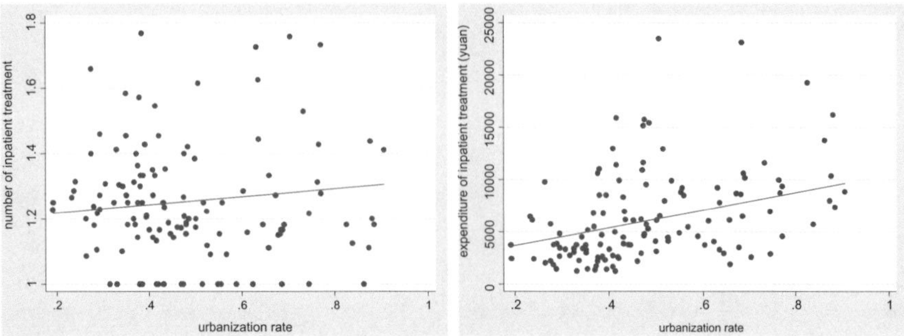

Figure 15.2 Urbanization and health service utilization.
***Source*: 2010 CFPS (Institute of Social Science Survey, 2010).**

result, their health should improve. On the other hand, the increased demand for medical services may be caused by lower health status due to problems such as environmental degradation during the process of urbanization. We do not know the direction of the causal relationship between medical consumption and urbanization. What is more, higher medical consumption might also be related to higher awareness of health issues as a result of promotion and increased diagnoses due to technological advances. However, our data demonstrates the basic fact that during the urbanization process, people have higher medical consumption, and a lower level of health.

As mentioned above, a highly concentrated population and increased industrial production are the major sources of urban pollution, which may have a negative effect on individual health. We collected air pollution data such as inhalable particles (PM10), sulfur dioxide (SO2) and nitrogen dioxide (NO2), and the fraction of days that air quality is second degree and above in a year in the capital cities of all provinces in China.[7] Figure 15.3 shows the relationship between urbanization and air pollution. Inhalable particles PM10, SO2, and

---

[7] Pollution data is from 2005 China Statistical Yearbooks. According to Air Quality Standard GB3095-1996, air quality is second degree if the following conditions are satisfied: annual average sulfur dioxide is lower than 0.06 mg/m^3; annual average nitrogen dioxide is lower than 0.04 mg/m^3; annual average inhalable particles (pm 10) is lower than 0.07 mg/m^3.

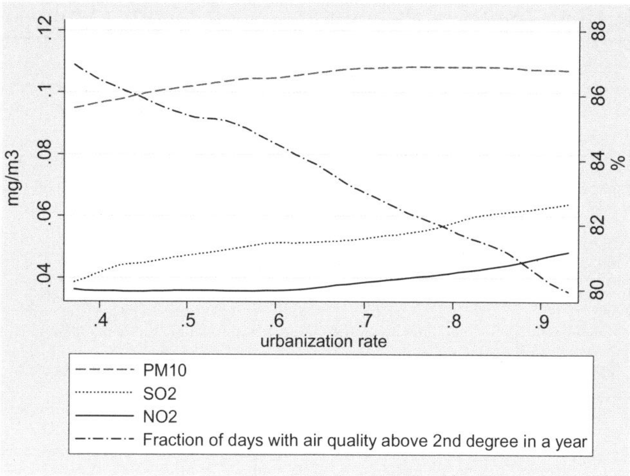

Figure 15.3 Urbanization and air pollution.
Source: **China Statistical Yearbooks (National Bureau of Statistics of China, 2011a)**

NO2 increase with the rate of urbanization. The fraction of days with good air quality (second degree and above) is lower when the index of urbanization is higher. For example, when the index of urbanization is 40%, the fraction of days with good air quality is 87%; when the urbanization rate is 90%, the fraction is 81%. We combined these indicators of air quality with the 2005 Inter-Census Population Survey to examine the impact of air quality on individual health outcomes.

Table 15.4 reports the estimated impact of air quality on self-reported health outcomes. Inhalable particles PM10, SO_2, and NO_2 all have significantly negative effects on health outcomes, while the fraction of days with good air quality is statistically positively related to health outcomes. These results indicate that air pollution has a negative impact on residents' health. People have a lower health status in a more polluted area. Pollution is the main reason that people's health worsens during urbanization.

In summary, we find a higher level of urbanization is associated with a lower level of health status for both urban and rural residents. The mechanisms of income, medical service consumption and pollution are discussed. We find that, during the process of urbanization,

Table 15.4 Impact of air pollution on self-reported health status

	(1)	(2)	(3)	(4)
PM10	–0.221***			
	(0.015)			
SO_2		–0.133***		
		(0.020)		
NO_2			–0.052**	
			(0.024)	
Fraction of days with good air quality in a year				0.001***
				(0.000)
Household annual income	0.013***	0.012***	0.012***	0.012***
	(0.002)	(0.002)	(0.002)	(0.002)
Age	–0.006***	–0.006***	–0.006***	–0.006***
	(0.000)	(0.000)	(0.000)	(0.000)
Male	0.004***	0.004***	0.004***	0.004***
	(0.001)	(0.001)	(0.001)	(0.001)
Married	0.119***	0.119***	0.119***	0.119***
	(0.001)	(0.001)	(0.001)	(0.001)
Have any health insurance	0.004***	0.004***	0.004***	0.004***
	(0.001)	(0.001)	(0.001)	(0.001)
Have access to clean water	0.000	0.002**	0.002**	0.001
	(0.001)	(0.001)	(0.001)	(0.001)
Education dummies	Yes	Yes	Yes	Yes
R-squared	0.233	0.232	0.232	0.233
Observations	472,587	472,587	472,587	472,587

Standard errors are shown in parenthesis. *significant at 10%; **significant at 5%; ***significant at 1%.

***Source*: 2005 Inter-Census Population Survey (National Bureau of Statistics of China, 2005)**

medical service provision and consumption increase. Pollution is the main reason that people's health worsens. The increase in income and health service consumption cannot overcome the impact of pollution.

15.4 Policy Recommendations and Concluding Remarks

China has been experiencing rapid urbanization since the 1980s, and the urban population now constitutes above 50% of the whole, this number expected to further increase in the coming decades. The overall urbanization impact on health seems to be mixed. The empirical analysis presented in this chapter demonstrates a negative relationship between urbanization and people's health status for both urban and rural residents, requiring the urgent attention of China's policymakers to mitigate the negative impact of urbanization on health. In this context, it is important for China to consider more pro-health policies as urbanization progresses, because better general health will provide vital human capital so necessary for the long-term development of China's economy. Combining both sets of our findings and the current health care reform in China, we propose three major policy recommendations as follows.

15.4.1 *Healthcare financing*

There has been a concerted effort by China's central government to establish universal health coverage (UHC), a basic service package through public financing (Pan *et al.*, 2014). At present, more than 95% of the total population in China is enrolled in one of the three major public health insurance programs. These three programs are the Urban Employee Basic Medical Insurance for the urban formal sector employees, the New Rural Cooperative Medical Scheme for the large rural population, and the Urban Resident Basic Medical Insurance that targets the remaining urban residents who are primarily the unemployed or those working in the informal sector.

These programs are administered by different government agencies, that is, the Ministry of Human Resources and Social Security manages the two urban programs while the National Health and Family Planning Commission (NHFPC) controls the rural program. A particular problem with such a management setting is that the three programs differ greatly in terms of eligibility, administration, and financing schemes. Thus, the lack of coordination and transferability among different programs and regions results in considerable fragmentation in China's health insurance systems. This in turn fails to accommodate the geographic mobility of migrant workers and significantly limits their access to care and the cost-effectiveness of insurance programs.

Given the huge and growing migrant population, there is a growing consensus in China to make stronger efforts to integrate the three public health insurance programs. As the first step, the central government has recently set the target for 2015, requesting all public insurance programs be mobile across different areas within each province by the end of 2015. This work should help extend further integration by removing some eligibility barriers, such as the local *Hukou* requirement as that currently prevents migrants from joining the Urban Resident Basic Medical Insurance. Moreover, an integrated system also means an important step in China's development towards a more harmonious society where public health coverage will be for all, without policy disparity between urban and rural populations.

15.4.2 *Healthcare delivery*

Rapid urbanization motivates millions of workers to emigrate from rural areas to cities. In the meantime, it creates millions of 'left behind' children and elderly in rural areas. The challenge is that the healthcare delivery system does not only need to expand rapidly, but also needs to become better customized to meet the demands of more heterogeneous populations.

Under the current state healthcare reform in China, one of the five major initiatives is to promote the equity of the basic public health services across different regions and populations. It is anticipated that as this policy initiative is being pursued, it will play a strong and positive role in offsetting the potential negative impacts of urbanization on these 'left-behind' groups.

Moreover, the literature indicates that the local government health expenditure is highly dependent on the level of local economic development and fiscal transfers from central government (Pan and Liu, 2012). Therefore, to equalize the local public health input among regions (one of the five health reform goals), there would also be a need for more central government interventions, such as increasing the share of special purpose grants for health, and formulating specific policies to allocate health resources based on the actual local health demand.

Furthermore, it is essential to improve the efficiency of the health delivery system to better meet the specific health demands associated with urbanization in China. Currently, the biggest problem in Chinese healthcare delivery is resource allocation (Pan and Hsieh, 2015), and this can be analyzed from both the institutional and personnel perspectives. At the institutional level, medical care providers have long been dominated by public hospitals, and the resources are allocated accordingly, following a top–down approach. In the tertiary, secondary and primary health care (the three-tier health care delivery system), the higher the tier a hospital is at, the more resources are available to them. At the personnel level, public hospital physicians are state employees, enjoying many system advantages and job security, which would be lost as an opportunity cost when seeking a medical practice outside the public system. As a result, medical resources, especially technologies and doctors, are highly concentrated in the hierarchical hospital-centered delivery system, which provides all types of services.

In contrast, primary care facilities and non-public providers are the weakest link in the health system in terms of resources and capacities. In response, Chinese patients follow resource allocation, and superior service delivery, seeking care from the best hospitals possible, for both primary care and tertiary care services, leading to a most inefficient and costly healthcare delivery system. It is clear that as urbanization continues, a large disease burden from chronic non-communicable diseases will grow, and this, coupled with an aging population, means the delivery system will have to make changes in the allocation of resources towards primary care and open market settings, or face increasing challenges from the unmet demand due to the present inequitable system. The current State health reform has laid out a promising roadmap with a good set of mechanisms for allocating resources towards more competitive and efficient market settings, including private healthcare providers entering the delivery system, multi-site medical practices, and for insurance to cover similar basic services in both the public and private systems.

15.4.3 *Further transition from medicine to health*

Among the determinants of health, behavior is the most important factor in explaining the variation in population health. Medical care should be the last step in the fight against disease. There is a wealth of evidence on the key role of behavior and behavior-related services in the promotion of health (McGinnis and Foege, 1993). A crucial difference between medical care and pro-health services is that the former is for patients with diseases, while the latter serves both the healthy and unhealthy populations. Compared to medical care, pro-health services play a more active role in contributing to population health, through multi-mechanisms such as strengthening healthy bodies, reducing catastrophic risks, preventing avoidable diseases, or postponing a disease onset. Such services and interventions may range from advice on healthy food, healthy environments, consultation care, and physical exercises, to health education and other public programs to promote healthy living. It is crucial to understand the inversely interdependent relationship between pro-health services and medical care, and the urbanization process with the relatively young population compounding such interdependency.

In October 2013, the Chinese government issued a major policy document on the development of a modern health service industry, a landmark policy initiative calling for provision of pro-health services (The State Council, 2013). A series of policy calls were made to stimulate changes in the support of market entry, investment, service supply, and insurance financing for pro-health services, which include wellness goods and services, medical care, and post-care services as well as products for healthy aging.

From a system perspective, while there might be a long way to go from the current disease-centered medicine to a pro-health system; we believe that such a system transition towards health promotion would make four major improvements.

First, it is believed that pro-health services would help improve the cost effectiveness of medical care, due to more appropriate use of resources for wellness and preventable conditions. Second, it would help improve the societal-environment conditions, resulting from a greater than usual investment in better health goals. Third, it would also help make a more harmonious society; this is partly because everything being equal, a healthier population would enjoy a better quality of life, leading to more healthy behaviors. Finally, it may well help China to pursue its economic transition for sustainable growth. From a Keynesian standpoint, it is widely believed among economists that the key to China's sustaining high economic growth is finding a greater source of consumption to substitute for the continued declining roles of both exports and investment as forces driving the economy.

According to the seminal work by Nobel laureate Robert Fogel (2008), based on his century-long observations among the Europeans and the Americans, in response to every 10% increase in income, people increased their health services spending over 16% accordingly, the largest component increase of all household consumption items. As such, it is highly recommended that China conduct more pro-health system reforms with stronger public and private support for greater gains in both population health and sustainable economic growth.

References

Alberini, A. and Krupnick, A. (1998). Air Quality and Episodes of Acute Respiratory Illness in Taiwan Cities: Evidence from Survey Data, *Journal of Urban Economics* **44**(1): 68–92.

Bauman, A., Allman-Farinelli, M., Huxley, R., *et al.* (2008). Leisure-time Physical Activity Alone May Not Be a Sufficient Public Health Approach to Prevent Obesity — A Focus on China, *Obesity Review* **9**(S1): 119–126.

Bell, A., Ge, K. and Popkin, B. (2001). Weight Gain and its Predictors in Chinese Adults, *International Journal of Obesity and Related Metabolic Disorders: Journal of the International Association for the Study of Obesity* **25**(7): 1079–1086.

Brajer, V. and Mead, R.W. (2003). Blue Skies in Beijing? Looking at the Olympic Effect, *The Journal of Environment and Development* **12**(2): 239–263.

Chang, D. and Wang, S. (2009). Status of Occupational Hygiene Safety and Health Hazards and its Intervention in Migrant Workers in China, *China Occupational Medicine* **4**: 28.

Chay, K.Y. and Greenstone, M. (1999). *The Impact of Air Pollution on Infant Mortality: Evidence from Geographic Variation in Pollution Shocks Induced by a Recession*, National Bureau of Economic Research Working Paper No. 7442. Available at http://www.nber.org/papers/w7442 [Accessed 2 March 2015].

Chen, J. (2011). Internal Migration and Health: Re-examining the Healthy Migrant Phenomenon in China, *Social Science and Medicine* **72**(8): 1294–1301.

Cheung, N.W. (2014). Social Stress, Locality of Social Ties and Mental Well-being: The Case of Rural Migrant Adolescents in Urban China, *Health and Place* **27**: 142–154.

Cohen, A.J., Anderson, H.R., Ostro, B., *et al.* (2004). Urban Air Pollution, *Comparative Quantification of Health Risks* **2**: 1353–1433.

Cole, M.A. and Neumayer, E. (2004). Examining the Impact of Demographic Factors on Air Pollution, *Population and Environment* **26**(1): 5–21.

Currie, J. and Neidell, M. (2004). Air Pollution and Infant Health: What Can We Learn from California's Recent Experience, National Bureau of Economic Research Working Paper No. 10251. Available at http://www.nber.org/papers/w10251 [Accessed 2 March 2015].

Dahly, D.L. and Adair, L.S. (2007). Quantifying the Urban Environment: A Scale Measure of Urbanicity Outperforms the Urban–Rural Dichotomy, *Social Science and Medicine* **64**(7): 1407–1419.

Dasgupta, P. (2004). Valuing Health Damages from Water Pollution in Urban Delhi, India: A Health Production Function Approach, *Environment and Development Economics* **9**(01) 83–106.

Ebenstein, A. (2012) The Consequences of Industrialization: Evidence from Water Pollution and Digestive Cancers in China, *Review of Economics and Statistics* **94**(1): 186–201.

Fogel, R.W. (2008). Forecasting the Cost of U.S. Health Care in 2040, National Bureau of Economic Research Working Paper No. 14361. Available at http://www.nber.org/papers/w14361 [Accessed 2 March 2015].

Fu, F.H. and Fung, L. (2004). The Cardiovascular Health of Residents in Selected Metropolitan Cities in China, *Preventive Medicine* **38**(4): 458–467.

Gong, P., Liang, S., Carlton, E.J., *et al.* (2012). Urbanisation and Health in China, *The Lancet* **379**(9818): 843–852.

Grumbach, K., Vranizan, K. and Bindman, A.B. (1997). Physician Supply and Access to Care in Urban Communities, *Health Affairs* **16**(1): 71–86.

Health Effects Institute (2004). *Health Effects of Outdoor Air Pollution in Developing Countries of Asia: A Literature Review*, Health Effects Institute, Boston.

Henderson, V. (2002). Urbanization in Developing Countries, *The World Bank Research Observer* **17**(1): 89–112.

Hong, Y., Li, X., Stanton, B., *et al.* (2006). Too costly to be ill: Health Care Access and Health Seeking Behaviors Among Rural-to-urban Migrants in China, *World Health and Population* **8**(2): 22.

Hu, G., Pekkarinen, H., Hänninen, O., *et al.* (2002). Commuting, Leisure-time Physical Activity, and Cardiovascular Risk Factors in China, *Medicine and Science in Sports and Exercise* **34**(2): 234–238.

Hu, G., Wen, M., Baker, T.D., *et al.* (2008). Road-traffic Deaths in China, 1985–2005: Threat and Opportunity, *Injury Prevention* **14**(3): 149–153.

Institute of Social Science Survey (2010). China Family Panel Studies. Available at http://www.isss.edu.cn/cfps/EN/ [Accessed 2 March 2015].

Ito, C. (2005) Urbanization and Water Pollution in China. Discussion Papers, Crawford School of Public Policy, ANU College of the Asia Pacific. Available at https://crawford.anu.edu.au/degrees/pogo/discussion_papers/PDP05-13.pdf [Accessed 2 March 2015].

Knudsen, A.B. and Slooff, R. (1992). Vector-Borne Disease Problems in Rapid Urbanization: New Approaches to Vector Control, *Bulletin of the World Health Organization* **70**(1): 1.

Krieger, J. and Higgins, D.L. (2002). Housing and Health: Time Again for Public Health Action, *American Journal of Public Health* **92**(5): 758–768.

Li, X.-H., Liu, J.-L., Gibson, V., *et al.* (2012). Urban Sustainability and Human Health in China, East Asia and Southeast Asia, *Current Opinion in Environmental Sustainability* **4**(4): 436–442.

Liu, G., Fan, M., Huang, Y., *et al.* (2014). Migrant Population's Health and Healthcare in China, Peking University CCHER Working Paper.

Liu, G.G., Wu, X., Peng, C., *et al.* (2003). Urbanization and Health Care in Rural China, *Contemporary Economic Policy* **21**(1): 11–24.

Liu, L., Ikeda, K., Chen, M., *et al.* (2004). Obesity, Emerging Risk in China: Trend of Increasing Prevalence of Obesity and its Association with Hypertension and Hypercholesterolaemia Among the Chinese, *Clinical and Experimental Pharmacology and Physiology* **31**(S2): S8–S10.

Mangyo, E. (2008). The Effect of Water Accessibility on Child Health in China, *Journal of Health Economics* **27**(5): 1343–1356.

McDade, T.W. and Adair, L.S. (2001). Defining the "Urban" in Urbanization and Health: A Factor Analysis Approach, *Social Science and Medicine* **53**(1): 55–70.

McGinnis, M., and Foege, W.H. (1993). Actual Causes of Death in the United States, *JAMA* **270**(18): 2207–2212.

Monda, K.L., Gordon-Larsen, P., Stevens, J., *et al.* (2007). China's Transition: The Effect of Rapid Urbanization on Adult Occupational Physical Activity, *Social Science and Medicine* **64**(4): 858–870.

Moore, M., Gould, P. and Keary, B.S. (2003). Global Urbanization and Impact on Health, *International Journal of Hygiene and Environmental Health* **206**(4): 269–278.

Mou, J., Cheng, J., Zhang, D., *et al.* (2009). Health Care Utilisation Amongst Shenzhen Migrant Workers: Does Being Insured Make a Difference? *BMC Health Services Research* **9**(1): 214.

National Bureau of Statistics of China (2010). *2010 Census Population Survey*, China Statistical Press, Beijing.

National Bureau of Statistics of China (2011a). *China Statistical Yearbook*, China Statistical Press, Beijing.

National Bureau of Statistics of China (2011b). *China City Statistical Yearbook*, China Statistical Press, Beijing.

National Bureau of Statistics of China (2005). *2005 Inter-Census Population Survey*, China Statistical Press, Beijing.

Neidell, M.J. (2004). Air Pollution, Health, and Socio-economic Status: The Effect of Outdoor Air Quality on Childhood Asthma, *Journal of Health Economics* **23**(6): 1209–1236.

O'Neill, M.S., Jerrett, M., Kawachi, I., *et al.* (2003). Health, Wealth, and Air Pollution: Advancing Theory and Methods, *Environmental Health Perspectives* **111**(16): 1861.

Ouyang, T., Zhu, Z. and Kuang, Y. (2006). Assessing Impact of Urbanization on River Water Quality in the Pearl River Delta Economic Zone,China, *Environmental Monitoring and Assessment* **120**(1–3): 313–325.

Pan, J. and Liu, G.G. (2012). The Determinants of Chinese Provincial Government Health Expenditures: Evidence from 2002–2006 Data, *Health Economics* **21**(7): 757–777.

Pan, J., Lei, X.Y. and Liu, G.G. (2015). Health Insurance and Health Status: Exploring the Causal Effects of a Policy Intervention, Health Economics, forthcoming.

Pan, J. and Hsieh, C.-R. (2015). Geographic Distribution of Hospital Beds Throughout China: A County Level Approach, unpublished working paper.

Phillips, M.R., Zhang, J., Shi, Q., *et al.* (2009). Prevalence, Treatment, and Associated Disability of Mental Disorders in Four Provinces in China During 2001–05: An Epidemiological Survey, *The Lancet* **373**(9680): 2041–2053.

Popkin, B.M. and Bisgrove, E.Z. (1988). Urbanization and Nutrition in Low-income Countries, *Food and Nutrition Bulletin* **10**(1): 3–23.

Pucher, J., Peng, Z.R., Mittal, N., *et al.* (2007). Urban Transport Trends and Policies in China and India: Impacts of Rapid Economic Growth, *Transport Reviews* **27**(4): 379–410.

Qin, X., Li, L. and Hsieh, C.-R. (2013). Too Few Doctors or Too Low Wages? Labor Supply of Health Care Professionals in China, *China Economic Review* **24**: 150–164.

SEPA (2006). *State of the Environment Report*, State Environmental Protection Administration, Beijing.

Shin, E., Hufschmidt, M.M. and Yok-shiu, F.L. (1997). *Evaluating The Economic Impacts Of Urban Environmental Problems: Asian Cities,*

Urban Management and Poverty Reduction, UNDP/UNCHS (Habitat), World Bank.

Social and Economic Investigation Team of National Bureau of Statistics, (2010). *China City Statistical Yearbook 2010*, China Statistical Press, Beijing.

Van de Poel, E., O'Donnell, O. and Van Doorslaer, E. (2012). Is There a Health Penalty of China's Rapid Urbanization? *Health Economics* **21**(4): 367–385.

Vigotti, M., Rossi, G., Bisanti, L., *et al.* (1996). Short Term Effects of Urban Air Pollution on Respiratory Health in Milan, Italy, 1980–89, *Journal of Epidemiology and Community Health* **50**(Suppl1): s71–s75.

Vlahov, D., Freudenberg, N., Proietti, F., *et al.* (2007). Urban as a Determinant of Health, *Journal of Urban Health* **84**(1): 16–26.

Wang, S., Li, Y., Chi, G., *et al.* (2008). Injury-related Fatalities in China: An Under-recognised Public-Health Problem, *The Lancet* **372**(9651): 1765–1773.

Wang, X., Ding, H., Ryan, L. *et al.* (1997). Association Between Air Pollution and Low Birth Weight: A Community-Based Study, *Environmental Health Perspectives* **105**(5): 514.

Wang, X. and Smith, K.R. (1999). *Near-term Health Benefits of Greenhouse Gas Reductions: A Proposed Assessment Method and Application in Two Energy Sectors of China,* Department of Protection of the Human Environment, World Health Organization.

Weng, X., Liu, Y., Ma, J., *et al.* (2007). An Urban–Rural Comparison of the Prevalence of the Metabolic Syndrome in Eastern China, *Public Health Nutrition* **10**(02): 131–136.

Wu, C., Maurer, C., Wang, Y., *et al.* (1999). Water Pollution and Human Health in China, *Environmental Health Perspectives* **107**(4): 251.

Yang, G., Wang, Y., Zeng, Y., *et al.* (2013). Rapid Health Transition in China, 1990–2010: Findings from the Global Burden of Disease Study 2010, *The Lancet* **381**(9882): 1987–2015.

Yu, W. and Zhou, A. (2004). Health Promotion in Companies, *Chinese Journal of Industrial Medicine* **17**: 3–4 (in Chinese).

Zhang, G., Yau, K. K. and Chen, G. (2013). Risk Factors Associated with Traffic Violations and Accident Severity in China, *Accident Analysis and Prevention* **59**: 18–25.

Zhang, J., Mauzerall, D.L., Zhu, T., *et al.* (2010). Environmental Health in China: Progress Towards Clean Air and Safe Water, *The Lancet* **375**(9720): 1110–1119.

Zhang, L. (2007). Investigation on Drinking Water Safety in China in 2006, *Journal of Enviromental Health* **24**: 595–597 (in Chinese).

Zhangtao (2010). Analysis on Occupational-Related Safety Fatal Accident Reports of China, 2001–2008, *Safety Science* **48**(5): 640–642.

Zheng, S. and Kahn, M. E. (2013). Understanding China's Urban Pollution Dynamics, *Journal of Economic Literature* **51**(3): 731–772.

Index